NURSING ISSUES:

PSYCHIATRIC NURSING, GERIATRIC NURSING AND NURSING BURNOUT

NURSING- ISSUES, PROBLEMS AND CHALLENGES

Additional books in this series can be found on Nova's website at:

https://www.novapublishers.com/catalog/index.php?cPath=23_29&seriesp=Nursing+-
+Issues%2C+Problems+and+Challenges

Additional E-books in this series can be found on Nova's website at:

https://www.novapublishers.com/catalog/index.php?cPath=23_29&seriespe=Nursing+-
+Issues%2C+Problems+and+Challenges

NURSING ISSUES: PSYCHIATRIC NURSING, GERIATRIC NURSING AND NURSING BURNOUT

CAITRIONA D. MCLAUGHLIN
AND
JAMIE N. DOCHERTY
EDITORS

Nova Biomedical Books
New York

Library of Congress Cataloging-in-Publication Data

Nursing issues : psychiatric nursing, geriatric nursing, and nursing burnout / editors, Caitriona D. McLaughlin and Jamie N. Docherty.
p. ; cm.
Includes bibliographical references and index.
ISBN 978-1-60741-598-5 (hardcover)
1. Psychiatric nursing. 2. Geriatric nursing. 3. Burn out (Psychology) I. McLaughlin, Caitriona D. II. Docherty, Jamie N.
  [DNLM: 1. Burnout, Professional. 2. Nurses--psychology. 3. Geriatric Nursing. 4. Mental Disorders--nursing. 5. Psychiatric Nursing. WY 87 N9757 2009]
RC440.N876 2009
610.73--dc22
2009048222

Published by Nova Science Publishers, Inc. ✦ *New York*

Contents

Preface

Psychiatric nursing, although advanced in areas of interpersonal skills and manpower management, have been sadly lacking in the area of research relating to practice. This book aims to provide empirical evidence in relation to understanding a fundamental aspect of the psychiatric nurses' role, namely what constitutes the therapeutic relationship. The problems nurses face in their approach to risk assessment and management, which is affected to a considerable degree by who defines that risk and how it is defined, are discussed. Furthermore, whether we like it or not, risk assessment and management is a regular and daily occurrence in health care. Using case vignettes from teaching and therapeutic research, the authors of this book explore ways in which inner and outer dialogues are at play as the mental health nurse attempts to make sense of the experiences of mental pain narrated by people in his/her case. In addition, work-stress and burnout complaints are increasingly leading to higher levels of absentee rates at work. Superimposed organizational demands, work overload and limited decision-making capacities are often associated with the development of occupational stress by nurses that eventually create a sensation of professional burnout. A comprehensive literature review relating to nursing burnout, an issue that has received increasing interest from researchers and healthcare administrators is explored in this book. Other chapters address individual work experiences, coping strategies and health decisions made by nurses for patient care.

Chapter I - Psychiatric nursing is invariably linked with a therapeutic role; however the question remains unanswered in relation to the extent psychiatric nurses perceive the importance of the constituents of the therapeutic relationship. The aim of this research is to ascertain the nature and comprehension psychiatric nurses assign this therapeutic role. The subject relates significantly to the role of the psychiatric nurses in relation to awareness of elements of the therapeutic relationship in his or her practice and the understanding and identifying this role clearly and unambiguously.

Grounded theory methodology was utilised to develop these conceptualisations to elicit a theory relating to what comprises the therapeutic relationship. Semi-structured depth interviews were conducted with 6 generic registered psychiatric nurses who have between two and ten years of experience.

The objective of the research was to formulate a theory relating to constituents of the therapeutic relationship to inform professional psychiatric nursing practice and to provide a theoretical framework to inform conscious psychiatric nursing practice in relation to forming therapeutic relationships. Strauss and Corbin (1990) describe one of the purposes of research is to guide practitioners' practices and to develop a basic knowledge. The aim of research was to fulfil this purpose; building theory implies interpreting data that must be conceptualised and the concepts related to a view of reality.

The main findings of the research related to how psychiatric nurses learn to form these relationships and what skills are utilised within the relationship. The research discovered that the therapeutic relationship is therapeutic, but the degree of positive change is difficult to measure. The study also highlighted that the learning that takes place in relation to the development of therapeutic relationships is an experiential process and begs the question is the focus of psychiatric nurse training, in relation to the therapeutic relationship, located appropriately.

Chapter II - This paper discusses individual constructs that form diathesis-stress models and formulates an adapted model for a corrections population. Diathesis-stress models are familiar within psychiatric nursing, but rarely discussed in the literature in their application to correctional population, or for their potential in guiding nursing practice in correctional settings. Of particular interest to this paper is the coping response of inmates to the stressors of incarceration and the implications for clinical care management.

Chapter III - Risk is discussed and defined in this chapter. Risk assessment and management are introduced along with the terminology, history and some assessment tools. Some tools are described with their associated major references to aid knowledge of this important area of practice. Issues related to the use of risk assessment instruments are discussed as aspects of clinical use, such as education and training, are important to understand.

Chapter IV - This chapter involves a comprehensive literature review relating to nursing burnout, an issue that is receiving increased interest from researchers and healthcare administrators over the past few decades. Maslach & Jackson (1981) developed the Maslach Burnout Inventory (MBI) to assess three aspects of the burnout syndrome: a feeling of emotional exhaustion; cynical attitudes toward one's clients (depersonalization); and the tendency to negatively evaluate oneself (low personal accomplishments). Certain conditions in the practice environment are shown to affect nurses' work lives by either contributing to or alleviating burnout. Also, individual attributes including demographic characteristics and personality traits can influence the development of nurse burnout; however, findings are inconsistent across studies. Nurse burnout has negative consequences of stress-related illness, absenteeism and turnover, which impacts quality of care, patient satisfaction and organizational cost. Incidence of nurse burnout is minimized in professional work environments that enable and encourage full scope of nursing practice. There is a critical need to create nursing work environments that support professional practice and put in place leadership development programs to ensure that high quality of patient care is provided. Managers should be aware that certain personality traits may predispose employees to workplace burnout. Clearly, as demonstrated by the evidence to date, the issue of burnout is one that requires policy attention from healthcare administrators, and one that warrants ongoing research toward a better understanding so new evidence can become available to inform future practice. Future research should involve more longitudinal studies and elaborated theoretical models to explain the causal mechanisms that link organizational features and processes of care, and how these factors affect outcomes relating to nurse performance and well-being, patient health and satisfaction, and how these outcomes then feed back into and impact the system at the organizational level and beyond.

Chapter V- The following chapter will endeavour to amalgamate the findings of this study with the evidence supplied in the available literature relating to the constituents of the therapeutic relationship in psychiatric nursing. The study objective was to explain how psychiatric nurses perceive the therapeutic relationship fits their role and what the relationship is comprised of. The previous chapter described the findings of the study. This chapter will be structured around the six categories identified in the findings. One comment of note is that due to the small scale of the study, tentative hypotheses are made; however the positing of a theory would be unreasonable. What the study does however is highlight the interpretations of the participants and compare these interpretations to what is described in the literature.

Chapter VI - In modern societies, work-stress and burnout complaints are increasingly leading to higher levels of absentee rates at work. Although burnout is not a classified psychiatric disorder, there is a large amount of co-morbidity with psychiatric disorders such as affective disorders. Therefore it is hardly surprising that mental health workers have developed treatment modalities for people suffering from these complaints. This chapter will describe two new developments in the treatment of burnout complaints at the Department of Psychiatry of the University Medical Center Groningen in the Netherlands.

1. In a research project, the effects of light in the treatment of the emotional exhaustion of the burnout syndrome were investigated. The preliminary conclusions of this small pilot study are promising: subjective energy levels increased.

2. At the clinic, a multidisciplinary day-care programme was developed to treat the burnout syndrome. Taking the principles of cognitive behaviour therapy and activation as a starting point, patients developed new coping strategies and social skills in order to become less vulnerable in their daily life and work situations. The effects of this programme were assessed during the programme and in a follow-up session a year later. A significant reduction in burnout symptoms was seen with 74.7 % of the participants being at work one year after having finished the programme.

Chapter VII - The mental health of an individual throughout the lifespan is influenced by a range of factors that can either protect the individual from mental health problems or make them more vulnerable to those problems. The interdependency between health issues and social/economic issues is most acutely experienced by people who are in poverty. In the USA this often involves communities of the non-white population .

An approach highlighted by the WHO to tackling the complex range of social, environmental and health issues is Community Development. The basic components of community development are outlined with reference to two community development projects; one in a third word country; the other in a western society. The projects are used to examine the inter-relationships between community involvement, empowerment and subsequent changes in living conditions and health status.

Promotion of, and barriers to, effective community development in the U.S. are explored in relation to the needs of the vulnerable members of society who live in poverty and who are at increased risk of developing mental health problems.

Chapter VIII - Superimposed organizational demands, work overload and limited decision-making capacities are often associated with the development of occupational stress by nurses that eventually create a sensation of professional burnout. In the current era of evidence-based practice, health organizations and regulatory bodies impose further demands on practicing nurses as to implement research evidence in practice setting. Also, evidence-based practice requires that nurses search the electronic literature as to find the best available evidence for practice. Lastly, in accordance to the traditional view of evidence-based practice, decisions relating to patient care are not the product of the practitioners' intellect, but the result of research findings deriving from randomized control trials that the practicing nurses merely implement. This traditional view of evidence based practice appears to create further organizational demands, work overload and limited decision-making potentials for practicing nurses that is bound to intensify the burnout feelings. Therefore, the current chapter will conclude that the traditional view on evidence-based practice needs to be abandoned as to avoid the perpetuation of burnout sensations in nurses. A more radical view will be proposed that conceptualizes evidence-based practice as an ideology of individual emancipation, where daily practice is based on the individual nurse's critical and reflexive analysis of singular situations and contexts taking into consideration the feasibility, appropriateness, meaningfulness and effectiveness of all types of evidence and developing a line of thought that has logical validity and argumentative coherence. This radical view will empower individual practitioners and enable them to undertake rational decisions based on the various types of knowledge that they possess leading to a notion of ownership of nursing praxis and a sense of professional fulfillment. Finally, this radical conceptualization of evidence-based practice not only fits in with the current trend in nursing, but also facilitates nurses to overcome the burnout feelings.

Chapter IX - Organisational and financial policies in the long-term care sector make it hard for caregivers to justify time away from caring for residents to participate in continuing education programs (Romanow, 2002). ELearning offers appropriate and useful methods to deliver convenient and flexible education that fits within the constraints of the healthcare workplace. The growing popularity of emerging technologies presents new opportunities for delivering engaging and effective learning. However, if these technologies are going to be used in education they need to be examined in that regard. Consequently, the purpose of this project was to explore the use of emerging technologies to develop an online learning resource for caregivers that require palliative care and collaborative practice expertise to care for terminally ill residents in long-term care homes.

Chapter X - Several studies analyze the importance that stress has on nursing professionals. However, several emotional variables, such as Emotional Intelligence, play a role in its impact. In this book chapter for *Nursing Burnout* we focus on the role that Emotional Intelligence has in Burnout. Specifically, we summarize a series of studies that analyze the modulator impact of emotional intelligence on nursing burnout, occupational stressors and their impact on the health of nursing professionals. Our studies show that those nursing professionals that have clear feelings about their emotions and situations that occur, and are capable of dealing with those emotions, have lower levels of stress in their work. Also, those nurses who show a high ability to curtail their negative emotional states and prolong positive emotional states show higher levels of overall health than those individuals who have trouble regulating their emotions.

The results imply that the emotional and cognitive dimensions related to emotional breakdown and burnout have to be taken into account in future training programs for nursing professionals.

Chapter XI - Caring for elderly and disabled people poses a challenge not only for society but for each person working in this domain. This study addresses individual work experiences, coping strategies and health behaviour of nurses in the elderly care.

Interviews (N = 52) were conducted and analyzed using qualitative content analysis (Elo & Kyngäs, 2008; Patton, 2002). The reliability of the developed category system was evaluated by providing interrater agreement which led to a very good result.

The interviews showed that daily routine in nursing homes was often made difficult by institutional standards and hampered by negative experiences with the residents. In addition to perceiving the hostile, egoistic and uncooperative behaviour of the residents as a burden, more than half emphasised time pressure and staff shortage as stressful. Positive working experiences were related to contacts with residents and their relatives who expressed gratefulness and appreciation but those experiences were outnumbered by unpleasant incidents. The most commonly mentioned coping strategies were taking exercises and seeking for social support. These strategies seemed to help reduce stress during leisure time. Coping with hassle during the working hours is mainly realized by communication with colleagues. On the other hand, delimitation which is defined as distancing oneself from the residents and work in general, plays an important role. About one third of the interview partners could only handle wearisome demands by taking (physical) revenge on the residents or sneering at them.

Health-risk behaviours such as smoking, unbalanced diet and high levels of drug use were frequently reported and multiple risk behaviour was observed. Eighty percent of the interviewed nurses were smokers and more than half of them reported the use of drugs in order to overcome working hours. Body mass index was between 19 and 41, most respondents were at least slightly overweight.

Work conditions in nursing homes seemed to lead to self-neglect and health-risk behaviour on the part of nurses and had negative impact on the interaction with the residents. Due to demographical changes in our society and the prospective increasing demand for nursing and health professionals, nursing homes should become a healthy workplace by focusing on workplace health promotion.

Chapter XII – Aims: This study examined whether prevalence of burnout is higher among community psychiatric nurses working under recently introduced job-specific work systems than among public health nurses (PHNs) engaged in other public health services. Work environment factors potentially contributing to burnout were identified. In addition, correlations of burnout with emergency patient referral systems and the feelings of PHNs providing mental health services were examined.

Methods: Two groups were examined. The Psychiatric group comprised 525 PHNs primarily engaged in public mental health services at public health centers (PHCs) that had adopted the job-specific work system. The Control group comprised 525 PHNs primarily engaged in other health services. Pines' Burnout Scale was used to measure burnout. Respondents were classified by burnout score into three groups: A (mentally stable, no burnout); B (positive signs, risk of burnout); and C (burnout present, action required). Groups B and C were considered representative of "burn-out". A questionnaire was also prepared to investigate systems for supporting PHNs working at PHCs and to define emergency mental health service factors contributing to burnout.

Results: Final respondents comprised 785 PHNs. Prevalence of burnout was significantly higher in the Psychiatric group (59.2%) than in the Control group (51.5%). Responses indicating lack of job control and increased annual frequency of emergency overtime services were significantly correlated with prevalence of burnout in the Psychiatric group, but not in the Control group. Also when analyzed in relation to several states of feeling of PHNs, prevalence of burnout among psychiatric PHNs was found to increase significantly as frequency of experiencing a feeling of restriction during overtime work.

Conclusions: Prevalence of burnout is significantly higher for community psychiatric nurses than for PHNs engaged in other services. Overwork in emergency services, lack of job control, and a feeling of restriction appear to represent work environment factors contributing to burnout. Inadequacy of emergency mental health service systems was identified as a cause of the high prevalence of burnout among these nurses.

Main Messages of this Chapter:

- Prevalence of burnout was significantly higher for community psychiatric nurses (prevalence 59.2%) than for PHNs engaged in other public health services in this nationwide survey.
- Excessive work demands, particularly for emergency overtime work, and low job control for community psychiatric nurses are work environment factors that appear to contribute to burnout.
- The work characteristics of community psychiatric nurses may be categorized as displaying "high job strain".
- Prevalence of burnout in community psychiatric nurses correlates significantly with frequency of a feeling of "restriction" during work.
- To implement de-institutionalisation that the national government has devised, establishment of a system that can not only accept discharged patients, but also cope with the emergency care needs of discharged patients is indispensable.
- Community psychiatric nurses will play a central role in any such system. Thus, countermeasures to improve the work environment and prevent burnout among nurses should be implemented.

In: Nursing Issues: Psychiatric Nursing, Geriatric Nursing…   ISBN: 978-1-60741-598-5
Editors: C. D. McLaughlin et al., pp. 1-82   © 2010 Nova Science Publishers, Inc.

Chapter I

Psychiatric Nurses Perceptions of the Constituents of the Therapeutic Relationship: a Grounded Theory Study

Adrian Scanlon
Dip Counselling, Ireland.

Abstract

Psychiatric nursing is invariably linked with a therapeutic role; however the question remains unanswered in relation to the extent psychiatric nurses perceive the importance of the constituents of the therapeutic relationship. The aim of this research is to ascertain the nature and comprehension psychiatric nurses assign this therapeutic role. The subject relates significantly to the role of the psychiatric nurses in relation to awareness of elements of the therapeutic relationship in his or her practice and the understanding and identifying this role clearly and unambiguously.

Grounded theory methodology was utilised to develop these conceptualisations to elicit a theory relating to what comprises the therapeutic relationship. Semi-structured depth interviews were conducted with 6 generic registered psychiatric nurses who have between two and ten years of experience.

The objective of the research was to formulate a theory relating to constituents of the therapeutic relationship to inform professional psychiatric nursing practice and to provide a theoretical framework to inform conscious psychiatric nursing practice in relation to forming therapeutic relationships. Strauss and Corbin (1990) describe one of the purposes of research is to guide practitioners' practices and to develop a basic knowledge. The aim of research was to fulfil this purpose; building theory implies interpreting data that must be conceptualised and the concepts related to a view of reality.

The main findings of the research related to how psychiatric nurses learn to form these relationships and what skills are utilised within the relationship. The research discovered that the therapeutic relationship is therapeutic, but the degree of positive change is difficult to measure. The study also highlighted that the learning that takes place in relation to the development of therapeutic relationships is an experiential process and begs the question is the focus of psychiatric nurse training, in relation to the therapeutic relationship, located appropriately.

Chapter One

The Research Problem

Introduction
This chapter begins with an overview of the research question and how this question is informed by previous practice. The question is contextualised by the historical influences on psychiatric nursing practice in relation to formation of therapeutic relationships and synthesising this with contemporary psychiatric nursing. The significance to psychiatric nursing practice and purpose of the research are also identified. Definitions of important terms used in the course of the study are made explicit.

The Research Problem
The growing emphasis on nurses to provide evidence to support best practice has been a major impetus for study in all areas of nursing. Psychiatric nursing, although advanced in areas of interpersonal skills and manpower management, have been sadly lacking in the area of research relating to practice. This study aims to provide empirical evidence in relation to understanding a fundamental aspect of the psychiatric nurses' role, namely what constitutes the therapeutic relationship.

While a positive therapeutic relationship is a necessary pre-requisite for a successful therapeutic outcome, it remains a largely unmeasured phenomenon that is not well understood. A review of the theoretical and empirical literature indicates that the elements of the therapeutic relationship in relation to interactive, subjective, dynamic components have been largely ignored (Weibe, 2002).

This study aims to explore the research in relation to the components of the therapeutic relationship elicited in the literature. Whilst this is of significance, I will attempt to bracket this knowledge and form a theory from the information provided by the participants. Psychiatric nurses intuitively form relationships with patients and these relationships invariably are stated to be therapeutic. Exploration of this phenomenon in a scientific sense is fundamental to understanding how and why psychiatric nurses perform his or her role. The early work of Peplau (1952) has acted as a catalyst for further study in this area and developments to advance psychiatric nursing practice have been significant. This study is designed to add to the growing evidence to promote conscious competence in psychiatric nursing.

Background to the research problem
Psychiatric nursing can be seen as occupying two care domains as indicated by the role or title; to nurse implies a doing activity and psychiatric nursing involves a competence and knowledge of conditions within the spectrum of the study and treatment of mental diseases (Rolfe, 1990). The role and function of mental health nurses has evolved from the custodial attendant to the inquiring professional practitioner. This evolution has necessitated a

fundamental shift from assisting medics in the care of inmates to autonomous therapeutic change agents (Chambers, 1998).

Fundamental to any research inquiry involving the discipline of psychiatry is the appreciation of the complexity and convoluted concept of the psyche or mind. Medical and natural sciences dominate medical practice and have influenced scientific inquiry in psychiatric nursing. Psychiatric nursing however has developed scientific respectability in its own right, as illustrated by Peplau (1952) who was one of the first scholars to locate psychiatric nursing within the American Neo-Freudian tradition of theorists. Contemporary psychiatric nursing therefore is based on the notion that therapeutic relationships are concerned with reactions of human beings to mental distress and illness and how individuals are assisted to cope or adapt to life experiences (Chambers, 1998).

The fact that psychiatric nursing and psychiatry is complex per se is reflected in the complexity of questions that are addressed by research, these questions are informed by human experiences of the psyche and outcomes are not easily measured and are epistemologically difficult to locate. Omery et al (1995) stated that when answering questions relating to human experiences nurses need to be assured in asserting the utilisation of less favoured research methodologies to refine, advance knowledge and understanding to improve the quality of care delivery. In this sense qualitative and naturalistic methods that are appropriate methods for certain research questions, and is the appropriate approach to answer the psychiatric nurses experiences of the constituent of the therapeutic relationship.

The literature seems to indicate two observations relating to psychiatric nursing knowledge; one proposes a biological basis of mental illness (Gournay, 1996), the second is a humanistic view concerned with social determinants of mental illness and subsequent relationship with the nurse (Barker et al, 1995). The approach of Humanistic Existentialism with a dual emphasis on suffering and care is seen as a natural maturational philosophy for the whole of nursing in the future. However with the emphasis on the psychological anguish of the existential dilemma it seems to be particularly suited to mental health nursing (Bevis, 1982). What humanism does do according to Bevis is to make it acceptable for individuals to deviate from these scientific norms and so enable the individual to choose about nursing care and medical treatment in accord with their own wishes and personal judgement. This fundamental shift enables nursing to move beyond the restrictions of practicing within the medical model.

The purpose of this study is to provide empirical evidence to support a claim that psychiatric nurses fully understand the components of therapeutic relationships. Barker (1998), Chambers (1998), Peplau (1952), Travelbee (1966) testify to the fact that the therapeutic relationship is "the rock" on which psychiatric nursing is built. Therefore a full and unequivocal understanding of what forms these relationships is paramount to performing the role of a psychiatric nurse.

The location of the therapeutic relationship within the role of psychiatric nursing therefore, as indicated in the literature, is an illusive concept (Barker, 1998, Gournay, 1996). Peplau (1972) was convinced of the centrality of this interpersonal and psychotherapeutic aspect in nursing. The Expert Review Committee on Psychiatric Nursing further emphasised the shift away from the medico-psychiatric model by highlighting four main areas of nursing: educational, technical, social and interpersonal, of which the interpersonal aspect was central to the task of the nurse (World Health Organisation, 1956). Travelbee (1966, 1969) additionally stressed the interpersonal or therapeutic relationship is a fundamental aspect of psychiatric nursing in his seminal works. He illustrated that without the therapeutic relationship psychiatric nursing could not have a therapeutic, healing or change agent role.

Altshul (1972) argued that some psychiatrists viewed nurses as occupying a therapeutic role as exceeding his or her authority in a service that continues to be dominated by the medical profession. A personal experience of this author on a psychiatric acute admission unit; overheard a conversation between two psychiatrists and a Director of Nursing, this conversation espoused the virtue of male nurses six foot two tall, well built and able to control patients physically. This conversation did not take place in the 19th century; it took place within the last five years, illustrating clearly where some psychiatrists locate contemporary psychiatric nurses.

Peavy (1996) described the need to determine and explore the paradigm shift from locating the therapeutic relationship within the paradigm of positivism, as being a scientific undertaking; to locating the therapeutic relationship within a culture of healing and describing activities as cultural practices. This shift would not only demystify the location of the therapeutic relationship within psychiatric nursing, it would also sociologically place interpersonal skills and the therapeutic relationship within the discipline of psychiatric nursing. Peavy (1996) argues that when individuals are experiencing pain or despair, some action is warranted either by the individual or by a concerned person; this action is an accepted justification for a therapeutic intervention. He additionally asserts that three essential ingredients have the capacity to support individuals in distress. These ingredients are to clarify aspects of his or her life world, offer hope and encouragement and provide comfort and support.

In addition to the afore mentioned paradigm shift Barker (1998) also proposes new and old paradigms; referring to the old paradigm of essentially rational, analytic, linear, objectifying, fragmenting, dismantling, disempowering and distancing approach of human distress. It is suggested that this paradigm is formed by predominantly masculine values and induces a patriarchal imbalance and fails to acknowledge the feminine values associated with post-modern society. The new paradigm acknowledges the value of balancing masculine and feminine values of post positivist methodology. The methodology and epistemology informing this new paradigm reflects qualitative research methods and this is fundamental to locate human factors within research. This paradigm shift has repercussions for the research of the constituents of the therapeutic relationship. Psychiatric nursing places large emphasis on the reciprocal nature of interpersonal relationships. If the emphasis of the relationship is reciprocal, the relationship from the perspective of the patient would necessitate more involvement and empowerment of mental health users. This increased involvement would enable an increased understanding of patient care issues from the care recipient.

These changing paradigms have initiated a debate in relation to the value of positivist and post positivist methodologies and how and indeed the rationale to measure mental health nursing interventions. Omery et al (1995) postulated one such aspect of the debate when espousing the notion of the chaos theory. Barker (1998) described the chaos theory as being the answer for researchers who seek a certainty principle to apply to research practice.

Chambers (1998) argues that whatever epistemology or grand theories are utilised to measure humanistic or components associated with interpersonal relationships, within psychiatric nursing, it may be of value to allow for spontaneous reactions between individuals. He argues that for the patients' value is placed on attitudinal and personality traits such as trust, genuineness, warmth and respect.

In addition to philosophical assumptions, theoretical conceptualisations and methodological identification psychiatric nurses are without a doubt professionally socialized to perform his or her role in certain ways. Chambers (1998) made reference to the fact that philosophical beliefs and values espoused by individuals are flavoured and influenced by socialization issues. Numerous studies have been conducted in relation to the socialization of nurses indicating that socialization factors are powerful and pervasive (Davies, 1993, Gerrish, 2000, Gray and Smith, 2000, Philpin, 1999). All these scholars conclude that the socialisation experiences of nurses affect clinical practice irrespective of educational experiences shaping practice.

The Research Question

Having identified the purpose and research problem a number of questions emerge which provide focus and direction to the phenomena under investigation. These questions are formed on a tentative basis that gives a philosophical direction to commence the study. Whilst appreciating that the method of study is dictated by the question and the emerging data influences resultant analysis, constant comparative method engages suitably with, both the question and the philosophical stance. The questions were:

1. How do psychiatric nurses form therapeutic liaisons with patients?
2. How do they differ from any other kind of relationship?
3. What makes therapeutic relationships therapeutic or curative?
4. How do psychiatric nurses learn to form these therapeutic relationships?
5. When do psychiatric nurses learn to form these therapeutic relationships?

Significance of the Study

Emphasis continues to be placed on the professionalisation of nursing and the necessity for nurses to practice firstly within his or her scope of practice and secondly utilising evidence based practice (An Bord Altranais, 2000, Hamer and Collinson, 1999). The notion that informs this study and what makes it a significant research endeavour is the questioning of the fundamental role of psychiatric nurses. Namely if psychiatric nurses claim to form therapeutic relationships with patients, are they doing this knowingly, with a complete understanding of why, how and when these relationships are formed? The findings of this study may advance an understanding and formulate a theory of the nature and constituents of the therapeutic relationship. The study may open a debate as to how psychiatric nurses perform their basic roles and how these are learned. A review of the literature indicated a dearth of studies on this particular subject; the findings may therefore advance further study into this fundamental aspect of psychiatric nursing care provision.

Definition of terms

For the purposes of this study *therapeutic relationship* refers to the relationship between psychiatric patients and psychiatric nurses. This relationship is stated to be therapeutic, however it is fundamental to the study to determine a difference between this relationship and other life relationships. *Therapeutic role* refers to some form of intervention on behalf of the psychiatric nurse to induce a positive or curative change by a psychiatric patient.

Summary

This chapter began by identifying the research problem, namely the clear, unambiguous understanding by psychiatric nurses of what constitutes the therapeutic relationship. A historical perspective was described in an attempt to contextualise a contemporary position. The study question focuses the research on the appropriate usage of therapeutic relationships in psychiatric nursing, whether it is intuitive or learned. The purpose and significance of the study are clearly stated and how the results may be further utilised is stated. An explanation of terms used in the study that the reader may not be familiar with is also defined.

What follows in chapter two is an introduction to relevant literature in the area relating to the therapeutic relationship in psychiatric nursing. The review covers published and unpublished material on the role identification in psychiatric nursing and how this relates to the therapeutic relationship. Related areas such as counselling and psychotherapy in nursing are also examined. Key studies are identified and critically analysed. The constant comparative method does mean however that the question and the findings will be constantly compared to the knowledge available. Chapter three will describe the research design and how and why the methodology is appropriate for the research question stated. Chapter four will explore in detail the findings of the study. Chapter five will discuss these findings and provide theoretical sensitivity in relation to the phenomenon under investigation, by locating the findings professionally, personally and with the a priori knowledge.

Chapter Two

Background to The Literature

Introduction

The review of the literature begins with a synopsis of the literature search strategy, followed by details of relevant published and unpublished material. Relevant literature related to the examination of meaning assigned to the therapeutic relationship in psychiatric nursing is reviewed. Examination of content and methods utilised to elicit meaning of therapeutic relationship is critically discussed. Whilst the author appreciates the need to review relevant research relating to the subject to situate the study, it is also pertinent to allow the emerging data to determine reality and to produce an informed theory. Commentary by experts in the field of communication, interpersonal skills, counselling and dynamics in human behaviour is discussed. Key studies are reviewed in detail including their aims, methodologies, findings and limitations. Any gaps in the knowledge relating to the therapeutic relationship and the understanding of its implementation are also examined. The chapter concludes with a summary of the material reviewed.

Review of the literature in naturalistic inquiry

Positivist research is probably the research most readers would be familiar with and this research process is a linear analytical process that dictates an extensive literature review to ascertain gaps, test hypotheses to contribute ideas to a body of knowledge. In contrast grounded theory research requires not reviewing any of the literature in the area under study. This statement is made in an understanding that the process of theory generation is not contaminated, constrained by, inhibited, stifled or otherwise impeded by influences other than the analysis of data (Glaser, 1992). To quote Glaser (1992 p32) *the researcher should not worry about covering the literature in the same field before his research begins, since it will always be there.* Hutchinson and Wilson (2001) maintain that a literature review is written before data collection and analysis to build a case for the proposed research. The literature review in grounded theory provides context to concepts and an awareness of gaps in the literature. Grounded theorists maintain a second literature review is required to link a priori knowledge and new theory or evidence (Hutchinson and Wilson, 2001).

Literature search strategy

The literature search involved exploring the published and unpublished material relating to the area of the therapeutic relationship. Most of the literature that was initially located referred to therapeutic relationships in the field of psychology, which although provided interesting reading and relevant, to a point, did not apply specifically to psychiatric nursing. Related areas of counselling, communication and interpersonal relationships were also examined. The searches involved utilisation of OVID databases and scanning library catalogues. The databases included Medline, Cinahl, Psych lit and other health related electronic databases. Keywords used during this exploration of the databases were therapy, therapeutic relationship, psychiatry, psychiatric nursing, nursing and in various combinations of these words.

Initial searches of Medline and Cinahl provided very few empirical studies relating to the area of the therapeutic relationship in psychiatric nursing. The associated area of counselling provided citations, mainly from the 1980s and 1990s, but unfortunately these had more relevance to the field of psychology. The emphasis of this study is psychiatric nursing practice and these studies do not apply to the area under investigation. What was evident during the search was a great deal of commentary, since the 1950s, was in relation to the changing role of the psychiatric nurse. This seems not coincidental with the publication of comment by Peplau (1952), who appears to have ignited this debate. Psych lit offered more promising research articles related to the phenomena under investigation. These articles seemed to be in two stages of publication. Firstly the 1950s and 1960s and secondly late 1990s to the present, perhaps fuelled by the requirement to perform utilising evidence based practice.

Although some of these studies were both relevant and provided interesting comment, none of the studies were specific to Irish mental health nursing. This disappointing dearth of empirical evidence is surprising due to the amount of anecdotal literature that is available in relation to interpersonal relationships and interpersonal communication. The search resulted in three significant studies relating to how psychiatric nurses perform their therapeutic role (Berkery, 1998, Evans, 1998, Weibe, 2002).

A search of libraries in University College Dublin, Waterford Institute of Technology and Waterford Regional Hospital provided a number of texts (Altshul, 1972, Burnard, 1994, Peplau, 1952, Travalbee, 1966). These texts proved to be important works to locate the phenomena under investigation in context. Although most texts are dated they provide seminal commentary by experts. These texts have been re-published on a number of occasions. The material utilised in the literature review were journal articles, both theoretical and empirical sources, fortunately most were available, some were located through inter-library loans and texts borrowed from various locations.

Literature search-historical context

The later part of the 19th century saw a slow transition from paternalistic management of patient care, to the utilisation of interpersonal skills, involving the development of change relationships between attendants and inmates. However medical dominance prevailed to restrict the development of therapeutic endeavours. The defining episode was the transition of roles from attendants to nurses that provided a platform for the development of a professional identity (Nolan, 1993).

It wasn't until the mid twentieth century, when nursing theorists (mainly from the United States) developed theories and conceptualisations of the therapeutic relationship between nurses and clients (Barker, 1998). The development of the therapeutic relationship enabled mental health nurses to view patient care beyond the restricting boundaries of the medical model of care and to empathise with the patients being treated.

The therapeutic relationship is a concept held by many researchers to be fundamental to the identity of mental health nurses (Altshul, 1972, Barker, 1998, Peplau, 1952). Research into the understanding of the therapeutic relationship has given nursing an evidence base and introduced theories in the middle of the last century. Its origins can be traced to attendants' interpersonal practices in the asylum care in the 19th century. The dominance of the medical practitioners' perception of mental distress, and the working-class status of asylum attendants, prevented the development of professional opinion and understanding of the therapeutic relationship from a discipline predominantly involved in the care of inmates in the asylums. It was the influence of Hilegard Peplau (1952, 1962, 1963, 1987, 1990) and other nursing theorists (Altshul, 1972, Orlando, 1961, Render and Weiss, 1959, Travelbee, 1966) who described mental health nursing as a therapeutic relationship.

The meaning assigned to therapy or therapeutic has evolved throughout the years into specific meaning, but the constituents of the relationship between carer and cared for has become obscured by rhetoric and political correctness. It is accepted that the nature of therapy has changed and in particular become less physical since the custodial care of 19th century asylums (Chambers, 1998, O'Brien, 2001, Wilshaw, 1997). Asylum care was characterised by paternalistic, authoritarian regimes and as a care regime therapy was custodial and based on physical restraint (Weir, 1992).

Background literature

The literature seems inclined to portray the therapeutic relationship as an elusive holy grail of psychiatric nursing endeavours. The contrary is actually the case, as the therapeutic relationship is the fundamental core and essence of the role of the psychiatric nurse (Altshul, 1972, Barker, 1998, Peplau 1952).

The literature indicates areas that require clarification from an evidence-based perspective and include attributes or attitudes, socialisation process, skills, curative factors and how the connection between nurse and patient is enactioned. These areas indicate the formation and intricacies within the relationship and how this process is defined as therapeutic. The literal definition of therapeutic is described as, contributing to the cure or soothing of a disease. Psychiatric nurses espouse practicing a therapeutic role and Peplau (1952), Altshul (1972), Forchuk and Brown (1989), Barker (1998) and Morrissey (2003) would maintain that the profession has embraced the role, but has not clearly identified in any sense the components of the relationship.

Scholars have quite clearly stated that the most appropriate approach to examine the therapeutic relationship is the interpretivist approach (Bevis, 1982, Chambers, 1998, Forchuk, 1991, Peavy, 1996). The theoretical process for examining the therapeutic relationship, which has emerged since the early work of Peplau (1952), emphasises the understanding and interpretation of human experiences. The experiences elucidated in the literature focuses on personal factors, skills, curative factors and how the relationship is developed, but from the literature more questions are asked than answers elicited (Chambers 1998, Sullivan 1998, Barker 1998). This study addresses these issues in an attempt to further the debate; the areas explored include how connection occurs in the therapeutic relationship, attitudes affecting the connection process, intuitive processes, curative factors and therapeutic skills used to develop the therapeutic relationship.

How connection occurs

Mental health care is delivered through a relationship between a clinician and a patient. Although this therapeutic relationship is of central importance for mental health care, it appears to be relatively neglected in psychiatric research. Empirical research has for the most part adopted concepts and methods developed in other disciplines such as psychotherapy and general medical practice.

Tickle-Dengen (2002) upon reviewing the available research suggested that communication functions within therapeutic relationships are fundamentally formulated in three concurrent and interlinked stages. These stages are, the development of rapport, the development of a working alliance and maintenance of the working alliance. These stages appear to be formed similar to the map of counselling espoused by Burnard (1994) (Appendix 1).

Rowan (2002) describes three approaches to therapeutic liaisons, instrumental, authentic and transpersonal. The instrumental approach is universal as a way of being. It is learned responses or developmental material that is reinforced by socialization agents such as the family or mass media. The authentic approach requires some kind of initiation, which is quite readily acquired through therapy. It involves dealing with certain closed or subconscious aspects of existence, all those aspects of ourselves that we are initially reluctant to recognize.

And the transpersonal approach also needs some kind of initiation, which has to be acquired through some of spiritual practice. It has to be some form of practice that teaches us, on an experiential level, that our boundaries are uncertain, that we do not live totally in isolation. It informs us that we are fundamentally divine, not limited by a narrow definition of our humanity.

Five types of therapeutic relationship were conceptualised by Clarkson (1994). These conceptualisations gave formal representation to the subjective experience of the therapeutic relationship within mental health nursing. The experiences are suggested to offer a theoretical framework to inform a working matrix fundamental to the relationship with patients.

The working alliance she describes as an agreement between carer and patient formulated to address a mutually agreed objective. The transferential or countertransferential relationship portrays a relationship during which essential issues described as dynamic that underpins the relationship itself and fundamentally forms the partnership. The developmentally needed relationship is described as initiating a corrective or informative function, during which identification of maladaptive interpersonal relationships are addressed. The I-Thou or person-to-person relationship is formed upon the subjective experience of the carer and the therapeutic essence is the product of the relationship itself, providing a forum for ventilation of experiences and emotions. The transpersonal relationship is described as factors extraneous to the relationship or spiritual elements of which quantification is limited and understanding in relation to what forms the relationship and how it operates is accepted as unknown or subconscious.

Psychiatric nursing is viewed by some to incorporate the role of developing therapeutic relationships (Gournay, 1996), whilst Forchuk (1991) views the therapeutic relationship as the essence and Peplau (1962) viewed it as the crux of psychiatric nursing practice. The relationship between psychiatric nurse and patient can be understood to be the development of self-awareness and healing for both parties (Peplau, 1952). A great deal is known about what psychiatric nurses are expected to do in forming therapeutic relationships, what is unsure is the meaning of this experience for the nurses. Most of the contemporary research on the therapeutic relationship has been conducted within a paradigm of positivist empirical research that emphasizes quantitative methods. While these investigations have provided vital information, they have been unable to capture the full intricacy of the factors of the relationship between nurse and patient. Therefore, the purpose of this research is to contribute to an increased knowledge of the meaning of the therapeutic relationship, from the perspective of psychiatric nurses.

Informed by the work of Peplau some scholars (Barker et al, 1995, Forchuk and Brown, 1989) have attempted to incorporate these conceptualisations into psychiatric nursing practice in the form of models and theories informing practice. Critics have argued that the ideologies and conceptualisations of the therapeutic relationship lack methodological objectivity and have encountered difficulty in measuring outcomes (Gournay, 1996).

Attitudes and attributes

The successful formulation of the therapeutic relationship is dependent upon attitudes peculiar to the individual therapist. Attitudes adopted will depend to some extent on the particular therapist and his or her training in interpersonal skills. Rolfe (1990) argued that the theorist most carers associated with identification of attitudes is the theories of Rogers (1981). He identified three essential attitudes namely, genuineness, respect and empathy. However Omer (2000) would argue against this general conception stating that desirable attitudes in relation to the formulation, exploration and sustaining of therapeutic relationships have no universal correct application.

Empathy, warmth, and the therapeutic relationship have been shown to have more impact in relation to patients' perspective or therapeutic effect than more specialized or technical interventions (Lambert, 2001). Decades of research indicate that the provision of therapy is an interpersonal process in which a main curative component is the nature of the therapeutic relationship.

Personal attributes are individual within individual relationship and are transient between each relationship. Attributes most associated with the formation of a therapeutic relationship include global statements relating to effective relationship formation described by Rogers (1981) and Egan (1994). The person centred approach postulated by Rogers is primarily a way of being that finds expression in attitudes and behaviours that create a growth-promoting climate. It is a basic philosophy rather than simply a technique or a method. These attributes include genuineness, respect and empathy. However what isn't answered is whether all these factors need to be present and what degree practitioners are aware of the application within the therapeutic relationship.

Intuitive processes

The research also shows that psychiatric nurses are at times practicing at an intuitive level; this begs the question, are psychiatric nurses practicing within his or her scope of practice? Conversely the therapeutic relationship is such an individualistic activity that some aspects of this relationship are described as immeasurable and need to remain such to allow spontaneity without measurement.

The influence of Peplau in relation to the issue of role identification and formalisation of conscious practice cannot be understated; almost all commentators and researchers refer to Peplau as a significant catalyst for the examination of the role of the psychiatric nurse in relation to the therapeutic relationship (Barker, 1998, Chambers, 1998, Higgins et al, 1999, Melrose and Shapiro, 1999, Morrissey, 2003, O'Brien, 2001, Stickley, 2002, Sullivan, 1998, Whalley and Patton, 1999).

If the essence or crux of psychiatric nursing is the development of therapeutic relationships between psychiatric nurses and patients, research must clearly identify the components of such relationships. It is difficult to identify these components due to a number of factors involved, the two main factors being the convolution of variables involved and the assumptions relating to the location of therapeutic liaisons within the role of psychiatric nursing.

Altshul (1972) postulated the development of therapeutic relationships between nurse and patient was the result of intuition and not a consciously competent theory driven process. Therefore if the essence of psychiatric nursing is the development of therapeutic relationships and these interactions are as a result of intuition, ergo psychiatric nurses are neither utilising evidence based practice nor are they performing their therapeutic role within the scope of professional practice.

Weibe (2002) described the therapeutic process as connection. Connection in this sense refers to the extent to, which a partnership evolves to address the therapeutic process. Connection occurs as a result of therapeutic techniques such as listening, questioning, clarifying, reflecting and interpreting. In addition to the afore mentioned skills or techniques the extra therapeutic or extraneous factors, which appear to be undeterminable for example need further study. These extraneous factors are factors said to be based on intuition of individual psychiatric nurse practising mainly as a result of the socialisation process.

Therapeutic skills

Heron (1974) postulated a matrix when conducting his studies into humanistic existentialism, namely a six category intervention analysis. Heron cited interventions made by therapists to enable personal growth as existing within the following categories:

- Prescriptive- Making suggestions or recommending.
- Informative- Gives new knowledge or information to the patient.
- Confronting- Challenges restrictive or repetitive attitudes, beliefs or behaviours of the patient.
- Cathartic- Helps the patient to release tension through tears, trembling, angry sounds or laughter.
- Catalytic- Helps draw out information from or encourages self-discovery in the patient.
- Supportive- Affirms the worth of and is supportive of the patient.

Techniques or skills identified as being fundamental to formulating, sustaining and advancing the therapeutic relationship are generally accepted to fall into listening, questioning, encouraging ventilation, reflecting on content and clarifying (Minishull, 1982, Burnard, 1994).

Listening or active attending seems and is so easy; to listen carefully to what the patient is saying verbally and non-verbally and also to listen to what the therapist and patient is saying internally (Egan, 1994). Burnard, (1994) suggests that active listening means taking cognisance of metaphors, the descriptions, the value judgements and verbalisations of the counsellor, as they are all indications of their personal world. Carkhuff, (1987) describes listening verbally and non-verbally as "attending" and this is the foundation of effective therapeutic relationships.

Any therapeutic intervention has to involve questions. Questioning has an important effect on therapeutic effectiveness, the number, type, intensity, open or closed and tone all have a bearing on the success or failure of the therapeutic relationship (Minishull, 1982). To some extent the skill of posing questions is allowing the individual to confront or challenge perspectives in their psyche. Researchers who agree that therapeutic relationships are helpful to the individual would concur that challenging or confronting the individuals' perceptions is a central component to the therapeutic nature of the relationship (Burnard 1991, Ellis & Dryden 1987).

The skill of encouragement is formed on the attitudes of the counsellor, being hopeful and supportive and conveying this attitude to the person. Encouragement is more than just a verbal exchange or a "pat on the back" (Tschudin, 1995). Encouraging a person to talk about their inner most fears, secrets, problems or anxieties, involves a range of attitudes including empathy, warmth, genuineness or transparency and as stated by Rogers (1981) unconditional positive regard.

The ability to attend and encourage ventilation in tandem with an ability to explore the verbalisations by echoing statements made during the conversation to encourage the extrapolation of issues is vital to continue the relationship. The issues themselves require a complete and clear understanding. Often a partial understanding of issues provokes anxiety for the patient and merely talking through them with a second party clarifies the issues for the person, without any intervention from the therapist (Nelson-Jones, 1993).

Curative factors

The notion of therapy implies some form of development or positive change in the individual. The notion of how individuals change is described by some commentators as curative (Berkery, 1998, Stickley, 2002), alternatively some scholars dispute the notion of a cure and would maintain the role of the psychiatric nurse is to optimise and maintain good health (Barker, 1998, Gournay, 1996).

To formulate a rationale to approach the understanding of the therapeutic relationship is partly located in research undertaken in the field previously. One such study identified seven elements related to change producing elements:

- The formulation of a relationship determined by real and fantasised qualities of carer and patient.
- The expression of emotional tension.
- Learning or development of understanding.
- Operant conditioning based on approval or disapproval and corrective responses during the therapeutic experience.
- Suggestion and persuasion, overt and covert.
- Development of self-awareness.
- Repeated reality testing and reflection.

(Marmor, 1982)

The fundamental principles described are all important elements of the therapeutic process within relationships. The formation of the relationship has been described as a journey with expectancy, outcomes and co-operation. The journey is in partnership and Berkery (1998) descriptively postulated a double helix to describe both therapist and patient travelling this journey together. What isn't described and is significant to psychiatric nursing practice are the components formulating this journey to ensure conscious competence in nursing practice. It isn't questionable whether the therapeutic relationship is the essence (Peplau 1951) or forms part of the role, what is imperative is that psychiatric nurses are aware of the significance of the therapeutic relationship within his or her role as mental health practitioners.

The curative elements described relate to how the psychiatric nurse engages with the patient and what elements of this engagement are curative or therapeutic. The curative elements can be described as engagement factors and developmental factors.

Key studies

Having reviewed the literature in relation to the therapeutic relationship and related areas of interpersonal relations and communication in psychiatric nursing a few relevant studies were discovered. These studies were determined to be of significance to this investigation due to the similarities of their aims and methodologies. The purpose of this study is to examine in detail psychiatric nurses perceptions of what constitutes the therapeutic relationship. The following section therefore reviews these studies in more detail.

Stickley (2002) although writing about counselling in mental health nursing describes one of the objectives of the study to explore mental health nurses experiences of the therapeutic relationship. The study research design was a grounded theory design involving five unstructured interviews of mental health nurses. The selection of nurses was psychiatric nurses qualified for less than two years, which would appear to this author insufficient time to gain exposure to the phenomena under investigation. What the study does describe is the role of the psychiatric nurse and discovers that psychiatric nurses are in a profession that is demanding and insufficiently trained to perform that role. This is significant to this investigation as one of the questions raised relates to the degree psychiatric nurses develop therapeutic relationships consciously and competently. The findings of the study produced four major themes:

- Mental Health Nursing is a stressful job.
- Nurse training did not equip them for one-to-one counselling.
- Effective supervision would assist counselling in psychiatric nursing.
- More effective training would benefit the nurse in this aspect of their work.

One unfortunate observation in relation to the study is the answers gleaned are more encompassing than the questions asked. The study makes a claim that changes in training methods are warranted, but these changes relate to counselling skills training. This is an aspect of psychiatric nurse training but the study does not apply this to how a psychiatric nurse utilises counselling in his or her practice. The study makes a claim that it illuminates a patient perspective and identifies what patient requirements may be. The study in general seemed far too broad ranging and as such appeared not to investigate in any detail any aspect proposed to be investigated.

Weibe (2002) studied the therapeutic relationship's essential yet elusive nature by exploring clients' and therapists' experiences of connection in the therapeutic relationship. Twelve participants were drawn from a Depression Project. Consistent with a two-person model of relationship, both clients and therapists in six therapeutic relationships were interviewed about their experiences of connection in actual videotaped therapy sessions. Interpersonal process recall (IPR) interviews were conducted in order to capture the here and now, subjective meaning and experience of connection for the participants. A grounded theory analysis was utilized in order to integrate both the clients' and the therapists' subjective experiences of connection. The resultant theory determined that connection in the therapeutic relationship is the experience of sharing a subjective world. The here and now experience of connection ranges from the ordinary to the profound, and it is grounded in the relationship in which it exists. Therefore, the experience of connection in the therapeutic relationship is unique. For both participants in the relationship, sharing a subjective world in the therapeutic relationship is coming to know, and interact with, the client's inner world. The mutual work of therapy is connecting, as is the interactive process of building the therapeutic relationship. The culmination of these choices is the experience, for both client and therapist, of connecting with the client's subjective world. For the therapist, this is the experience of meeting and sharing another's inner world. For the client, this is the experience of knowing his/her own inner world. Therefore, in connecting with another, one ultimately connects with oneself. This is the significance of connection in the therapeutic relationship.

The study although rigorous and describing vividly the nature of how patient and nurse engage in the therapeutic relationship, what it does not do is to posit a theory as described by Glaser and Strauss (1967) or Strauss and Corbin (1990). It is as described by Priest et al (2002) analytic description. Methodologically the study is open to criticism due to the selection of participants and the conditions of data collection. Videotaping of the interviews under real life situations is difficult, if not impossible due to the Hawthorne effect. This relates to how the participant who is knowingly being studied alters his or her behaviour to produce a more favourable view of them in the study. The question is posed therefore how authentic is the data collected due to the fact the participants may have altered his or her natural behaviour due the awareness they are being studied.

Berkery (1998) studied nurse psychotherapists' experiences of the meaning of the therapeutic relationship. Ontological hermeneutics was the mode of inquiry used to explore the meaning of this human experience. An interpretation of the meaning of being in a therapeutic relationship was derived from in-depth unstructured interviews with five experienced nurse psychotherapists. The interpretation of meaning was achieved through a process of continuous dialogue and reflection with the text. The interpretation revealed shared practices and common meanings among the therapists. Two constitutive patterns and seven themes emerged. The first constitutive pattern "In the Trenches or Lost in Stories" and the three themes that constitute it, describes the ways the therapists travelled with their clients on the journey of psychotherapy. The second constitutive pattern, "The Begging Bowl: Allowing an Opening for Possibilities" describes the how of the therapeutic relationship and consists of four themes. The therapeutic relationship is described as a journey, and pictured as moving in the shape of a double helix. The therapist and client travel side-by-side bound together by the bonds of the therapeutic relationship. It is clear that the therapists were not distant objective observers in the relationship; they were intimately and actively committed to their clients and their journey together. The relationship is not one way; the relationship is healing for the therapists as well and they grow in their ability to provide care authentically. The intent of this interpretive research was not to gather facts, but rather, to initiate a dialogue about experiences with therapeutic relationships in the practice of nurse psychotherapists. This research raised many questions that can only be addressed by continuing dialogue among nurse clinicians, educators and researchers.

Evans (1998) study was to investigate patient and therapist perceptions of the therapeutic relationship and to develop a theory about the relationship based on these findings. An existing model of the therapeutic relationship was explicated and used as point of comparison to the findings of this study. A book co-written by therapist Irvin Yalom and his patient was used as the data source for this analysis. This book contained narratives written by both therapist and patient after each therapy session over the course of their twenty-month therapy. These narratives contained patient and therapist perceptions of their experiences in therapy. The text of these narratives was analysed qualitatively based on established procedures of grounded theory analysis. This method yielded 482 meaning units, which were thought to depict central relationship themes over the course of therapy. A hierarchical categorization structure was developed from these meaning units, in which categories were established to explain relationships among items and to illuminate core themes that emerged from the data set. The three categories of "Third-Party Participants in the Relationship," "Patient Participation in the Relationship," and "Therapist Participation in the Relationship" formed the core categories within which all other categories were grouped. Based on the findings, a theory of the therapeutic relationship was developed that sought to explain the possible dynamics from which the categorization scheme emerged. A comparison was made between an established theory of the relationship and the findings yielded by this study.

This study claims to be a grounded theory method, although the methods of analysis were utilised, the philosophical assumptions informing grounded theory were lacking. This can be illustrated by the method of data collection and analysis; complete emersion in the data is advocated in grounded theory (Glaser, 1992), however half the data is collected through a hermeneutic analysis of a previous therapeutic relationship by Irvin Yalom. Grounded theory is also informed by human interaction and analysis of symbols this study is an analysis of text and therefore methodologically questionable.

Gaps in the literature
The review of the literature indicates that the therapeutic relationship, although the essence of psychiatric nursing (Peplau, 1952) is not understood to any great extent. Attempts have been made to empirically locate aspects of the therapeutic relationship in nursing epistemology (Berkery, 1998, Evans, 1998, Stickley, 2002, Weibe, 2002). On the whole comment on how psychiatric nurses perceive their role in relation to developing therapeutic relationships has been as result of the location of psychiatric nursing within the American neo-Freudian tradition by Peplau (1952). This study offers the opportunity to provide empirical evidence to explore the phenomena in Irish psychiatric nursing, hither to unexplored.

Summary
A common theme identified in a great deal of the literature relating to the therapeutic relationship is that psychiatric nurses are practicing at an intuitive level (Altshul, 1972, Barker, 1998, Morrissey, 2003, Weibe, 2002). This intuitive development of the therapeutic relationship is not merely the use of personal experience; it is an application of developmentally acquired knowledge relating to human experience and the addition of acquired knowledge relating to interpersonal skills. The degree of understanding attributed to

the constituents of the therapeutic relationship is minimal (Barker,1998, Gournay, 1996, Stickley, 2002). Perhaps the reason for this is, to fully understand and adjust practice in the light of research findings would fundamentally challenge psychiatric nursing practice which is seen as a profession based on common sense and intuitive practice (Altshul, 1972).

As provided by the evidence in the literature interpersonal relationships and the therapeutic process within psychiatric nursing relationships has been the subject of discourse for approximately three decades. It is not coincidental that Peplau postulated her ideas at this time however consensus of opinion suggests that components formulating the therapeutic relationship have not been fully extrapolated (Barker, 1998, Forchuk, 1991, Stickley, 2002).

What is clearly stated is the most appropriate research methodology is located within the interpretivist paradigm (Altshul, 1972, Barker, 1998, Peplau, 1990). If psychiatric nurses consider the positivist perspective appropriate to explore human experiences and relationships. This may be a reflection of professional insecurity and as cited by Bevis (1982). Nurses should be confident to utilise appropriate, but less favourable approaches to research to advance knowledge and nursing science. The purpose of this study is to explore psychiatric nurses' perceptions of the constituents of the therapeutic relationship and the evidence supplied by the literature would indicate possibly the most appropriate method would be a grounded theory approach as the therapeutic relationship is a circumstance driven process. One of the aims of grounded theory research as described by Strauss and Corbin (1990) is to guide practitioners' practice and to develop a basic knowledge. What the literature is also generating is a need to advance an epistemological basis for the exploration of professional practice and relate this issue to the impact on the clarification of the role of the psychiatric nurse.

Findings of key studies indicated that it is important when developing therapeutic relationships that the various players in the relationship are aware of who does what, why and how (Evans, 1998). What was also clearly identified in the key studies was that this is a partnership between psychiatric nurse and the patient and this partnership is a journey into the world of the patient (Berkery, 1998). Weibe (2002) describes vividly the nature of how connection occurs between patient and nurse and describes this relationship as an equal partnership. What is described illuminates the debate surrounding the nature of the therapeutic relationship, what it does not do is concretely dissect and explain the components of the therapeutic relationship that is the objective of this study. Appendix 2 indicates how the literature review has significance in this study to enable the sensitising of concepts and to highlight gaps in the literature.

Chapter three, which follows, explains the theoretical perspective, method and methodology of the study. A detailed description of how a grounded theory investigation is appropriate to study the stated phenomena is discussed.

Chapter Three

The Study Design

Introduction

This chapter begins with the methods and methodology used to explore psychiatric nurses perceptions of the constituents of the therapeutic relationship. The first section of the chapter begins with a discussion of the naturalistic paradigm in relation to social science research. This is discussed in relation to nursing epistemology. The discussion informs the rationale for the choice of methods for this investigation. Grounded theory design is explained in detail and relates the method to the research question. The sampling processes are examined and the negotiation of access procedures explained. The process of data collection and data analysis are described in detail. Ethical considerations are discussed in relation to the study.

Naturalistic paradigm in research

Identifying the approaches informing research methods is crucial to maintain authenticity, rigour and appropriateness. Ontology refers to assumptions made in relation to what constitutes reality (Guba and Lincoln, 1994). Reality in naturalistic inquiry is referred to in relation to this study when choosing a research approach. It identifies whether reality is external to the individual or a result of the persons' consciousness.

Epistemology refers to the way in which the knowledge of reality is constructed, it considers how and what is knowledge and describes the relationship between researcher and what may be known (Blaikie, 1993).

Research in psychiatric nursing and nursing in general is predominantly within the field of social sciences. Social science research exists within two research paradigms. These research paradigms differ fundamentally in relation to the most effective means of generating knowledge.

The positivist paradigm considers there to be an objective truth that is independent from the subject. Positivist research is linear, analytical, deductive and tests hypotheses. Research within this paradigm is concerned with the measurement of observable data and manipulation of the data to discover universal laws (Paley, 2000).

The naturalistic paradigm considers there is no single objective reality and that reality is constructed by the interpretation of each individual, including the researcher (Schumacher and Gortner, 1992). The presenting phenomena are studied in their own context and are specific to circumstance. Naturalistic inquiry seeks to gain knowledge through understanding how individuals interpret their own circumstances (Treacy and Hyde, 1999). To this end data are collected by interviewing and observing participants in situ. The three main naturalistic methods of research are ethnography, phenomenology and grounded theory.

Grounded theory is informed by the constructionist research paradigm, that emphasizes social reality is produced and reproduced by social actors (Norton, 1999). As a result the constructionist perspective maintains there are many constructions of reality. The constructionist research paradigm understands researchers are inseparable from formation of social realities, due to the fact researchers construct the worlds they research. In constructionist research ontology and epistemology merge due to the knower being inseparable from whatever can be known within the overall construction of a particular reality (Annells, 1996).

Within the constructionist paradigm individuals are perceived not to encounter phenomena and identify meaning singularly. Humans moreover are introduced to a world of meaning and enter a social sphere and describe an environment of significant symbols. In relation to the proposed study, psychiatric nurses enter the field of psychiatric nursing and are socialised into particular practice and the culture reveals meaning in relation to reality. Ergo, constructionists view all meaningful reality is socially constructed and to identify meaning would necessitate epistemology to be within the culture of psychiatric nursing and constructed from interactions between actors (Crotty, 1998).

In this sense what is maintained to be reality is the meaning attributed to social interactions in the context of culturally adapted phenomena. Constructionists suppose that society is actively and creatively encountered and emphasised by individual players within social settings.

The three notions of ontology, epistemology and methodology are reciprocally related in that ontology defines epistemology and methodology is informed by both ontology and epistemology. Grounded theory is located in the interprevist approach of constructionism, which informs the theoretical framework of symbolic interactionism.

Naturalistic inquiry is the most appropriate approach to use in this study. The research question is what determines the method of research adopted and in this case the research question seeks to ascertain what psychiatric nurses perceive to be the constituents of the therapeutic relationship. Naturalistic inquiry accepts that there are many perceptions of what constitutes reality and the objective of this study is to explore perceptions of psychiatric nurses perceptions of what forms the relationship between nurse and patient and what makes this relationship therapeutic.

Choosing a research approach

The objective of this research is to develop a theory to inform conscious psychiatric nursing practice in relation to forming therapeutic relationships. To date research described as grounded theory has been largely descriptive. As stated by Glaser (1992) and Priest et al (2002) research described as grounded theory utilising well-known analytical methods falls short of the formation of theories and is merely analytical description.

Strauss and Corbin (1990) describe one of the purposes of research is to guide practitioners' practices and to develop a basic knowledge. In this study the objective is to form a theory relating to constituents of the therapeutic relationship to inform professional psychiatric nursing practice. Building theory implies interpreting data that must be conceptualised and the concepts related to a view of reality. This view of reality is formed upon results of data analysis that provides a framework to develop a theory. The process of analysis leading to the postulation of a theory is a systematic approach to build on existing knowledge and to integrate a priori knowledge with new knowledge.

A grounded theory study is derived inductively by studying the phenomenon produced in the study area. Significantly the two founder fathers of grounded theory Barney Glaser and Anselm Strauss differed in relation to analysis of data Glaser (1992) maintaining that emergence relied purely upon the participants' views of reality. However Strauss and Corbin (1990) posited that to formulate a theory with any meaning it must be formed through evidence from literature, professional experience and personal experience and to some extent 'force' the formulation of a theory. The following section identifies the theoretical background informing grounded theory.

Theoretical perspective informing grounded theory research

Social psychologists Mead (1934) and Blumer (1969) postulated theories relating to human interaction, defining social interaction in terms of symbols or language. Symbolic Interactionism holds three basic assumptions:

- Human beings act toward things on the basis of the meaning that things have for them.
- The meaning of things in life raises out of the social interaction that a person has with others.
- Meanings are modified through an interpretive process in which people engage when they deal with things that they encounter.

(Blumer, 1969)

Benzies and Allen (2001) maintain that symbolic interactionism is also influenced by Darwin's theory of evolution, citing that the environment is dynamic and human behaviour is determined by adapting to the environment. Symbolic interactionism extracts from this theory that the individual and the environment have a dependant relationship through formation of relationships.

This philosophy underpins the symbolic interactionist perspective, proponents of which argue that the socialisation process is not just about individuals learning about their society but is also a process whereby they develop the ability to think and to absorb information and shape it according to their needs (Ritzer, 1996). In this way, social life is defined by the meanings that we attach to objects. For symbolic interactionists the role of language is of central importance as they regard language as an enormous set of symbols.

Because of human beings ability to understand symbols, people can adjust the behaviour they will employ as, amongst other things, they are aware of the potential consequences of any action, or can learn what the consequences are likely to be. Erving Goffman, who famously interpreted social action as a dramatic performance, further developed this understanding of human behaviour, as a series of symbolic interactions (Goffman, 1961).

The objective of this study is to explore psychiatric nurses' perceptions of the constituents of the therapeutic relationship, the method chosen answers this question as the perceptions of their reality is the research objective. The methodology chosen, namely grounded theory allowed a systematic, dense, explanatory theory to be developed (Preist et al, 2002).

Sample

This section of the study seeks to identify a rationale for the chosen sample. The section will explore how access to the participants was obtained. The section will also identify a rationale for including certain participants and not including others and provide clear criteria for making these decisions. The section will review how the sample was selected and review the process to achieve this selection.

Negotiating access

The research was conducted in an Irish psychiatric hospital setting; the identified participants were sufficiently exposed to the research phenomenon. Access to conduct the research was negotiated with a number of gatekeepers before the commencement of the study. These gatekeepers included the Director of Psychiatric Nursing Services, the Programme Manager, Ward Managers and the Individual nurses involved in the study. The researcher must seek to gain ethical approval to conduct the study from appropriate authorities. Formal ethical approval was sought and granted by the Director of Nursing (appendix 5, appendix 8). Formal approval to conduct the study is paramount to good practice in research, protecting the researcher and the participant (Mason, 1996).

Inclusion criteria

The sample nurses was generic psychiatric nurses with no post registration training in counselling or related courses that could bias the data towards a counselling orientation. The research refers to psychiatric nurses' perceptions of the constituents of the therapeutic relationship that could be biased by extra training in counselling. The size of the sample was determined by saturation of theoretical codes (Strauss and Corbin, 1990). Saturation occurs if the researcher can use the data to answer questions in relation to cause, context and consequences of a code. In this study it was assumed that saturation would occur with a sample of six participants. Saturation was not achieved in this particular study due to the small sample size and the limited amount of time to reach a conclusion to the study. In relation to time constraints, the sample size of six balances saturation and expediency. To locate a purposive sample, the inclusion criteria in this study required:

- Voluntary participation.
- Registered on the psychiatric division of nurses.
- Nurses who have been registered longer than two years and no longer than ten years.
- Nurses who have no additional training in counselling or related field.

The sample of psychiatric nurses was post registration nurses of between two and ten years. The assumption was that nurses trained over two years would have sufficient exposure to form an educated opinion. The ten-year threshold is identified due to; nurses trained beyond this period would have been educated in a different curriculum.

Sample selection

Having located the research question and identified research methods it is incumbent upon the researcher to define and access a sample. The sample for this study was a purposive sample of six psychiatric nurses. The rationale for Purposive sampling as opposed to any other form of sampling lies with the selected methodology. Grounded theory requires information to be obtained from a particular research population this population must hold the information required. In this study the information required is located in psychiatric nurses who are post qualification between two and ten years, this would ensure sufficient exposure to the phenomenon of the therapeutic relationship, without crossing educational differences. The Assistant Director of Nursing department were requested to furnish me with a list of names of nurses who fulfil the inclusion criteria. Nurses who met the inclusion criteria were selected from the list. The nurses who were selected to participate were requested to on the basis of the research question and the notion that they hold the required answers to this research question.

Sample selection process

Upon receiving the list of nurses who fulfil the selection inclusion criteria I began to invite individuals to participate in the study. In this study the target population was a purposive and volunteer sample. The participants' involvement in the study was qualified by an explanation of the research question and their role in the study. The initial contact was made with each participant by telephone. One identified nurse decided not to participate in the study due to prior commitments and one other prospective participant could not find the time to participate in the study.

Following the initial contact I arranged interviews on an individual basis and arranged to meet each participant half an hour before each interview. This initial interview was to informally clarify objectives of the study, inform participants of their rights of participation and to gain informed consent. The negotiation of access was required to be explicit in relation to study objectives. Approval or informed consent was required from the authorities and from the participants. This study identified a clear agenda and the ethical approval for the study was made explicit (Appendix 5). Informed consent was sought from each participant, disseminating explicit information in relation to future use of the material, researcher's right to publish the results of the study and the participants right to withdraw consent (Maykut and Morehouse, 1994). Each participant was asked to read an informed consent form and sign to express approval and understanding of their rights (Appendix 4).

As consistent with a grounded theory method of research, theoretical sampling or purposive sampling was adopted. This process involves deciding on the sample size and type prior and during the research. This purposive sample is based on the type of questions requiring to be answered by participants and information required to be collected to answer the question. Appendix two indicates that the process of grounded theory requires clear purposive sampling or theoretical sampling as in this study.

Data collection

The framework of data collection was semi-structured depth interviews; the topic guide will include themes identified by the background literature. Appendix 3 identifies themes in relation to the research question elicited from the literature. The interviews were transcribed and analysed as identified by Strauss and Corbin, (1990). A pilot of the proposed interviews was undertaken prior to the study to unsure the interview is focused, fits the study, is timed well and is conducted under the exact arrangements as the actual interviews.

Access to the tapes and transcripts were strictly limited to the researcher and relevant academic staff supervising the researcher. The study has been reported in the first person as the researcher is co-participant in the research process. The interviews were six interviews of fifty to sixty minutes duration, to best enable saturation of data, whilst cognisant of expediency and time constraints.

Saturation refers to completeness of theoretical information and no new concepts are emerging. New descriptive data may be added but without altering codes the data will be exhausted and repetitive. The researcher by repeating questions of emerging data eventually acquires a sense of closure.

The Interview guide (appendix 3)

An interview guide was developed informed by the available literature and upon my own experiences as a psychiatric nurse. It comprised open questions and was used as a reference to prompt me during the interviews, as I am a novice researcher. It was sufficiently structured to allow me to deviate from the guide to explore the participants' world and to expand on important information that was emerging. The guide was amended regularly, following information gained from previous interviews, but the main tenants of the guide remained constant.

A GANT chart (appendix 6) outlines the sequence of events through the research process. Resources identified for the study are detailed in appendix 7 and include technical and manpower issues.

Pilot study

Pilot studies are small representations of the proposed investigation. They are performed in an attempt to determine any problems in the research design in relation to data collection procedures. By undertaking a pilot of the proposed study the researcher can make modifications to the data collection process, informed by the lessons from the pilot exercise (Polit and Hungler, 1995). In this investigation the objective of the pilot study was to test the interview schedule and to ascertain whether the answers given and the data collected were appropriate to answer the research question. In addition to testing structural and logistical requirements the pilot study aimed to allow the researchers to practise interactive skills such as listening skills, asking questions and interpersonal skills (Keats, 2000).

The pilot interview was a useful exercise in this particular study, to identify repetitions in the original interview guide, these where altered in subsequent interviews. I also learned that the timing of the interview was good and gave sufficient scope to explore areas as they emerged from the participants. I changed one particular question that was attempting to explore perceived attitudes of the patient towards developing therapeutic relationships. This question in hindsight was inappropriate and difficult for the nurse to answer. Subsequent studies examining the therapeutic relationship from the perspective of the patient may address this anomaly.

The interviews

Individual semi-structured interviews were chosen as a method of data collection. This method enabled a flexible approach to data collection and fits with grounded theory methodology (Morse and Field, 1985). More structured data collection methods would not be consistent with a grounded theory approach, as it would not allow the participants the opportunity to expand on their responses to the questions posed in the interview. Prior to the interview commencing I sought permission to record the interview and to take notes as required, each participant granted this. I reassured each participant of the commitment to maintain confidentiality and anonymity prior to each interview. Six depth interviews were conducted.

Procedural issues

Arranging interviews seems and sounds an easy process, however in practice a great deal needs to be considered. The process initially involved searching the staff records system for the purposive sample as specified. The names of nurses identified in the search had to be liased with to arrange appropriate times and venues. Extraneous variables such as identified in one particular case had to be considered. This particular nurse was on night duty at the time and I had to consider would the fact they were on night duty impact on the results of the study. I needed to consider would an interview at night although convenient and expedient, would it be different in any way to the remainder of interviews conducted during the day. My conclusion was to allow the individual to complete their night duty and conduct all the interviews under similar conditions.

The interviews generally went well and following the pilot interview the question were amended slightly in the light of the data emerging. The data and the nature of the findings produced in the pilot interview were sufficient to be included in the general data collection. The interviews were conducted in the participants' place of work, in a quiet area, undisturbed. Each participant volunteered and co-operated with the ethos of the study and provided a substantial amount of significant data. The following chapter is an analysis of the emerging data.

The interviews generally went well and the interview guide (appendix three) assisted in keeping me focussed. My confidence increased as I became more confident and familiar with the interview guide and the emerging information. Each successive interview added to information from the previous interview and I began to synthesise the emerging issues to the previous issues. Prior to each interview the equipment was checked including, spare batteries and the microphone was functioning. The interviews took place in the participants' place of work. The reason for this was to ensure that most interviews were consistent and that the individuals involved were comfortable in the environment. In addition, if granted permission for an hour away from the work place the participants may be encouraged to engage more fully.

The transcribing of the interviews was very much underestimated; it was very tedious and time consuming. The interviews on average lasted between fifty minutes and one hour, these interviews took approximately nine to eleven hours to transcribe onto a text document. The interviews were hand written from listening to the tape over and rewinding. These notes written by hand were then transcribed to a text document and adjusted appropriately. The quality of the tape recordings was sufficient to enable me to easily transfer the data from verbal to written material. This was significant as it meant no data was lost.

Following the interviews the data was transcribed and analysed. This analysis is discussed in the following section. Interviewees or participants can be identified in the findings by reference to participant and the page of the transcript, for example p1.2.

Data analysis

Analysis of the data was according to methods described by Strauss and Corbin (1990); namely grounded theory. This is a constant comparative method, best described as a cyclical process involving inductive and deductive processes. The following section describes how the data were dealt with upon being collected, the analysis process to the formulation of a theory. The objective of this research is to provide a theory in relation to psychiatric nurses' perceptions of the constituents of the therapeutic relationship.

Handling the data

When the interviews were transcribed any names reference to names or places was erased or references were coded to maintain anonymity. When the data was transcribed the tapes were played simultaneously to readings the transcripts to verify the content as correct. These transcripts were copied and stored in a locked draw; the original documents were used for analysis. When the interviews were typed there was a total of thirty nine thousand eight hundred and three words in the six interview transcripts. This wordage amounted to fifty four pages of text only format in courier font.

Analysing the data

Grounded theory method states that the development of theory should be as a result of analysis of data and not prior knowledge (Glaser, 1992, Glaser and Strauss, 1967). This process should be a clear consistent process that reveals the analytical process. In grounded theory two positions have been adopted by the two founders, namely Anselm Strauss and Barney Glaser. Glaser (1992) maintains the development of theory should be grounded in the data and the theory should emerge.

Strauss and Corbin (1990) posited that the method should not merely be descriptive, but should explain phenomena elicited from the data (Stern, 1994). This fundamental difference explains the rationale for adopting either a 'Glaserian' or 'Strausserian' approach. Having conducted a review of literature and the notion that a priori knowledge will influence the 'forcing' of a theory to explain psychiatric nurses' perceptions of the constituents of the therapeutic relationship, Strauss and Corbin's (1990) explanation of grounded theory best suited the study.

Grounded theory has four fundamental criteria to ensure the appropriate application of theory to phenomenon.

- Fit- describes the realities under study in the eyes of the subject.
- Understanding- explains the major variations in behaviour in the area.
- Generality- if it fits and has understanding the grounded theory has achieved generality.
- Control- the theory provides a conceptual framework elucidated in a structured empirical method, it can be described as having control.

(Glaser and Strauss, 1967).

The method of theory generation was a constant comparative analysis. This is an inductive and deductive process, best explained as a cyclical analysis from the general to the particular. Generating data, analysis of data, comparison with a priori knowledge, re-generation of data and formulation of theory to explain the themes or codes emerging from the data. Constant comparative analysis is collecting and analysing data simultaneously, it requires data collection, categorising codes in respect of emerging concepts and identifying core categories. The method involves returning to the field cyclically to eventually produce a theory. The constant comparative method was achieved in this study by constantly returning to the data, moving between open coding and axial coding, comparing codes with categories, categories with sub-categories and constantly cycling between these areas. This constant cycling allowed me to engage fully with the emerging data and to provide concepts to explain phenomenon.

Coding is a process by which data are analysed, conceptualised and re-formulated in previously unidentified ways. This process is fundamental to the whole generation of grounded theory. The procedures of grounded theory are designed to:

- Build a theory, not test a hypothesis.
- Ensure the research process is rigorous.
- Help researchers overcome biases and assumptions that can be introduced to the research process.
- Provide the grounding needed to develop rich, explanatory theory that relates to the reality it represents.

(Strauss and Corbin, 1990).

The coding system in grounded theory incorporates three sets of coding procedures to assist the researchers to dissect the data, conceptualise it and re-build it in new ways (Priest et al, 2002). These three coding phases are termed open coding, axial coding and selective coding.

Open coding

Open coding is the first phase of the analytical process involving fracturing or taking the data apart and analysing the data for differences and similarities (Strauss and Corbin, 1990). Data refers to sentences or paragraphs of transcripts of speech from interviews. Examples of questions the researcher should consider when analysing the data should include; what is the basis for this point of view? Do other participants hold this belief or similar? Is there any relation between themes or concepts? These questions were constantly being asked throughout the research process and as the researcher I was constantly being drawn into debate with the data as to what formed a particular opinion and why. The aim of open coding was to define concepts that form units of analysis. The list of concepts were sorted into groups of related phenomena to became categories.

The interview transcripts were examined to totality, to obtain an overall sense of the content and a flavour of the responses by the participants to various issues. Each transcript was read several times to enable me to engage with the emerging data. Coding began with a sentence-by-sentence, word-by-word analysis. As the data were presenting some of the words or phrases appeared meaningful and these were highlighted. These highlighted words or phrases were labelled by the use of memos and written on index cards. The words or phrases were not allocated any interpretation at this stage. Strauss and Corbin (1990) suggest the use of in vivo codes to avoid early interpretation of the emerging data. These codes are a direct representation of the words used by the participants.

Initially there were a total of one thousand one hundred and seventy four in vivo codes; many of these codes were repeated throughout the six transcripts, examples of open codes from participant one can be observed in appendix 9. Similar codes were amalgamated and index cards were used to identify sub-categories linking codes with similar codes. The index cards were moved re-moved and grouped and re-grouped until sub-categories emerged that seemed fit the codes that were produced. I visited the data on a daily basis for a prolonged period to enable me to filter the data and the sub-categories. There were a total of twenty-three sub-categories on completion of the open coding. The sub-categories translated into concepts by amalgamating groups of ideas or sub-categories. This notion advances open coding to the next phase axial coding.

Axial coding

Axial coding in contrast seeks to compare and connect categories and sub-categories. This phase seeks to identify rationale to define categories, such as conditions that influence phenomenon and to contextualise the data (Strauss and Corbin, 1990). Strauss and Corbin use the terms context, conditions and consequences to analyse the emerging phenomenon. The researcher must consider the context in which the phenomena occurred, what conditions were present and what the consequences of the actions that arose. At this stage as patterns in the data emerge, it is possible to generate tentative hypotheses or make statements of similarities and differences between the emerging phenomena.

The process of amalgamating sub-categories and codes was commenced tentatively at the beginning of the analysis. The process as stated is a constant comparative method and referring to the codes sub-categories and memos, I began to link sub-categories with concepts or ideas that encapsulated the amalgamated sub-categories and codes. The categories that were produced encapsulated the open codes represented more abstract definitions of the sub-categories. Sub-categories were allocated to categories as they emerged and seemed to describe the resultant data. This was a very challenging stage of the research process, as decisions I made were my own responsibility and as a result of my own plausible interpretation of the emerging data. Six categories emerged on completion of the axial coding process. The categories although linking the data, were distinct and separate entities with properties incorporated by the codes and sub-categories.

Selective coding

The objective of selective coding is to discover core categories to which all categories have a relation. The researcher identifies the main theme from the emerging categories. The core category has six essential characteristics:

- It recurs frequently in the data.
- It links data together.
- It explains much of the variations in data.
- It has implications for a more formal or generalised theory.

- As it becomes more intense it advances the theory.
- It permits optimal variation in analysis.

(Strauss, 1987)

This final phase is the most challenging aspect to grounded theory as it seeks to integrate codes, as opposed to many studies proposing to be grounded theory, merely presenting themes. Selective coding makes alterations and integrates codes and categories into a true grounded theory (Priest et al, 2002). The limited time frame and the small sample size prevented the progression to the selective coding process.

The process of grounded theory was eloquently presented by Hutchinson and Wilson, (2001) in the form of a flow chart (appendix 2). This diagram shows clearly the process from primary review of the background literature to contextualise the research question to the positing of a theory. This particular model informed this study and aspects of the model were adhered to, given time constraints and the small scale of the study. What I did not do was to produce a basic sociological and psychological process or achieve selective coding, due to the small scale of the study and the time limitations. The secondary literature review was conducted following the analysis of the findings to provide theoretical sensitivity and place this study in context with existing knowledge relating to the understanding of the constituents of the therapeutic relationship.

Memos

To induce a grounded theory the analysis of data must be elicited at a theoretical level. Memos should be a part of this procedure to apply principles of constant comparative analysis, in the form of index cards, journal recordings or on a computer to establish connections between the data. The emphasis is related to identifying ideas or concepts. Ideas are identified and can be recalled with ease due to the code or codes that they describe with each memo (Strauss and Corbin, 1990). Questions the researcher needs to ask when memoing include:

- Are they separate codes?
- Is one code a property or a phase in another?
- What are the conditions that influence a code?

Through repeated questioning of memos and codes a theory is developed. The basic sociological psychological process emerges and the data becomes integrated. The conditional matrix forms a pictorial representation of an analysis of levels of the world and society we engage with. The picture is presented as a set of circles with the inner circle concerned interactions most closely related (actions pertaining to the phenomenon. The outer ring represents issues pertaining to an international level (issues such as international politics or governmental regulations). The conditional matrix has various levels between these extremes including national, community, organisational/ institutional, group or individual and interaction level. The conditional matrix as described by Strauss and Corbin (1990) was conducted in this study in the form of contextualising the data within national and international psychiatric nursing, however the basic sociological and psychological process was not fully extrapolated due to the small scale of the study.

Rigour

The pursuit of excellence in research is referred to as rigour; this involves accuracy, discipline and adherence to detail. Within the naturalistic paradigm certain steps should be taken to ensure scientific rigor. Sandelowski (1986) describes four aspects of trustworthiness promoting rigor within the naturalistic paradigm. These four criteria refer to credibility, applicability, consistency and confirmability. These four principles of trustworthiness have been upheld throughout the research process.

Credibility

The credibility of the study is increased when scholars and readers of the study identify with the phenomena having read the study. Recording of the interviews was the first step to maximise credibility, this action ensured that all the data were collected and no information was lost. The data and the interpretations were presented to two of the participants to verify the findings. The two participants were asked to comment on the accuracy of the stated categories, in addition two psychiatric nurses independent of the study were asked to comment on the findings of the study. Feedback from these individuals can be observed in appendix twelve. Member validation is a process to check the information presented is accurate and that varying perspectives are encountered (Seale, 1999).

Consistency

The audit trail of the researcher is an important consideration to ensure consistency of the study. Consistency from this study would be clear if another scholar would find similar results from the same data given similar circumstances (Sandelowski, 1986). I attempted to make explicit my decision trail by stating a rationale informing all decisions. This transparency extends to decisions relating to participants, data collection and analysis. Appendix eleven describes the decisions made during the research process and provides evidence to support the claim that the study is consistent and other researchers would have made similar decisions.

Confirmability

Confirmability in this study refers to the research loop described by Sandelowski (1986), returning to the participants to verify results. In addition the confirmability is reinforced in this study by the production of research notes made during each interview (appendix 10) and the transparency of the decision trail. Notes were taken during each interview to assist in the data collection process and to assist in the data analysis.

Applicability

Guba and Lincoln (1994) posit that the notion of applicability is confirmed when the hypotheses can be transferred between contexts depending upon the degree of fit, that describes the realities of the study in the eyes of the subject (Glaser and Strauss, 1967). Candidates who volunteer to participate in research projects are often the more articulate and informative, a treat to applicability can occur when members of a population are not well represented (Sandelowski, 1986). This study incorporated a purposive and volunteer sample and therefore the sample is a fair representation of the population.

Ethical considerations

Ethics are concerned with issues of right and wrong, good and bad and doing no harm. In research ethical consideration must be maintained at all stages of the process. During this study the researcher has been cognisant of the ethical principles and these have been applied throughout the study. Thuroux's five principles apply these principles to a research scenario and are applied under similar forms as follows:

- Value of life
- Goodness and rightness
- Justice and fairness
- Honesty
- Individual freedom

Cited in Tschudin, (1995)

When undertaking research in social sciences, particularly a nursing study, cognisance must be given to a possible role conflict between, the nurse as an advocate and the nurse as a researcher.

Ethical approval to conduct the study was sought from the Director of Nursing and Regional Manager. The aim of the study was to involve psychiatric nurses and, as cited by Bell (1993), approval from authorities governing nurses is sufficient to gain ethical approval. A full informed consent procedure (appendix 4) was completed by each participant and a copy informed consent form was enclosed to the Director of Nursing and Regional Manager, in addition to a letter requesting ethical approval (appendix 5). Reply (appendix 8). A coding system was used to maintain anonymity and this was conveyed and made explicit to the participants in the form of informed consent.

Confidentiality was considered in relation to ethical considerations, it is based on the right to anonymity and linked to the ethical principle of the respect of person. Informed consent was given in the light of the following and could be withdrawn at any stage of the research process:

- Clarity of the purpose of the study and justification.
- Description.
- The benefits.
- The risks.
- Right to withdraw.
- Confidentiality.
- Who to contact for further follow-up.

(Polit and Hungler, 1995)

Responsibility for disclosure or maintenance of confidentiality rests with the individual moral agent. There can be no breach of confidence if information is not regarded as confidential or secret and is already in the public domain. A coding system was utilised in the research. Confidentiality was maintained throughout the entire research and it was explained to each participant that the results of the study will be presented in the form of a dissertation and this is alluded to in the informed consent procedure (appendix 4).

Summary

This chapter described a range of methodological aspects in relation to this investigation. Issues relating to research paradigms and how this study is located in relation to the naturalistic paradigm were discussed. A rationale for the choice of research methodology informed, by this research paradigm was described. The research method chosen was discussed in detail, including data collection and data analysis methods. Ethical considerations were discussed and an explanation of how these principles relate to this investigation given. Chapter four, that follows, gives details of the findings of the study. The final chapter then discusses in detail the research analyses.

Chapter Four

FINDINGS

Introduction

This Chapter describes in detail the findings of the study and presents the research results systematically using grounded theory methodology. It begins with a brief description of procedural issues relating to the study. A description of participants involved in the study follows, including a rationale for their inclusion. This is followed by a presentation of the findings by discussing the analysis of the emerging data. The findings are presented in categories and sub-categories. These findings are a plausible interpretation of the data, it is not a definitive interpretation, as previously discussed, naturalistic inquiry has many interpretations of reality. The findings are not generalisable, however they do represent the views of the participants involved in the study.

Description of participants

The participants in the study were six psychiatric nurses employed in various areas of the psychiatric nursing service in a region in the South of Ireland. The sample nurses were generic psychiatric nurses with no post registration training in counselling or related courses that could bias the results towards the discipline of counselling. The research refers to psychiatric nurses' perceptions of the constituents of the therapeutic relationship, these perceptions could have been biased by additional training in counselling.

The sample of psychiatric nurses was composed of post registration nurses with between two and ten years experience. The assumption is that nurses trained over two years will have sufficient exposure to form an educated opinion on the topic of interest. The ten-year threshold is identified due to; nurses trained beyond this period would have been educated in a different curriculum. The six nurses were equally divided between the genders.

Results

The results of the study outline the perceptions held by psychiatric nurses in relation to the therapeutic relationship. The categories that emerged are formed by the opinions of the participants. The categories are related; to how psychiatric nurses combine a therapeutic role with a service provision role, how the process of therapy is identified in practice, how do psychiatric nurses learn to develop therapeutic relationships, time is an important influence on the success or failure of the therapeutic relationship, what skills are required to form therapeutic relationships and how attitudes affect the formation of therapeutic relationships. The findings of the study are presented in the form of categories and sub-categories that emerged from the data.

Schematic representation

The following section discusses the data supplied by the participants of the study and provides context to the data. This process is best summarised in the form of a schematic matrix. The matrix contextualises the data and as indicated by Strauss and Corbin (1990) provides a theoretical framework to produce findings. The framework begins with professional or role conflicts, indicates the processes necessary to develop therapeutic relationships, examines how learning occurs, examines the nature of time limitations and culminates in the influences personal and attitudinal factors affect the development of the therapeutic relationship.

Category	Sub-category	Context
Nursing is providing	Professional aspects	Psychiatric nursing is an activity located in a professional role; how
a service	of care	does this affect the therapeutic relationship?
	Individualised care	Psychiatric nurses espouse individualised care; is this possible and how does it affect the therapeutic relationship?
	Working in a team	The participants of this study highlighted nursing is mostly performed
		in teams Positive and negative aspects of this are discussed.
	The helping aspect is	Providing help or care was an aspect of the psychiatric nurses' role
	based on a caring approach	highlighted by the participants.
	The nature or the therapeutic	The degree and type of intervention is governed by the psychiatric
	relationship is dependent	condition of the patient.
	upon illness.	
The Process of therapy	The impact of personal	Personal issues have an inevitable influence on how and why
	life issues	therapeutic relationships are formed.
	Therapeutic framework	What guides practice and how do relationships begin, develop and
		end?
	Therapeutic factors	What is therapeutic? What makes it different from any other
		relationship?

Category	Sub-category	Context
	Curative factors	How do people cope and what changes circumstances to enable this
		coping?
	Dependency level	The normalising process decreases the dependency on nurses. How does
		this influence the therapeutic relationship?
Learning in the	Experiential learning	
therapeutic relationship	How do psychiatric nurses' learn to develop therapeutic relationships?	
	Intuitive learning	
Developing therapeutic	Incremental nature of the	To develop a relationship with an individual in any therapeutic sense
relationships is limited	therapeutic relationship	takes time. How is this compromised by the psychiatric nursing role?
by time		
	The nurse' minute	Often psychiatric nurses' have to prioritise workload how does this
		impact on relationship development?
	Role diversity	Psychiatric nursing is very diverse and has many demands.
Skills required to form	Trust	
therapeutic relationships		
	Humour	Skills identified by the
		participants of the study.
	Conscious decision-making	
	Providing information	
Attitudes	Therapeutic boundaries	How do nurses compromise therapeutic distance and professional
		boundaries?
	Different personalities	How do personality conflicts affect the development of the
		therapeutic relationship?
	Non-judgemental attitude	Does this exist. Is it possible in psychiatric nursing?

Nursing is providing a service

This category is comprised of five sub-categories relating to the dichotomous relationship between therapy and the provision of psychiatric nursing services. The five sub-categories are; professional aspects of care, individualised care, working in a team, the helping aspect is based on a caring approach and the nature of the therapeutic relationship is dependent upon illness and class. The category suggests that the diversity of psychiatric nursing results in a ' jack of all trades- master of none' scenario. Psychiatric nurses have so many tasks and duties to perform that, to perform any task to the optimum results in detracting from another area.

Professional aspects of care

This sub-category indicates that psychiatric nurses have a responsibility to conduct themselves in a certain manner. This manner is dictated by a code of conduct augmented by personal morals and ethics.

You feel somewhat obliged to help your clients. You're there, they are there for help. You should be in a position to help. You have knowledge. You are part of a profession (P 4.3).

This professional aspect of care relates to how psychiatric nurses change their approach within relationships and what makes these relationships professional and therapeutic. Therapeutic relationships differ from any other kind of relationships due to the fact psychiatric nurses are bound by a code of conduct and also a duty of care.

But with regard to professional, again it comes down to that balance of getting as close as you can to a patient but keeping your distance (P3.2).

This statement indicates that the involvement between patient and nurse is close enough to develop a therapeutic role and distant enough to remain within the professional code of conduct and preserve the altruistic, professional and caring nature of the relationship.

It is a relationship that is a professional relationship that you would build up with a patient. You can't get too close or too friendly. But there again you don't want to be cold and too hard on them. You have to find a balance of the friendly side of it but yet the side where you have to have an element of control and discipline with the patient…It is hard to find a balance with some patients. With psychiatry, you get a lot of manipulative patients that will try and manipulate you through getting really friendly with you and trying to evade getting personal with patients. Keeping it professional is important (P3.1).

These professional aspects of care sometimes restrict the nature of therapeutic interventions. The professional responsibilities interfere with the natural, maturational development of relationships in terms of therapeutic endeavour.

Take for instance someone with a personality disorder a lot of their behaviour is attention seeking and what you want to say to them is to get a grip, but you can't say that because it is not professional (P2.2).

The sub-categories detailed in this section indicate that psychiatric nurses are often called upon to make decisions in the patients' best interest. These decisions are often in conflict between are therapeutic rationale and the provision of care in a professional sense. This dichotomy between therapy and service provision affects how psychiatric nurses engage in therapeutic relationships.

Individualised care

This sub-category relates to the approach psychiatric nurse have towards patients and how they treat each patient according to their needs. This treatment is dictated by how nurses identify patient needs and approach this treatment in different ways.

they are all different. They are all very much totally different from one another. All their needs are different as well. I suppose somebody might need a bit of help or somebody to listen to or chat to and somebody might not need that at all (P5.3)

Individualised care in relation to how psychiatric nurses perceive the therapeutic relationship also describes a process of care provision in relation to continuous care by a team of nurses. Continuity of care is significant in relation building therapeutic relationships, due to the relationship development being beyond the control of the individual nurse.

staffing levels play a lot in it. I think it definitely does. To a certain degree, it must affect the relationship. You have a patient that is looking at you from admissions and saying right this is my man in here. If I have anything wrong, I will go to this man. If anything is bothering me, I go to this man. You come down the road two days later and he comes up to you and you say 'look I'm not actually dealing with you. Dr. x is dealing with you today. That is John's job, go and talk to John'. John has to start two days later to build up a relationship with the patient. And John could only be on it for a day or two, and then it is somebody else (P3.5).

As indicated by these codes individualised care is possible in theory, however continuity of individualised care is harder to achieve. In relation to the therapeutic relationship the implication is that the relationship building is staccato and inconsistent.

Working in a team

As indicated nursing on the whole is an activity performed in teams, inter-disciplinary teams and multi-disciplinary teams. The result is that any therapeutic relationship developed is dependent, not only on individualised factors, but also factors between individuals and between disciplines. This sub-category describes the relationship between teamwork and developing the therapeutic relationship. The notion of responsibility and the degree nurses feel empowered within the multi-disciplinary team significantly affects the development of therapeutic relationships.

In so far as giving care to the patients, my part in the multi-disciplinary team is kind of limited in ways, in so far that I'm not allowed opinionate things. It's limited in ways I find it is only a personal thing that you are still kind of answerable to doctors (P3.1).

In any therapeutic scenario the therapist would exhibit a degree of unconditional positive regard, but this theory is exposed when describing relationship development and teamwork. Personality difficulties and ability to develop rapport is compromised when the psychiatric nurse is involved in a particular method of care delivery. Primary nursing for example, in a real sense, involves nurses working with a group of patients, but the degree of choice and development of rapport is questionable.

You are working with a certain sector or doctor and you have those clients and that is it. You have no choice. There is going to be personality clashes (4.4).

The positive aspect of teamwork is illustrated by the learning that is undertaken by psychiatric nurses from and between nurses. Psychiatric nurses would describe learning their role predominantly experientially. Traditionally psychiatric nurses have learned their role by clinical placements augmented by 'block periods' in a school of nursing. This study as previously stated is undertaken with this cohort of traditionally trained nurses and reflects this phenomenon.

when you have your colleagues that are working with you as well, if there's problems happening needless to say you can ask somebody what they think, what they would do, or can you help me out with this one (P5.4)

The helping aspect is based on a caring approach

The nature of nursing is presented at times as a helping or caring profession. The codes identified in this sub-category support this statement. The sub-category presents codes relating to how nurses have a role to help others.

this is my job , I love it…so the relationships I form here they need help, they need help in some shape or form. They need help, you have help to give them (P1.3)

Nursing in general, but particularly in psychiatry is dominated by the desire to help or care for fellow human beings. This altruistic notion is of course diluted by the personality traits and attitudes of the individual nurse.

Some people make better nurses than others. I think there has to be an element of care in every nurse. There has to be some element of wanting to help people (P4.3).

Helping or caring is the domain of psychiatric nursing that historically has been the area most emphasised when psychiatric nurses describe their role. It is however the area possibly least studied empirically and other disciplines have provided the evidence to support practice. This evidence does not easily translate between disciplines, as psychiatric nursing is a specific discipline with specific aspects forming the role.

The nature of the therapeutic relationship is dependent upon illness and class

This sub-category describes how the development of the therapeutic relationship is dependent upon the nature of the patients' illness or disorder. The type of illness in conjunction with individual factors mitigate to impact on the formulation of the therapeutic relationship.

its just that if somebody was psychotic or quite paranoid you might approach them differently. That somebody elated say or quite depressed you'd take more of a slower approach with them or may be more of a one to one (P1.1).

In addition to types of illnesses or disorders encountered in psychiatric nursing, patients are representatives of various social strata. The sociological influences upon individuals also affect the nature of the therapeutic relationship.

If you dealing with a solicitor or doctor, which I suppose we all have at times, I suppose you are not going to speak in the same way as you are to somebody who has not received a full education. So language-wise, you try and bring yourself to their standard as you perceive it without talking down to certain people or talking up to others…You put it into basic kind of terms, if you are trying to explain illnesses or problems they may have. As in you'd feel a bit high rather than tell them they are in a manic phase (P4.4-5).

Psychiatric nursing is perhaps unique in relation to forming relationships determined as therapeutic. This unique situation is manifested by the requirement to form relationships with patients who on occasions have been admitted to hospital involuntarily.

The other side of it is hard in acute psychiatry to build up a relationship with a patient is when you have temporary admissions. And then, turn around and try and develop a nurse/patient relationship with them (P3.6).

The sub-category emphasises that psychiatric nurses on occasions have to form therapeutic relationships with people who may not have anything in common with the nurse, or the person has been entered into the therapeutic milieu under duress.

The contradiction between therapy and service is summarised by a professional accountability, responsibility to the public and providing a service; balancing with the necessity to develop a close yet distant and individualised relationship. It seems by the evidence supplied in this study that the balancing of these factors are inextricably linked and are opposing phenomena.

The process of therapy

This category describes the way therapy is fluid and transient and the factors that distinguish a therapeutic relationship as opposed to other relationships developed in peoples lives. The process of therapy is dependent upon a number of factors and these are reflected in the five sub-categories that are incorporated in this category. These five sub-categories are; the impact of personal life issues, therapeutic framework, therapeutic factors, curative factors and dependency levels.

The impact of personal life issues

This sub-category describes the affect personal feelings, prejudices personalities and attitudes has on the forming of therapeutic relationships. Psychiatric nurses are professional people however they are people, with the same expressions of emotions and feelings as the people they are treating. This is reflected in confusion in relation to the degree of personal experiences they should or should not express to the patients. The question is; would my experiences burden the patient further or would an insight into handling the situation in a different way benefit the patient?

the emphasis of the relationship is on the patient, you allow them to deal with issues that they want to deal with without burdening them (P4.4).

The confusion extends to an ability to express in an articulate way the difficulty of therapeutic boundaries and clearly locating themselves within this relationship.

when I said distance earlier on I meant as in not distant as in physical distance, I meant closeness as in I'd never discuss my private life with a patient (P1.6-7).

The role of a psychiatric nurse is to treat patients who have psychological illnesses and disorders of the mind. Part of this treatment is to enable the patient to develop life skills to cope with life events. What needs to be borne in mind is that in addition to being patients and staff the relationship is a more intimate relationship.

you are a person and they are a person... (P2.5)

This more intimate relationship is reflected in the expression of parity in a relationship and respecting the professional aspect of the care relationship.

I'm only human, I'm a human being at the end of the day and we all have our ups and downs in work, we have maybe bad days in work, good days in work and in your personal life as well... (P1.5).

This sub-category indicates the difficult decision psychiatric nurses need to make in relation to the type and extent of personal information they divulge to patients to enhance the therapeutic nature of the therapeutic relationship. These decisions are made in relation to professional aspects of the nurses' role and taking account of personal morals.

Bridges could be built an awful lot quicker if you were going to be very open about who you are, what you do, as in where you come from, you know, personal situations...I just think myself I would hold back on any information outside work. I feel that it doesn't need to come into the patient/nurse relationship (P5.7).

This sub-category emphasises that although psychiatric nurses aspire to bracket personal life influences it is at times impossible to disown life experiences. These life experiences significantly influence how psychiatric nurses develop therapeutic relationships.

Therapeutic framework

This sub-category describes how the therapeutic relationship develops and how psychiatric nurses can and do formulate a loose plan to address forming these relationships. These frameworks are not formally recognised structures but are personal plans that individual nurses adopt to give structure to their everyday practice in relation to forming therapeutic relationships.

you know, I'd always introduce myself, shake their hand in situations where you can do that you know, I'd never be stand offish with a patient, if they'd let me sit in the chair beside them you know, kind of go through their property with them…I'd always talk through what I was going to do with them as well. (P1.6)

The frameworks nurses adopt are based on good mannerly behaviour that any individual may adopt on meeting a person for the first time. The difference between any mannerly individual and a psychiatric nurse is the extent the nurse goes to, to enable the individual to 'feel at home' or 'feel comfortable' with their illness or disability.

You initially introduce yourself and bring the patient to a quiet environment where you can speak without interruption. Sit down face to face, just try and speak calmly and let them know what is happening, what the next steps are. Maybe do something simple like offer them a cup of tea to help them feel more relaxed. And then once you see that they are starting to relax, initiate more conversation on their problems. The best thing to do in a therapeutic relationship is to explain (P2.2-3).

The framework of therapeutic intervention is a loose expression of how each nurse controls their practice and gives a degree of structure to an everyday activity. This framework is an individual expression of their practice and becomes so second nature even to describe it is difficult.

Therapeutic factors

This sub-category describes the participants' perceptions of what factors are therapeutic in the therapeutic relationship and how these relationships differ from other relationships. These factors are a combination and collection of factors described as contributing to a therapeutic scenario. The first code describes the nurse's role in providing care to needy individuals.

caring for somebody who can't provide it for themselves (P1.8).

Therapeutic factors within therapeutic relationships relates to how the patient reacts to the interventions offered by the nurse. This reaction is typified by the notion of a rapport between the patient and the nurse. The rapport refers to the affinity and emotional closeness between two individuals and how this is recognised and used in a therapeutic way.

a rapport you can develop with the patient (P1.1).

The affinity and closeness between nurse and patient is only a portion of the relationship, other aspects include, what nurses do with the information gleaned in the therapeutic milieu. The relationship between nurse and patient must be a relationship held in confidence to enable the patient to feel confident in sharing their inner world, this was one of the clearer aspects understood by the participants. This understanding may be due to the fact nursing and therapy share the common notion of confidentiality.

therapeutic and confidential relationship. You have to be non-biased (P2.1).

The participants in this study recognised that nurses at times need to be advocates for patients and make appropriate decisions for the patients. The nurses also need to make authoritative decisions and act in the patients' best interest, which at times causes conflict.

control and discipline with the patient (P3.1).

Therapeutic factors identified in this sub-category are the perceptions of the participants of the study. The factors described indicate the factors necessary to engage, sustain and develop a positive change in the patient.

Curative factors

This sub-category differs slightly from the previous sub-category in relation to the level and degree of permanency in lifestyle changes and coping with illness or disorder.

Our role is to help people get better. Our role is to make their life as comfortable as possible (P4.1).

A notion in therapeutic relationships that is reflected in this study is the notion that to cure a patient in psychiatric terms is a misnomer and that the illnesses displayed by patients are managed or coped with. When describing curative factors in this study I am referring to a change of circumstances for the patient to improve their condition. This improvement can be as a result of a lot of factors and this study is interested in the improvement attributed to the therapeutic relationship. One of the curative factors identified by the participants of the study was an interpersonal statement reflecting the personality differences and how this affects the improvement that patients make.

You will either draw somebody out of themselves or you won't (P5.1).

Nurses often don't acknowledge their abilities or achievements but some of the participants of this study recognised that they do have a significant role to play in the improvement of the patients' conditions.

We have some answers; we don't have all the answers (P2.2).

The curative factors outlined in this sub-category identify what positive change may be made in the patient and how the psychiatric nurse acts as a change agent. The codes identified by the participants describe the role of the nurse in this change and the role of the patient.

Dependency levels

This sub-category describes the relationship between nurse and patient and how this relationship changes as the patient becomes 'better' and more able to deal with their illness or disorder. The nurses' role in this scenario is to enable the patient to understand the facets of their disability and enable them to cope better. The therapeutic relationship is the vehicle to drive this process and the end product is a normalisation and a return to independence.

they need to conduct their normal day to day living then when things start back on the increase they slowly regain their independence you know for themselves where they come in they might be more dependent on nursing staff, even on medication or something you know where they felt that they needed to use that as a crutch but as they progress in their mental health or as the recovery process progresses their become more independent. (P1.9).

Recognition of this normalising process is the marker to indicate the therapeutic positive movement or change. It is vital for the psychiatric nurse to recognise this positive development in the patients' recovery process, as this is an indication that the therapeutic process is therapeutic or not. The relationship between nurse and patient changes as the therapeutic process progresses and it is subtle change from a dependent relationship to a more shared relationship.

they are moving from a stage of dependence to independence, and part of that process is that the relationship becomes more equal, from being one-way to being more of a shared process (P4.8).

The process of therapy therefore is a progressive cyclical relationship with the emphasis on understanding from the point of view of the nurse and the patient. The patient needs to learn how to deal with whatever ails them. The nurse needs to understand how the patient improves to enable them to reproduce similar therapeutic processes in the future. These change processes are both professional and personal factors that influence the connection between patient and nurse.

Learning in relation to the therapeutic relationship

How psychiatric nurses learn to practice is a significant factor in reproduction of appropriate methods to treat patients. If we understand how learning was produced we can amend future learning to tailor psychiatric nursing practice with the hindsight gained through examination of current trends. Two forms of learning were identified in this study, reflected in two sub-categories: experiential learning and intuitive learning.

Experiential learning

This sub-category describes how psychiatric nurses learn aspects of their role through a process not necessarily formal, but just as pervasive as the formal curriculum. This process of learning experientially is driven by a natural curiosity of the person learning. It stems from the motivating factors intrinsic to each individual learner. These motivating factors are described in the codes and relate to practical, social, personal and research problems of interest to the psychiatric nurse.

learned about forming therapeutic relationships, it was through observing what other members of staff were doing, tailoring your own processes and learning and putting that into action yourself, based on what you had observed. So it wasn't anything you learned academically in the school (P5.4).

In relation to learning about the therapeutic relationship and how this is located in the role of a psychiatric nurse, this process is a socialisation process that involves all learning, both formal and informal. This process of learning from an experiential point of view is displayed by participants in the study constantly referring to learning their role by watching, absorbing and adopting aspects of how senior colleagues perform their duties.

you would watch other nurses and see how they relate to patients and you would pick up how some people don't relate very well and how some people relate very well. And you get tips from more experienced staff...(P2.1) the therapeutic relationship is a very real thing, it is between two people. It is very different to read about and put it on a piece of paper. It is more of an experience based, almost an apprenticeship (P6.5).

This sub-category describes the participants' opinions of how they learn to form and develop therapeutic relationships. The sub-category describes learning through experience and how this learning is incremental and practical experience of the therapeutic relationship.

Intuitive learning

This sub-category describes how psychiatric nurses sometimes act on instinct as opposed to any learned methods. The learning involved in intuitive caring is in the form of life experience in combination with experience collected through exposure to the role.

after a few years of working, you start to pick up on non-verbal cues. You start to see things that maybe, of course they are not always there, but that you think there is something going on with the client which you just feel isn't the same as it was the day before. Maybe their mannerisms have changed...that sixth sense that kind of, that there is something there that they are not the same as they were the day before maybe... (P4.2)

Psychiatric nurses appreciate that they must behave within accepted standards but have difficulty explaining with any degree of coherence what this process is or how decisions are reached informing this behaviour.

I mean you have your own intuition which I would call it your gut instinct...intuition if you were in a situation and you kind of thought there was something just not right (P1.7)

The intuition described therefore by the participants is an application of human skills by a knowledgeable professional. The application of skills developed through a socialisation process within the remit of a professional nurse.

I gathered a body of knowledge about subjects that I use in my professional life, which I use in liaison with interaction skills. The human skills are the foot in the door and then I proceed to try and pass across the information... I could have human skills and no knowledge to back it up and it would be pretty useless, or I could have huge knowledge and no human skills (P6.5).

Intuitive learning is significant in relation to how psychiatric nurses develop skills, this sub-category describes how the participants of this study learned to develop and utilise knowledge and skills relating to the therapeutic relationship. This learning is described as intuitive, but different interpretations of the meaning of intuition are expressed.

Developing the therapeutic relationship is limited by time

Time in relation to any therapeutic intervention is crucial and to identify how much time is allocated to these activities in psychiatric nursing is difficult, due to the diversity of role function. In any other therapeutic relationship, outside the discipline of psychiatric nursing, time is negotiated and it forms a crucial part of the contractual arrangement with the patient. This category explores the affect time can have on forming and maintaining therapeutic relationships in psychiatric nursing. The category is made up of three sub-categories describing the participants' interpretation of how time influences the therapeutic relationship; namely the incremental nature of the therapeutic relationship, the nurses' minute and role diversity.

Incremental nature of the therapeutic relationship

This sub-category describes how forming the therapeutic relationship takes time and it is important that the nurse realises the timing process. The participants in this study showed that the timing of interventions depends on the relationship factors and illness factors and these are very much individualised.

if they come into hospital in the evening time or you know that they're too distressed and upset and tearful and anxious and angry and all the kind of emotional aspects that comes with an admission to hospital but think it's from the next day from like when they're reviewed the next day when they're calmed down a little bit when the realisation hits…(P1.5)

The difference in interpretation of how long it takes to form therapeutic relationships is interesting. Participants had different views about how long it takes to form effective relationships, however this maybe reflects the difference between different personalities and different interpersonal skills development.

A relationship isn't going to develop within twenty minutes, an hour or a day even. It does take at least three or four days to build up a genuine good relationship with a patient, in so far as they trust you (P3.2)

This sub-category emphasises that the development of the therapeutic relationship does not happen immediately and requires time to develop. The participants of this study describe the therapeutic relationship being built and factors in the relationship being cumulative.

The nurses' minute

This sub-category illustrates the emphasis on genuineness and openness in the relationship between nurse and patient. This genuineness is emphasised by the way in which the nurse performs his or her duties and how this is conveyed to the patient. For example, if a nurse states they will do a particular task for a patient, this task is performed and not forgotten due to this prioritisation process.

The nurses minute again, getting back to that. That you do have time for them even though you have twelve other clients or whatever it is, that you do make certain time for certain people during the day. If they ask you to do something, you do it. That you don' do it the next day. If you are writing reports or a care plan at the time, that you can put it down for a few minutes at least (P4.5)

This sub-category emphasises that nurses often have to prioritise use of their time. The participants of this study expressed a willingness to be genuine to the patients by fulfilling stated tasks. There is a realisation however that this is not always possible and prior tasks are a priority.

Role diversity

The profession of psychiatric nursing is multi-facetted as indicated previously and the nurse is drawn in many directions. This sub-category indicates how the many and different roles impact on the forming of the therapeutic relationship.

quite often you would feel you don't have enough time to give to patients because you have so many other things to do. You have, like, you now take on students as preceptor. There are so many other jobs you have to do and you are often caught short-staffed as well, so you don't always have the time for patients that you would like to have and you find yourself saying that I'll come back to you and you're hoping you will have the time to come back to them but you don't always have the time. But you can prioritise. You know, sometimes people say we have to make the beds or we have to do things that aren't as important as sitting down with a patient. Some things can wait, so you just have to prioritise (P2.3).

The category indicates the importance of time constraints on the development of therapeutic relationships and how the participants of this study perceive these constraints. The loose formation of contracts between the nurse and the patient is an important pre-requisite for the development of therapeutic relationships.

Skills required to form therapeutic relationships

Skills involved in forming therapeutic relationships require interpersonal skills that can be learned but the learning tends to be in the form of learning about oneself. The field of counselling and psychotherapy have embraced this principle, psychiatric nurses are however more reluctant and describe this as detracting emphasis from the needs of the patient. This category describes the interpretation the participants have of skills required to form therapeutic relationships. The category is made up of four sub-categories illustrating what participants perceive to be skills required to develop therapeutic relationships. These sub-categories are: trust, humour, conscious decision making and providing information.

Trust

This sub-category indicates that psychiatric nurses place a huge emphasis on the development of trust and feel that the skills required to form a trusting relationship are understated. The first aspect of the trusting relationship is enabling the patient to feel safe and secure and how this is conveyed to the patient.

build the trust over a period of time but if the patent doesn't get a sense of kind of security and safety when they come in or that they can't confide in you, you know you're missing out on a whole, kind of, you know, therapeutic sense where they might feel they can't engage with you or they wont ventilate if they've any concerns...(P1.1).

Conveying safety and security to the patient is important and equally important is the ability to convey understanding of the patients' point of view. The participants of this study refer to this understanding as empathic understanding. The ability to put oneself in the other persons' shoes is important when trying to treat a person with respect and dignity.

You have to look at it from the patients' point of view, they are expecting something from you. They are expecting you to be able to help them (P2.2).

Sometimes acting as a confidante and listening to the patient is sufficient to enable the patients to unburden themselves and feel less isolated in their despair. This ability to allow the patient ventilate their despair is often referred to in nursing reports, but the skill is more intricate than merely listening. It is a process enabling the patient to feel the centre of attention and to listen to what they are telling you without passing judgement. If this can be achieved the patient will develop trust and be able to rely on the nurse.

I suppose if a patient confides in you, you must have done something right in their eyes. They found in themselves to approach you and confide in you (P3.9)

If the nurse can convey trust in the form of safety and security, empathic understanding and acting as a confidante then the therapeutic relationship will be enhanced and the relationship said to be therapeutic. These factors need not be present in any other form of relationship and are specific to the therapeutic nature of psychiatric nursing relationships.

Basically, being a confidante, doing what's right for a person you are dealing with and having their best interests at heart. Being honest (P5.2).

This sub-category indicates that trust is an important component in developing therapeutic relationships. The participants of this study clearly emphasise developing a trusting relationship would enhance a therapeutic outcome.

Humour

An understated skill that most psychiatric nurses have is the ability to use humour as a means of developing relationships with patients. This use of humour has rarely, if at all, been recognised as a feature in psychiatric nursing practice. However this sub-category clearly illustrates that participants in this study utilise humour in various ways and for varying reasons. Firstly the use of humour to develop a pathway to engage further with the patient and make them feel at ease.

well it helps to sit down and make them comfortable and to sit in front of the person and use eye contact. To smile at them I suppose. Maybe if you could even make a little joke it would help them relax as well (P2.4).

The use of humour enables the relationship to be more inclined towards the friendly relationship as opposed to the professional relationship that was discussed previously. Humour assists in the development of rapport and the collapsing of any hierarchical restrictions to the therapeutic nature of the relationship.

I think it makes it easier and the relationship is formed quicker if the person is outgoing and able to chat away, or crack a joke and have a banter beforehand (5.11).

The relationship between nurse and patient initially involves interpretations and misinterpretations. The feelings experienced by patients are based on past experiences and media expressions of the nurses' role. Participants in this study differentiate between the friendly relationship and the authoritarian relationship and associate the development of a therapeutic relationship with friendliness and the use of humour as a vehicle or skill to achieve the therapeutic relationship.

I find joking with them works an awful lot better rather than being serious with them. You know, having a friendly relationship rather than an authoritarian one (P4.4).

The role of a psychiatric nurse is to deal with stress and tension expressed by patients everyday. Participants expressed the view that a bit of humour can at times diffuse difficult situations and clear the air, particularly when patients are experiencing stress or anxiety provoking situations.

a smile or wink or even a bit of black guarding. Even cracking a small joke eases the stress and the tension (P5.9).

This sub-category, although on the surface, describes the use of humour as a positive and beneficial activity that most of the participants would describe as ice-breaking, diffusing or increasing friendliness. The reverse can be true and the use of humour can be belittling and demeaning, particularly between nurses. For example jokes about patients between nurses with no malice intended but an undertone of mocking the patients.

Conscious decision-making

This sub-category indicates how the participants of this study perceive their role in relation to the development of therapeutic relationships in terms of a conscious decision making process. The scope of professional practice for nurses indicates that nurses should perform their duties within their sphere of competence. The participants in this study questioned whether or not they perform this particular aspect of their role consciously or not.

it's kind of a conscious effort or whether I do it naturally I think I always kind of if somebody comes in, more so with the obviously female patients (P1.6).

Nursing in general is an activity that is performed in the spur of the moment with nurses reacting to situations and these reactions are based on how they reacted previously and how they were taught to react. This results in nurses often having to 'talk to themselves' to stop and think before reacting.

I think you often have to stop and think before you actually say something or before you make plans on the care of the patient. You really have to stop and think which would be the right way to go and you have to maybe involve other people, other members of the team, before you make a decision (P2.2).

You have a professional distance as well. You have to have some distance in yourself and stand back and look at the situation differently (P6.2).

This sub-category indicates that although developing relationships with patients and with people in general is a natural process. The development of relationships in a therapeutic sense is a more conscious process.

Providing information

This sub-category relates to the way nurses have an educative role and patients are sometimes looking for advice (maybe to affirm what they think anyway). Giving advice or providing information is tricky; how do nurses know the advice they are giving is good advice. Participants in this study described giving information in a factual way about unequivocal topics such as what processes the patient will be undergoing.

You would always be conscious of explaining what you are going to do for a patient and learn them to ask questions. To give them the answers when they ask questions, not to be fobbing them off. Try to give them answers as close as possible (P2.3).

The communication process is the giving of a message and the reciprocal returning of that message. This communication process in psychiatric nursing as described by the participants in this study is described as a more informal process, with a hidden agenda of giving and gaining information.

I think people are more forthcoming with information when they are not asked directly. You probably get a truer picture and you can actually assess them by just chatting and asking them the same questions but in a more conversational type setting (P5.11).

In addition to the type of information given to patients the clarity of the delivery of the information is important. This code emphasises the importance of how the information is conveyed to the patient.

Simple short sentences, certainly initially. People have difficulty sometimes in taking in information, especially in a stressful time, like an admission to hospital or suffering from an illness (P6.4).

This category describing skills identified by the participants reflects how the communication process is utilised in a more understanding and understood relationship. The human relationship is about social animals in social settings behaving appropriately. In this study it is identified that this human behaviour is produced in a therapeutic setting and if a degree of trust and rapport is evident then the relationship will flourish, if it is not it will perish. These skills are shown to be life skills as opposed to any learned or professional skills.

Attitudes affecting the development of the therapeutic relationship

This category describes the different attitudes that patients and nurses may have and how these attitudes impact on the therapeutic relationship. The category is divided into three sub-categories namely: therapeutic boundaries, different personalities and non-judgemental attitude. These sub-categories reflect the personality difficulties nurses and patients experience, how nurses try to bracket these difficulties and what a therapeutic distance means. Psychiatric nurses involved in this study identified these attitudinal factors as affecting the development of helping relationships.

Therapeutic boundaries

This sub-category illustrates the confusion that exists in relation therapeutic distance or how close a psychiatric nurse feels they can become engaged with a patient. This closeness or distance is governed by the individual personalities involved and the degree of professionalism exhibited by the nurse.

it comes down to that balance of getting as close as you can to a patient but keeping your distance. They don't need to know a lot of personal information about you. The best way is get as close as you can and build up a good enough relationship with a patient that they trust you. Keep your professional distance from them, without getting too familiar with them or anything like that (P3.1).

The relationship is developed on the basis of what the patient requires, and is patient focussed. The participants in this study felt the need to detach themselves from the relationship in relation to keeping a professional boundary. Maintaining these boundaries is necessary to maintain an emotional distance between nurse and patient, to ensure appropriateness of behaviour.

But in the therapeutic relationship, there is a kind of distance and a barrier that you don't cross…that is purely to help the patient, purely to keep that detachment there. It is not there that you don't open yourself up to them. You don't want to throw your problems as well back on the patient (4.3)

Maintaining therapeutic boundaries in the formation of the therapeutic relationship results in mutual respect by the patient and the psychiatric nurse. This mutual respect is based on that fact that the nurse respects the difficulties the patient may be experiencing and the patient respects the attitudes and skills the psychiatric nurses displays.

when you are in work , I think you have to maintain some degree of , I won't say standing back or not getting too close to somebody, because I think you have to have, I won't say respect for each other but, there has to be some level of boundaries (P5.5).

This sub-category reflects the opinions of the participants of this study in relation to how close or distant the patient and the psychiatric nurse are required to engage in the therapeutic relationship

Different personalities

This sub-category presents the participants views relating to how personality differences or difficulties can impinge on the development of therapeutic relationships. The first code presents the view that the psychiatric nurse must bracket opinions or biases formulated in their own lives and treat the patient on face value.

You have to talk to yourself before you go into the patient and tell yourself you have to approach them in a certain way. You can't be judgemental towards them. They are coming for help, they are coming into your care. You have to remain professional no matter what your opinion is (P2.5).

In this sense, by bracketing their own personality traits or learned prejudices the nurses are betraying their own personality and presenting an artificial front to the patient. This is contrary to the formation of therapeutic relationships, in the sense that, there is a requirement in a therapeutic sense to be genuine in forming relationships with patients.

You would be more inclined, I think, to leave a patient ventilate a little bit more than you would with your friends...You would leave them get so far, certainly further than you would with your friends...(P4.4)

The attitude of the nurse plays an important role in how a patient perceives their involvement in the relationship. The nurse's personal history, professional development or personal maturity may impact on the development of the relationship.

As a child I would have been very, very open. A lot of it wouldn't even be job specific, in that my own personality would be somewhat open and perhaps I fit my personality around the job. I don't think you can take on the persona of a nurse (P6.4).

Factors of the nurse's personal and professional life influence the way their personality is formed. In addition the degree of job satisfaction and burnout would affect the degree of involvement or degree of interest the nurse has in their job and hence the involvement with the patient.

I think a lot of it has to do with personality as well. If you have somebody who has no interest as well and will probably just gauge someone with the bare minimum and see what has to be done. I think patients pick up on that too. Whereas if you have someone who is happy in what they're doing. Maybe some of it can be learned, maybe some of it is who you are to a certain extent. Maybe some people find it easier to get in on a conversation than others (P5.8).

This sub-category indicates that to engage in any therapeutic relationship the personality differences and difficulties affect this engagement.

Non-judgemental attitude

The attitudes of the nurses and the patients were discussed previously in this study, however one specific attitude that was mentioned on a number of occasions by numerous participants was a non-judgemental attitude. This sub-category is significant in relation to how nurses hold personal opinions and do not act or display these opinions to the patient.

Just say if a patient came in that I'd never - to me attitude means non-judgemental in kind of hand in hand that's to me I'll never judge a patient no matter what situation they came in no matter how much it bothered me or annoyed me or whatever, you'd never let that show when you're dealing with a patient (P1.7)

The participants were at variance in describing the affect personal opinion or attitudes affect the development of the therapeutic relationship. Some participants' described being able to successfully detach themselves from these attitudes when dealing with patients, other participants felt that non-judgemental attitude is a fallacy that nurse can never detach themselves from attitudes developed over their lifetime. Opinions about individuals are formed from the very moment the nurse meets the patient and this is an unavoidable natural result of human inquisitiveness.

To a degree, you can be non-judgemental but a lot of people, and I suppose it's human nature, you make up a small part of your mind on someone on appearance, which is wrong. You look at someone, oh, he could be such and such. And you look at another person and you say he looks nice, he could be pleasant. You know, you shouldn't, but you do. I won't say you 100% make your mind up on appearance alone, but it does go a small part of it (P3.8).

you can't be non-judgemental because everyone makes decisions about people every second of every day. You don't act on your judgements or certainly your personal judgements shouldn't affect your professional behaviour (P6.5).

This category illustrates quite clearly that the attitudes that patients hold and the attitudes that nurses hold affect the development of any relationship, but particularly the forming of therapeutic relationships. These attitudes are formed through life experience and are so pervasive that to even abandon them for a temporary period is challenging for the professional psychiatric nurse.

Summary

In this chapter I have attempted to present a plausible explanation of the information gleaned from semi-structured interviews in relation to the participants' perception of the constituents of the therapeutic relationship. The findings presented are an interpretation of views expressed by six psychiatric nurses. The method to analyse the data was a grounded theory approach as defined by Strauss and Corbin (1990). The key categories identified in the study were: how the process of therapy is identified in practice, how do psychiatric nurses learn to develop therapeutic relationships, time is an important influence on the success or failure of the therapeutic relationship, what skills are required to form therapeutic relationships and how attitudes affect the formation of therapeutic relationships. The following and final chapter is an analysis of the findings in relation to a priori knowledge. Strauss and Corbin (1990) refer to this process as theoretical sensitivity, taking account of existing literature, personal and professional factors to synthesise the study to existing knowledge in relation to the therapeutic relationship.

Chapter Five

Disscusion

Introduction

The following chapter will endeavour to amalgamate the findings of this study with the evidence supplied in the available literature relating to the constituents of the therapeutic relationship in psychiatric nursing. The study objective was to explain how psychiatric nurses perceive the therapeutic relationship fits their role and what the relationship is comprised of. The previous chapter described the findings of the study. This chapter will be structured around the six categories identified in the findings. One comment of note is that due to the small scale of the study, tentative hypotheses are made; however the positing of a theory would be unreasonable. What the study does however is highlight the interpretations of the participants and compare these interpretations to what is described in the literature.

Review of the findings

The findings of the study identify the perceptions held by psychiatric nurses in relation to the therapeutic relationship. The categories described the views of the participants in relation to; to how psychiatric nurses combine a therapeutic role with a service provision role, how the process of therapy is identified in practice, how do psychiatric nurses learn to develop therapeutic relationships, time is an important influence on the success or failure of the therapeutic relationship, what skills are required to form therapeutic relationships and how attitudes affect the formation of therapeutic relationships.

The first thing to recognise from the study is the identification of how the therapeutic relationship is located in the role of a psychiatric nurse. Barker (1998) and Peplau (1962) described the therapeutic relationship as the essence of the psychiatric nurse. If the essence or crux of psychiatric nursing is the development of therapeutic relationships between psychiatric nurses and patients, research must clearly identify the components of such relationships. It is difficult to identify these components due to a number of factors involved, the two main factors being the convolution of variables involved and the assumptions relating to the location of therapeutic liaisons within the role of psychiatric nursing. The participants in this study however quite clearly identify the therapeutic relationship as one of the many diverse roles of the psychiatric nurse. This therapeutic relationship role is identified as an intervention, the fact that it is imperative that nurses engage in therapeutic relationships is none the less a facet of their role. This theoretical position is supported in the literature by Gournay (1996) who views psychiatric nursing as incorporating the role of developing therapeutic relationships within their overall psychiatric nursing role.

Nursing is providing a service

The first category identified in this study described psychiatric nursing as providing a service to the public and patients. The role of a nurse is first and foremost to provide a service to the patients and the public in general. Part of this role as stated is to develop therapeutic relationships. These relationships are therapeutic due to the patient requiring help from a state of despair and the professional nurse has an onus to provide this service or care. The problem of the nurse providing this service is that the psychiatric nurse has so many functions to perform that to provide therapy within a relationship is ultimately so time consuming and intricate that the nurse can not fully commit to the therapeutic relationship. The fundamental premise as described by Fealy, (1995) is that a professional nurse develops a caring relationship with a client/patient, as determined by organisational dictums and professional codes of conduct, assuming the person being cared for has an illness, crisis or unable to care for themselves. The role of the psychiatric nurse as described in this study highlights the fact that all nursing is performed in teams of some shape or form, whether multi-disciplinary or inter-disciplinary teams. This emphasises that psychiatric nurses have responsibilities primarily to the patients, but also have responsibilities to fellow nurses and nursing students. In relation to forming therapeutic relationships this is significant, as indicated by the findings of this study in relation to how nurses learn to develop therapeutic relationships. The requirement to form therapeutic relationships as indicated in this study is described therefore as a balancing of therapeutic factors and the provision of a nursing service. Stickley (2002) describes the role of the psychiatric nurse and discovers that psychiatric nurses are in a profession that is demanding and insufficiently trained to perform that role. This is significant to this investigation as one of the questions raised relates to the degree psychiatric nurses develop therapeutic relationships consciously and competently. Having stated that the dichotomy exists between therapy and service provision and how this impacts on how and why psychiatric nurses develop therapeutic relationships, it is still an important role of the psychiatric nurse to engage in therapeutic relationships. The following section describes the process of therapy and how this process is dependent upon numerous factors.

The process of therapy

Weibe (2002) determined that connection in the therapeutic relationship is the experience of sharing a subjective world. Connection within the therapeutic relationship relates to the degree to which the patient and the nurse become engaged and it is grounded in the relationship in which it exists. Therefore, the experience of connection in the therapeutic relationship is unique. In this study the cyclical nature of the therapeutic relationship is explored and the participants would concur that the connecting features and the process of therapy is dependent upon personal and professional factors. The mutual work of therapy is connecting, as is the interactive process of building the therapeutic relationship.

Five types of therapeutic relationship were conceptualised by Clarkson (1994) these types of relationships were reflected in the responses by the participants in this study. These responses concurred with Clarkson (1994) that differing approaches needed to be taken at different times to different problems.

The working alliance she describes as an agreement between carer and patient formulated to address a mutually agreed objective. The participants in this study would agree that some common goal is warranted, however the process mitigated against the formulation of a contractual arrangement. What exists in the majority of cases is a common goal that is loosely stated between nurse and patient. The developmentally needed relationship is described as initiating a corrective or informative function, during which identification of maladaptive interpersonal relationships are addressed. This study highlighted that the psychiatric nurses in this study identified a clear role in relation to providing information to patients. This role was separated into the type of information and the method of delivery. The I-Thou or person-to-person relationship is formed upon the subjective experience of the carer and the therapeutic essence is the product of the relationship itself, providing a forum for ventilation of experiences and emotions.

Marmor (1982) identified seven elements described as change producing; these were identified within the frame of this study, but expressed more explicitly by the following elements:

- The formulation of a relationship determined by real and fantasised qualities of carer and patient.
- The expression of emotional tension.
- Learning or development of understanding.
- Operant conditioning based on approval or disapproval and corrective responses during the therapeutic experience.
- Suggestion and persuasion, overt and covert.
- Development of self-awareness.
- Repeated reality testing and reflection.

(Marmor, 1982)

Rowan (2002) describes three approaches to therapeutic liaisons, instrumental, authentic and transpersonal. The instrumental approach is universal as a way of being; it is learned responses or developmental material that is reinforced by socialisation agents such as the family or mass media. The findings of this study indicate that the participants of this study recognise that learning about the therapeutic relationship is an experiential process fuelled by the natural curiosity of the individual nurse. The authentic approach requires some kind of initiation, which is quite readily acquired through therapy. The initiation of some form of intervention is as a result of a professional duty of care. The participants of this study would confirm this view and most stated that nursing is dominated by the desire to help and if this was not the case people would not enter nursing. It involves dealing with certain closed or subconscious aspects of existence, all those aspects of ourselves that we are initially reluctant to recognize. And the transpersonal approach also needs some kind of initiation, which has to be acquired through some of spiritual practice. It has to be some form of practice that teaches us, on an experiential level, that our boundaries are uncertain, that we do not live totally in isolation. It informs us that we are fundamentally divine, not limited by a narrow definition of our humanity. The learning of the therapeutic relationship is explored in more detail in the following section and illustrates from the literature supplied by the participants in this study that it is akin to a socialisation process.

Learning in relation to the therapeutic relationship

Participants in this study identified two forms of learning or understanding how to form and develop therapeutic relationships. The participants on the whole described learning about the therapeutic relationship through a socialisation process. Numerous studies have been conducted in relation to the socialisation of nurses indicating that socialisation factors are powerful and pervasive (Davies, 1993, Gerrish, 2000, Gray and Smith, 2000, Philpin, 1999). All these scholars conclude that the socialisation experiences of nurses affect clinical practice irrespective of educational experiences shaping practice. The participants in this study would confirm that most of the learning in relation to developing therapeutic relationships is conducted in the form of a socialising process. Experiential learning or the socialisation process is described by the participants in this study as a process of developing skills by participant observation. Experience and intuition it that sense are interlinked but are also separate identities. Carper (1978) first described ways of knowing in nursing and legitimised different forms of knowledge and development of knowledge. Heath (1998) drawing on the theories of Carper described intuitive knowledge as an accumulation of past experiences by the expert nurse who get to the heart of the problem. The participants in this study refer to gut instinct at times governing decision-making and action plans. Pyles and Stern (1983) also identified the importance of clinical experience in the development of gut feelings and suggested that intuition was an integral part of comprehensive patient care.

Altshul (1972) postulated the development of therapeutic relationships between nurse and patient was the result of intuition and not a consciously competent theory driven process. Therefore if the essence of psychiatric nursing is the development of therapeutic relationships and these interactions are as a result of intuition, ergo psychiatric nurses are neither utilising evidence based practice nor are they performing their therapeutic role within the scope of professional practice. The evidence shared by the literature and the participants of this study suggest that intuition is a combination of experience and personal knowing (Carper, 1978, Pyles and Stern, 1983, McCutcheon, 2001). Intuition is therefore a skill that affects the effectiveness of the therapeutic relationship and intuition must be acknowledged in the scope of practice and its use documented.

Developing the therapeutic relationship is limited by time

The role of the psychiatric nurse as stated previously is diverse and due to the service provision aspect they are pulled in many directions. This factor alone necessitates a prioritisation of the use of time. As stated by the participants in this study the priority the majority of the time is to provide care. Boykin and Schoenhofer, (1993) proposed the notion or philosophy of caring as a nurturing process and caring reflects the human mode of being. The basis of this philosophical perspective is extended from the works of theorists, such as Roach (1984) concurrent with the view that caring is a human experience and a reflection of morality and the ethical principle of respect of the person.

They view the act of nursing as a reaction to needs and maintain that nurses are caring individuals whose assignment is to promote health and welfare, through caring actions. It is also stated that similar to Roach, (1984) caring is not exclusive to nursing, however, caring is a unique expression within the profession of nursing.

Tickle-Dengen (2002) upon reviewing the available research suggested that communication functions within therapeutic relationships are fundamentally formulated in three concurrent and interlinked stages. These stages are, the development of rapport, the development of a working alliance and maintenance of the working alliance. These stages appear to be formed similar to the map of counselling espoused by Burnard (1994). The participants in this study identified that no formal process or framework exists to formulate the therapeutic relationship. This process is individual and depends upon time with no formal contracts.

Due to the fact that developing the therapeutic relationship is incremental in nature, do nurses have time to formulate these relationships? The conclusion drawn in this study is no; due to time restrictions, the diverse role, the impact of personal factors, the affect of illness and the affect personality difficulties have on forming these relationships. Having stated the difficulties psychiatric nurses face in their everyday encounters with patients and prioritisation, the following section describes the skills necessary to develop therapeutic relationships. The literature assumes that nurses have skills and time to formulate therapeutic relationships (Barker, 1998, Burnard, 1994, Marmor, 1982, Weibe, 2002). This study emphasises that psychiatric nurses do not have time or the appropriate skills to competently develop therapeutic relationships.

Skills required to form therapeutic relationships

Participants in this study are at variance with the available literature (Rogers, 1981, Burnard, 1994, Marmor, 1982). The skills developed and utilised in therapeutic relationships is an application acquired human skills accompanied by knowledge of how to intervene when patients are in distress. The ability to develop these skills is individual and an expression of the personality and moral development of the individual and not a demonstration of skills acquired through any academic exercise. Humanistic psychology that influences nursing curricula emphasises that interpersonal skills can be learned (Heron, 1974). These skills however relate to intervention skills identified in the six category intervention analysis (Heron, 1974). These intervention skills are part of how the therapeutic relationship is performed. Participants in this study identify intervention skills and personal and professional development as key components to competently form therapeutic relationships. One point of note was the regularity the participants of this study stated that the use humour was a skill that they used in their day-to-day interventions with patients.

The use of humour in the therapeutic relationship was a common feature identified by most of the participants of this study. The use of humour was felt to be a skill most psychiatric nurses possess. Humour was described in this study as a pathway to further dialogue, assisting in the development of rapport, a therapeutic tool to alleviate stress and devolving the professional relationship to a friendly level. Most of the participants of this study felt the use of humour benefited the relationship in some way. Sayre (2001) would not agree with this position, in a study of 59 psychiatric nurses she identified two forms of humour used by psychiatric nurses, whimsical and sarcastic. Sayre (2001) identified that psychiatric nurses engaged more in sarcastic humour and suggested that recognition of detrimental effects of joking behaviours should be an area of concern. The participants in this study remarked on the beneficial effects of joking behaviours, but this was from the perspective of the nurse and untested from the perspective of the patient.

Therapeutic interventions are described as caring actions undertaken by nurses such as, attentive listening, teaching or educating patients, touch, presence, technical competence or indeed all interventions to promote health and well-being (Morse et al, 1990). Techniques or skills identified as being fundamental to formulating, sustaining and advancing the therapeutic relationship are generally accepted to fall into listening, questioning, encouraging ventilation, reflecting on content and clarifying (Minishull, 1982, Burnard, 1994). The literature therefore would suggest that the development of the therapeutic relationship is founded on trust (Burnard, 1991, Rogers, 1981, Tschudin, 1985), this was a feature of the findings of this study.

Attitudes affecting the development of the therapeutic relationship

The successful formulation of the therapeutic relationship is dependent upon attitudes peculiar to the individual therapist. Attitudes adopted will depend to some extent on the particular therapist and their training in interpersonal skills. Rolfe (1990) argued that the theorist most carers associated with identification of attitudes is the theories of Rogers (1981). He identified three essential attitudes namely, genuineness, respect and empathy. However Omer (2000) would argue against this general conception stating that desirable attitudes in relation to the formulation, exploration and sustaining of therapeutic relationships have no universal correct application. The findings of this study would lean towards agreeing with Omer (2000) as the diversity, complexity and individuality of psychiatric nursing and in particular the therapeutic relationship mitigates to form therapeutic relationships on a day-to-day individualised basis.

Empathy, warmth, and the therapeutic relationship have been shown to have more impact in relation to patients' perspective or therapeutic effect than more specialized or technical interventions (Lambert, 2001). Decades of research indicate that the provision of therapy is an interpersonal process in which a main curative component is the nature of the therapeutic relationship. This study indicates that participants were at a loss to clearly articulate a meaning for non-judgemental. Although all the participants stated that to form therapeutic relationships psychiatric nurses needed to be non-judgemental, some felt that being non-judgemental was a misnomer. This position was formed by the notion that their own developmental psychology influenced prejudices that were so pervasive that being non-judgemental was not possible.

Limitations

The objective of the study was to examine in more detail the constituents of the therapeutic relationship, to this end the objectives were realised, however no research is entirely flawless (Sandelowski, 1986). This particular study although examining the phenomena in detail only examines the question from a nursing perspective. The therapeutic relationship is a reciprocal relationship and no account is given from the patient perspective. This position is partly as a result of the limited time frame to conduct the study. The study is also limited in the type of methodology utilised, as the findings are not generalisable to a larger population (Mason, 1996). However the findings are of significance as these opinions cited by the participants are supported by a priori knowledge. The study is also limited due to the fact that it was a small-scale study and the researcher a novice researcher. The study is also limited by the size of the sample; due to the sample being small the research selective coding process and the basic psychological and sociological process could not be completed.

The study was limited by the fact interviews were the method of data collection; ideally a combination of interviews and observation would be a better way to affirm the findings (Field and Morse, 1985). In relation to the study findings what was not addressed which is of significance was the notion of measuring the degree of therapeutic change.

As previously stated the purpose of the study is to extract meaning from an activity that is undertaken by psychiatric nurses every day of his or her working life. However this activity as previously stated is a two-way reciprocal relationship and the study is addressing the phenomena from the psychiatric nurses perspective. As previously stated, the nature of the relationship between mental health workers and mental health users is changing. Mental health users are actively encouraged to be involved and empowered in care provision. This changing dynamic necessitates further research beyond this study to ascertain the full picture incorporating the perspective of the patient.

Recommendations

The recommendations from the study are that:

For research

- The study could be repeated on a larger scale.
- The study could be a pluralistic study to identify a tool to measure the degree of therapeutic change or improvement. For example the study could incorporate qualitative and quantitative methodology, enable measurement of change and analysis of perceptions.

For practice

- The study could take into account the perspective of the patients to draw conclusions in relation to effectiveness of interventions.

For Managers

- Psychiatric nurses sometimes need direction and assistance to organise and prioritise their care provision. The participants of this study identified the need to accept the therapy and service provision roles and to acknowledge the difficulty in fulfilling these roles completely.

For Clinicians

- Understanding the role of the psychiatric nurse is difficult, as it is such an individual activity, however psychiatric nurses need to be sure that what they are doing is both therapeutic and consciously performed. Further study into how psychiatric nurses are aware and consciously develop therapeutic relationships could benefit psychiatric nursing practice.

Conclusion

The results of the study indicate that the process of developing therapeutic relationships is a combination of a learned experience through the acquiring of interpersonal skills, however these skills are redundant if the individual has not acquired sufficient life experience to intuitively appreciate the therapeutic aspect of the relationship. Intuition was a major feature of the findings from the study and the understanding of how this intuitive caring was learned was spurious. The constituents of the therapeutic relationship are clearly convoluted and interlinked with one aspect affecting and influencing the operationalisation of another. What is clear is that the skills, attitudes and knowledge learned in relation to the therapeutic relationship is learned through a socialising process or through experiential learning. This has significance in relation to forming a nursing curriculum, and in particular the assessment of clinical competence. The nurses need to develop these skills and demonstrate application of acquired life attitudes in the form of appropriate interventions. This demonstration can only be performed in the clinical area and therefore developed and assessed there also. This chapter examined the findings of the study and integrated these findings with the available literature in the field. The study identified components associated with the therapeutic relationship, as identified by the participants of this study.

As provided by the evidence in the literature interpersonal relationships and the therapeutic process within relationships has been the subject of discourse for approximately three decades. It is not coincidental that Peplau postulated her ideas at this time however consensus of opinion suggests that components formulating the therapeutic relationship have not been fully extrapolated.

What is clearly stated is the most appropriate research methodology is located within the interpretivist paradigm. If psychiatric nurses consider the positivist perspective to explore human experiences and relationships, may be a reflection of professional insecurity and as cited by Bevis (1982), nurses should be confident to utilise appropriate, but less favourable approaches to research to advance knowledge and nursing science. The question posed refers to perceptions of the constituents of the therapeutic relationship and the evidence supplied by the literature would indicate possibly the most appropriate method would be a grounded theory approach as the therapeutic relationship is a circumstance driven process. What the literature is also generating is a need to advance an epistemological basis for the exploration of professional practice and relate this issue to the impact on the clarification of the role of the psychiatric nurse.

The research also shows that psychiatric nurses are at times practicing at an intuitive level; this begs the question are psychiatric nurses practicing what he or she espouses to practice or is it a paper exercise? The flip side of this scenario is that the therapeutic relationship is such an individualistic activity that some aspects of this relationship are described as immeasurable and need to remain such to allow spontaneity without measurement.

References

Altshul, A. (1972). A Study of interaction patterns in acute psychiatric wards. *Edinburgh, Churchill Livingstone.*

An Bord Altranais. (2000) Scope of Nursing and Midwifery Practice Framework. Dublin, *An Bord Altranais.*

Annells, M. (1996). Grounded theory method: philosophical perspectives, paradigm of inquiry and postmodernism. *Qualitative Health Research., 2, 4,* 375-391.

Barker, P. (1998). The future of the theory of interpersonal relation? A personal reflection on Peplau's legacy. *Journal of Psychiatric and Mental Health Nursing., 5,* 213-220.

Barker, P., Reynolds, B. & Ward, T. (1995). The proper focus of nursing: a critique of the 'caring' ideology. *International Journal of Nursing Studies., 32,* 386-397.

Bell, J. (1993). Doing your research: A guide for first time researchers in education and social science. Milton Keynes, Open University Press.

Benzies, K. M. & Allen, M. N. (2001). Symbolic interactionism as a theoretical perspective for multiple method research. *Journal of Advanced Nursing., 33(4),* 541-547.

Berkery, A. C. (1998). What it means to be in a therapeutic relationship: a hermeneutic interpretation of the practice of nurse psychotherapists. Unpublished Dissertation, Adelphi University, USA.

Bevis, E. O. (1982). Curriculum building in nursing- a process, 3rd ed. St Louis, CV Mosby.

Blaikie, N. (1993). Approaches to social enquiry. *Cambridge, Polity.*

Blumer, H. (1969). Symbolic interactionism: perspective and method. Englewood Cliffs, NJ, Prentice-Hall.

Boykin, A. & Schoenhofer, S. (1993). Nursing as Caring: A model for transforming practice. National League for Nursing, New York.

Burnard, P. (1991). Acquiring minimum counselling skills. *NursingStandard., 5(46),* 37-39.

Burnard, P. (1994). Counselling Skills for Health Professionals. (2nd Ed). London, *Chapman and Hall.*

Carper, B. (1978). Fundamental patterns of knowing in nursing. *Advances in Nursing Science., 1(1),* 13-23.

Chambers, M. (1998). Interpersonal mental health nursing: Research issues and challenges. *Journal of Psychiatric and Mental Health Nursing., 5,* 203-211.

Clarkson, P. (1994). The psychotherapeutic relationship. In The Handbook of Psychotherapy, Clarkson P. and Routledge M eds. London.

Carkhuff, R. R. (1987). The Art of helping. (6th Ed). Amherst, *Human Resource Development Press.*

Crotty, M. (1998). The foundations of social research: meaning and perspective in the research process., London, Sage.

Davies, E. (1993). Clinical role modelling: uncovering hidden knowledge. *Journal of Advanced Nursing., 18, 4,* 627-636.

Egan, G. (1994). The skilled helper (5th ed). Pacific grove, California, Brooks/Cole.

Ellis, A. & Dryden, W. (1987). The Practice of Rational *Emotive Therapy.*, New York, Springer.

Evans, K. J. (1998). Therapist and patient perceptions of the therapeutic relationship: A grounded theory. Unpublished Dissertation, University Microfilms International, Auburn University, USA.

Fealy, G. M. (1995). Professional caring: the moral dimension. *Journal of Advanced Nursing.*, *22*, 1135-1140.

Field, P. A. & Morse, J. M. (1985). Nursing Research: *the application of qualitative approaches.*, London, Croom Helm.

Forchuk, C. (1991). A comparison of the works of Peplau and Orlando. *Archives of Psychiatric Nursing.*, V, 38-45.

Forchuk, C. & Brown, B. (1989). Establishing a nurse-client relationship. *Journal of Psychosocial Nursing and Mental Health Services.*, *27*, 30-34.

Gerrish, K. (2000). Still fumbling along? A comparative study of the newly qualified nurse's perception of the transition from student to qualified nurse. *Journal of Advanced Nursing.*, *32(2)*, 473-480.

Glaser, B. G. (1992). Basics of grounded theory analysis: emergence vs forcing. *Mill Valley, California.*, Sociology Press.

Glaser, B. G. & Strauss, A. (1967). The discovery of grounded theory: strategies for qualitative research. New York, Aldine de Gruyter.

Goffman, E. (1961). Asylums. New York, Doubleday Anchor.

Gournay, K. (1996). Schizophrenia: a review of the contemporary literature and implications for mental health nursing theory practice and education. *Journal of Psychiatric and Mental Health Nursing.*, *4*, 441-446.

Gray, M. & Smith, L. (2000). the qualities of an effective mentor from the student nurse's perspective: findings from a longitudinal qualitative study. *Journal of Advanced Nursing.*, *32*, *6*, 1542-1549.

Guba, E. G. & Lincoln, Y. S. (1994). Competing paradigms in qualitative research. In Handbook of Qualitative research, Eds Denzin NK and Lincoln YS. London, Sage.

Hamer, S. & Collinson, G. (1999). Achieving evidence based practice: *A handbook for practitioners.*, London, Bailliere Tindall.

Heath, H. (1998). Reflection and patterns of knowing in nursing. *Journal of Advanced nursing.*, *27*, *5*, 1054-1059.

Heron, J. (1974). The peer learning community. Guildford, University of Surrey.

Higgins, R., Hurst, K. & Wistow, G. (1999). Nursing acute patients: A quantitative and qualitative study. *Journal of Advanced Nursing.*, *29(1)*, 52-63.

Hutchinson, S. A. & Wilson, H. S. (2001). Grounded theory: the method, In Nursing research: A qualitative perspective 3rd ed, (Ed Munhall PL). London, Jones and Bartlett.

Keats, D. M. (2000). Interviewing: a practical guide for students and professionals. Buckingham, Open University Press.

Lambert, M. J. (2001). Research summary on the therapeutic relationship and psychotherapy outcome. Psychotherapy: *Theory, Research, Practice, Training.*, *38(4)*, 357-361.

Marmor, J. (1982). Change in psychoanylitic treatment. In Curative Factors in Dynamic Psychotherapy, Slipp S ed. New York, Magraw Hill.

Mason, J. (1996). Qualitative Researching. London, Sage Publications

Maykut, P. & Morehouse, R. (1994). Beginning Qualitative Research: *A philosophic and practical guide. London.*, The Falmer Press.

McCutcheon, H. (2001). Intuition: an important tool in the practice of nursing. *Journal of Advanced Nursing., 35(3)*, 342-348.

Mead, G. H. (1934). Mind, self and society. Chicago, University of Chicago Press.

Melrose, S. & Shapiro, B. (1999). Student's perceptions of their psychiatric mental health clinical nursing experience: a personal construct theory exploration. *Journal of Advanced Nursing., 30(6)*, 1451-1458.

Minishull, D. (1982). Counselling in psychiatric nursing Part 1. *Nursing Times., 78*, 1201-1202.

Morrissey, M. V. (2003). Becoming a mental health nurse: a qualitative study (part 1). The *International Journal of Psychiatric Nursing Research., 8(3)*, 963-971.

Morse, J. M., Solberg, S. M., Neander, W. L., Bottoroff, J. L. & Johnson, J. L. (1990). Concepts of caring and caring as a concept. *Advances in Nursing Science., 13(1)*, 1-14.

Nelson-Jones, R., (1993). Practical counselling and helping skills, How to use the lifeskills helping model (3rd ed). New York, Cassell.

Nolan, P. W. (1993). A history of the training of asylum nurses. *Journal of Advanced Nursing., 18*, 1193-1201.

Norton, L. (1999). The philosophical bases of grounded theory and their implications for research practice. *Nurse Researcher., 7(1)*.

O'Brien, A. J. (2001). The therapeutic relationship: historical development and contemporary significance. *Journal of Psychiatric and Mental Health Nursing., 8*, 129-137.

Omer, H. (2000). Troubles in the therapeutic relationship: A pluralistic perspective. *Journal of Clinical Psychology., 56(2)*, 201-210.

Omery, A., Kasper, C. E. & Sage, G. G. (1995). In search of nursing science. London, Sage Publications.

Orlando, I. J. (1961). The dynamic nurse-patient relationship. New York, G.P. Putnam's Sons.

Paley, J. (2000). Paradigms and presuppositions: the difference between qualitative and quantitative research. Scholarly Inquiry for Nursing Practice: *An International Journal.*, 14, 2.

Peplau, H. E. (1952). Interpersonal relations in nursing. New York, Putnam.

Peplau, H. E. (1962). Interpersonal techniques: The crux of psychiatric nursing. *American Journal of Nursing., 62*, 50-54.

Peplau, H. E. (1963). The heart of nursing: interpersonal relations. *The Canadian Nurse., 61*, 273-275.

Peplau, H. E. (1972). The nurse as counsellor. *Journal of American College Health.*, 35, 11-14.

Peplau, H. E. (1987). Interpersonal constructs for nursing practice. *Nurse Education Today.*, 7, 201-208.

Peplau, H. E. (1990). Interpersonal relations: Theoretical constructs and applications in psychiatric nursing practice. In Psychiatric and Mental Health Nursing: Theory and Practice. (eds Reynolds W. and Cormack D.). London, Chapman and Hall.

Peavy, R. V. (1996). Counselling as a culture of healing. British Journal of Guidance Counselling., *24(1)*, 141-150.

Philpin, S. M. (1999). The impact of Project 2000 reforms on the occupational socialisation of nurses. *Journal of Advanced Nursing.*, *29(6)*, 1326-1331.

Polit, D. & Hungler, B. (1995). Nursing research: Principles and methods (5th Ed). Philadelphia Pa, Lippincott.

Priest, H., Roberts, P. & Woods, L. (2002). An overview of three different approaches to the interpretation of qualitative data. Part 1: theoretical issues. *Nurse Researcher.*, *10*, 1, 30-42.

Pyles, S. & Stern, P. (1983). Discovery of nursing Gestalt in critical care nursing. The importance of the Gray Gorilla Syndrome. Journal of Nursing Scholarship. 15(2), 51-58.

Render, H. W. & Weiss, M. O. (1959). Nurse-Patient relationships in psychiatry, 2nd ed. New York, McGraw-Hill.

Ritzer, G. (1996). Sociology theory (4th ed). New York, McGraw Hill.

Roach, S. (1984). Caring: the human mode of being. University of Toronto, Toronto.

Rogers, C. (1981). Client-centred Therapy. London, Constable.

Rolfe, G. (1990). The assessment of therapeutic attitudes in the psychiatric setting. *Journal of Advanced Nursing.*, *15*, 564-570.

Rowan, J. (2002). The three approaches to a therapeutic relationship: Instrumental, authentic, transpersonal. *Counselling Psychology Review.*, *17(4)*, 3-10.

Sandelowski, M. (1986). 'The problems of rigor in qualitative research. *Advances in Nursing Science.*, *8(3)*, 27-37.

Sayre, J. (2001). The use of aberrant medical humor by psychiatric unit staff. *Issues in Mental Health Nursing.*, *22*, 669-689.

Schumacher, K. & Gortner, S. (1992). (Mis)conceptions and reconceptions about traditional science. *Advances in Nursing Science.*, *14(4)*, 1-11.

Seale, C. (1999). Researching Society and Culture. London, Sage Publications.

Stern, P. N. (1994). Eroding grounded theory, in Critical issues in qualitative research methods, ed Morse JM. Thousand Oaks, CA, Sage.

Stickley, T. (2002). Counselling and mental health nursing: a qualitative study. Journal of *Psychiatric and Mental Health Nursing.*, *9*, 301-308.

Strauss, A. (1987). Qualitative data analysis for social scientists. Cambridge, Cambridge University Press.

Strauss, A. & Corbin, J. (1990). Basics of qualitative research. Newbury Park CA, Sage.

Sullivan, P. (1998). Therapeutic interaction and mental health nursing. *Nursing Standard.*, *12*, *45*, 39-42.

Tickle-Dengen, L. (2002). Client-centered practice, therapeutic relationship, and the use of research evidence. *American Journal of Occupational Therapy.*, *56(4)*, 470-474.

Treacy, M. P. & Hyde, A. (1999). Nursing Research Design and Practice. Dublin, University College Dublin Press.

Travelbee, J. (1966). Interpersonal aspects of nursing. Philadelphia, F.A. *Davis Company*.

Travelbee, J. (1969). Intervention in psychiatric nursing. Process in the one to one relationship. Philadelphia, F.A. Davis Company.

Tschudin, V. (1995). Counselling skills for nurses. (2nd Ed). London, Baliere Tindall.

Whalley, J. & Patton, H. (1999). 'Freedom of speech': promoting the use of counselling skills. *Mental Health Nursing.*, *19(1)*, 20-23.

Weibe, L. M. (2002). Connection in the therapeutic relationship: Sharing a subjective world. *Unpublished dissertation.*, University of Toronto.

Weir, R. J. (1992). An experimental course of lectures on moral treatment for mentally ill people. *Journal of Advanced Nursing.*, *17*, 390-395.

Wilshaw G. (1997). Integration of therapeutic approaches: a new direction for mental health nurses? *Journal of Advanced Nursing.*, *26*, 15-19.

World Health Organisation (1956). First report of the expert committee on psychiatric nursing. Geneva, WHO.

Appendix One

Map of counselling
(Burnard, 1994)

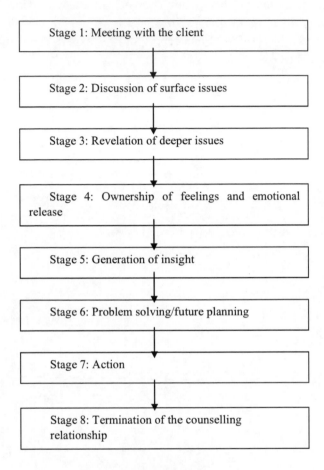

Stage 1: Meeting with the client

Stage 2: Discussion of surface issues

Stage 3: Revelation of deeper issues

Stage 4: Ownership of feelings and emotional release

Stage 5: Generation of insight

Stage 6: Problem solving/future planning

Stage 7: Action

Stage 8: Termination of the counselling relationship

Appendix Two

Process	Product
Primary literature review	Discovery of sensitising concepts,
	gaps in knowledge
Data collection: interviews,	Masses of narrative data
	observations, documents
Coding: coding paradigm, axial	Level I codes- called in vivo
coding, constant comparative	or substantive
	method
	Level II codes- called categories
	Level III codes- called theoretical
	constructs

Appendix Two (*Continued*)

Process	Product
Memoing	Theoretical and methodological ideas
Theoretical sampling	Dense data that lead to the illumination
	and expansion of theoretical constructs
Sorting	Basic social psychological problem and
	or process (BSP)- a central theme
	and/or
	basic social structural process (BSSP)-
	a central theme
Selective coding based on	Theory delimited to a few theoretical
BSP, BSSP	constructs, their categories and properties
Saturation of codes, categories	A dense, parsimonious theory covering
and constructs	behavioural variation; a sense of closure
Secondary literature review	Discovery of literature that supports,
	illuminates or extends proposed theory
Writing the theory	A piece of publishable research
(Hutchinson and Wilson, 2001)	

Appendix Three

Research questions/Topic guide

Semi-structured depth interview

Warm up Questions

1). Please describe your role as a psychiatric nurse?
2). Where do you work?
3). What kind of patients do you nurse?
4). What do you understand by the term therapeutic relationship?

Socialisation process

5). How did you learn about forming therapeutic relationships?

Learning- what learned	Socialisation	
	When	Intuition
	How	Academia

How connection occurs

6). How does this relationship differ from other relationships?
7). Are there any differences in how you feel?
8). Are there any differences in the way you think?
9). Are there any differences in the way you behave?
10). How do you go about developing the therapeutic relationship in your day-to-day practice?
11). Do you use a particular framework to guide you?

Skills Identified/ Used to form Therapeutic Relationships

12). Could you describe skills you use in developing therapeutic relationships?

    a).   Language
    b).   Behaviour

13). Where did you learn or develop these skills?
14). How did you learn or develop these skills?

Attitudes

15). How do attitudes affect relationship building?

    a).   Give examples of your own relationships
    b).   Previous experience-Individual
    c).   Previous experience-patient/knowledge

16). Do personalities affect forming therapeutic relationships?

Identify curative factors

17). How do you identify positive therapeutic change or movement in the individual?
18). What factors are therapeutic in the relationships?
19). How do you know these factors are therapeutic?

Appendix Four

Informed consent form - Therapeutic relationship research

1. *Purpose*: You are being asked to participate in a research study in which you will be asked to describe your thoughts, interpretations, perceptions and feelings as a practicing psychiatric nurse. The reason for conducting this study is to advance an understanding and develop a theory in relation to the constituents of the therapeutic relationship.

2. *Procedure:* The study will consist of 5-6 interviews that the investigator will conduct over a two-month period. The interviews will last approximately 60 minutes. You will be asked to respond to questions relating to your experiences in relation to utilisation and forming of therapeutic relationships. The interviews will be tape-recorded and the tape recordings will be erased once the tapes have been transcribed. At your request the interview may be terminated at any stage and the tape recorder turned off.

3. *Risks*: There are no anticipated physical risks involved by participating in this study. If you feel that the content of the interview is causing you feelings of stress or emotional discomfort please know that you may end the interview.

4. *Benefits*: There is no direct benefit to you for participating in this study. The results of this study, it is hoped, will assist psychiatric nurses to formulate a deeper understanding of what are the constituents of the therapeutic relationship and hence a more informed level of practice.

5. *Confidentiality*: Names will not be used in the reporting of any information you tell the researcher. All information that refers to, or can be identified with you, will remain confidential to the extent permitted by law. The study will be reported in a dissertation presented to University College Dublin.

6. *Participation is voluntary*: Your participation in this study is voluntary. If you decide to participate and later decide that you do not wish to continue, you may at any time withdraw your consent and stop your participation.

7. *Whom to contact for answers*: If there are any questions at any time regarding this study or your participation in it, you are free to consult with the researcher

8. I have read and received a copy of this informed consent form.

_____   _____

signature of the researcher, date   signature of participant, date
date_____

Appendix Five

Researcher
Address
17th February 2004

Director of Nursing
Address

Re: Ethical approval to conduct research into what psychiatric nurses perceive to be the constituents of the therapeutic relationship.

Dear Mr

I am seeking ethical approval as stated above. The research is proposed to involve 5-6 psychiatric nurses, with between two and ten years experience.

The study is proposed to be conducted as outlined in the enclosed informed consent form. The benefits and risks are explained to each participant.

I propose to utilise taped depth interviews of 60 minutes duration and the methods to conduct the research will be a grounded theory approach, as described by Strauss and Corbin (1997).

I would appreciate a reply as soon as possible to enable as much time as possible to analyse the findings.

I will make a copy of my research available when the research is complete.

Yours faithfully

Researcher
cc. Regional Manager, Special Hospital Programme, Address.

Appendix Six

Gant chart

		Sep	Oct	Nov	Dec	Jan	Feb	Mar	Apr	May	Jun	Jul	Aug	Sep
Prelim reading														
Lit review														
Research Prop														
Ethical Approval														
Interviews (pilot)														
Interviews/field work														
Transcribing														
Open coding														

		Sep	Oct	Nov	Dec	Jan	Feb	Mar	Apr	May	Jun	Jul	Aug	Sep
Axial coding	Constant comparative analysis													
Selective coding														
Analysis of data														
Writing up dissertation														
	Time line													

Appendix Seven

Resources and Study Management

The management of the research should include a timetable, citing a realistic agenda for the whole process, from conception or feasibility to completion.

Equipment needed would include:

- Computer
- Printer
- Office space
- Telephone calls
- Tape recorder and microphone
- Photocopier
- Paper and general stationary

General administrative costs are projected to include travel expenses, photocopying, telephone calls, paper, tapes, binding the study and printing.

Appendix Eight

Letter of Reply from the Director of Nursing Services

BF/JP

9th March 2004

Mr Adrian Scanlon

> Re: Ethical Approval to conduct Research into what psychiatric nurses perceive to
>   Be the constituents of the therapeutic relationship

Dear Mr Scanlon,
I am in agreement for ethical approval to allow you to proceed with this research. I wish you well in your studies.
Yours sincerely

Director of Nursing

Appendix Nine

Open coding- Participant 1

Categories	Codes	Comments	
Attitudes affecting	Not stand-offish	Contradiction in emotional	
development of	don't ever presume	involvement	
TR.	all good intensions		
	A distance		
	Approach in different ways		
	Closeness		
Categories	Codes	Comments	
	Sense of trust		
	Warm feelings		
	Make myself open		
	Different personalities		
	Never judgemental		
	Respect privacy		
	Non-judgemental		
	Not take concerns lightly		

Appendix Nine (*Continued*)

	Psychiatry words		
	own free will		
	own way of working		
	treat each intervention differently		
	affecting their care		
	plan in your mind		
	admit that they have problems		
	approach differently		
	boundaries		
	open conversation		
	level like mates		
Trust	safety & security:	build trust	trust staff links with
	Actually come to me	experience and	
Rely on staff with you	teamwork		
	In a vulnerable position		
	Building on a bit of trust		
	Confidence in you: confide		
Categories	Codes	Comments	
	No one else to turn too		
	Trust from word go		
	To trust me I'd be open and honest		
	Empathy:	put yourself in their position	
		Trying to get patient to talk back	
Skills required to form TR	Patient	personal	
	Different approaches	support	
	Different approaches require	2 way	reassuring
	different skills	conversation	encouraging
	different nursing styles	self confidence	
	acquire different skills	down to your	
	Non-threatening	confidence	
	Duty of care is to encourage		
	Competence		
	Relaxed and calm approach		
	Not to be confrontational		
	Female nurses are able to		
	get around male patients		
	let them know		
	talk normally		
	hand gestures		
Nursing is providing	Providing a service		
a service	aiming for service satisfaction		
	different services		
	working with colleagues		
	mightn't converse with a patient		

	Responsibility: to get tasks done		
		More responsibility more authority	
		You're in charge	
		Would affect my TR	
		Responsible for own actions	
	Same nurse		
	Role		
	Hospital not a nice experience		
Duty of care: providing care for those who can't provide it for themselves			
	Role changes with experience		
	When it's quieter on the ward		
Experience	Learn through practice		
	Experience: learn over time		
	Choice of therapies		
	Colleagues step in		
	Learn when a student		
Categories	Codes	Comments	
	All the experience		
	Learn skills through experience		
	My own framework		
	Never learn from a book		
	Students can't say too much in case say wrong thing		
	Learn so many things from different colleagues		
	Reading the situation		
	It's my experience		
	Watching colleagues		
	I think it's just practice		
	Take the situation as I see it		
	You'd know the next time		
Intuitive nature of TR	learned		
Conscious effort versus	use intuition		
Naturally performed	your own intuition		
	Your gut instinct		
	Never the same situation		
	Words I'd use		
	In my head		
	I would have known anyway		
	If you have intuition		
	Gut instinct		
	Go with the flow		
	Niggling you		
	I ride the waves		
Helping or caring aspect	causing stress if ventilating		

Appendix Nine (*Continued*)

Of the TR	you have help to give them		
Quite distressed			
	They're distressed		
	They need help		
	Addresses you with their problem		
	Mightn't get anywhere		
	What is hoped to be achieved		
	Providing support for them		
	What kind of help I can provide		
	What I have to give		
	That will help them		
Process of therapy	Therapeutic factors	Curative factors	
	Slow gradual change	Kind of treatment	
	Answers questions	put it into the TR	
	Caring	medication	
	Engage the mind	counselling	
	Compliance	there for them	
	Advice	care for people	
Categories	Codes	Comments	
	Diffuse the situation	talked down the person	
	Need some kind of treatment	more independent	
	Not physical distance	use that as a crutch	
	Patient opens up	slowly regain independence	
	Adopt a different approach	hospital environment	
	Giving something to the patients	supportive network	
	Distraction	Little niche of various patients	
	List of questions	they're not going to open up	
	Know questions I want to ask		
Professional aspects to	Conduct yourself in a professional manner		
TRs	have to be professional		
	Pointing the finger		
	Wouldn't be my place		
	There is plenty of other staff for them		
	What my role is		
	Professional in work		
	Professional person		
	Professional all the time		
	Stepping over the work		
	Go through it with them		
	Right decision		
	Professional people		
	A standard		
	It is policy or procedure		
	Right way to address somebody		

Categories	Codes	Comments	
	Cycle of treatment		
	Dependent on nursing staff		
	Supportive role of the nurse		
	It is a more professional kind of relationship		
Providing information to patients	On the level		
	give them options		
	give answers to questions		
	give to the patient		
	I've seen research on it		
	Pinpoint		
	I leave the issues		
Impact of personal life on the TR	I don't bring it home with me		
	problems/involvement left at work		
	less involved		
	never bring problems into work		
	have ups & downs		
	human being at the end of the day		
	only acting as somebody else		
Categories	Codes	Comments	
	straight living		
	conduct self as in life		
	never discuss private life		
	not discuss problems		
	my actions		
	only natural		
	it could be you or a member of your family		
	they're human, you're human		
Nature of the TR is Dependent upon illness	A situation		
	A low ebb		
	Such a disturbed degree		
	Opportunity		
	Acute		
	Buried so deep		
	It is very frightening		
	Pacing the floor		
	Disruptive		
	Anxious		
	Not willing to engage		
	Their mental state		
	Lot of emotionally charged feelings		
	Too distressed and upset		
	Practically catatonic		
	Stuperous state		
	Psychotic depression		
	Massive weight loss		
	Tearful		
	No appetite		

	Pacing the floor		
Conscious decision making	Really have to stop and think		
	Stand back		
	Before you make a decision		
	Think before you actually say something		
	Watch what you do or say		

Appendix Ten

Interview notes

Participant 1- Date: 28 – 4 – 04 Time: 3.30pm
Role
Acute
Various 18 – Geriatric
Slower Approach
Intuition – prior to
Rapport – engage -   Two way   Relaxed
Open   Calming
Personal -   safety security
Studying – school
Experience – Rogers
Responsibility –
Help – give help, treatment
Boundaries
Important – more in personal life
Distant
Emotionally charged – same rapport
Different in different circumstances.
Skills – Normally –
Layman's Language
Reassurance
Reward – Encourage
Responsibility
Praise
Open – Closeness
Intuition – Socialisation
Gut instinct
Duty of Care
Noise
People looking in
Conversation – confides

Trust – Rapport

Participant 2- Date: 5-5-04 Time: 3.15pm

Acute – Role Various

TR – Getting to know patients

Time

Watch other nurses –

Differences experience

Lesson the problem

Training read counselling skills role play

Respect – confidentiality – non-biased

Job to do – expecting help.   Health professions – rules – problems opinions respected.

Stop and think.

Introduce –

Explain – ask questions

Reassurance Time

Understanding – thinking feeling

Skills – clear – tone voice

Rationale – open question

Looking at other nurses

Attitudes – non-judgemental

- re – attitudes/personalities

Continuity of care

Responding – independent – prompting

Scales – mood thoughts

Like – expand – honesty

Informed consent

Response – lye – genuineness

Participant 3- Date: 6-5-04 Time: 3.00pm

Care – limited – answerable to doctors

Therapy used – personal level.

Medical decision undermining nursing role.

16 – Geriatric

Professional build up balance friendly control and discipline

Distance – Trust

Confidential Non judgemental – personal issues

Classroom – learn properly

Mistakes – good? bad?

Level – impersonal approach

Rapport

Experience – socialisation

Love – different – bond

Different approach – things in common

Goal

Professionalism again – job
Giving care – more one sided relationship
Altruistic
Boundaries
Limitations – Relaxed
Codes of Practice
Friendly – not for granted – stigma
Continuity of Care – staffing levels
Set questions – suicide questions
Temporary admissions –
Personal – suicide
Friendly – professional. Shake not hug.
Codes – dress policies
On ward – mistakes – socialisation
Watch other nurses – adapt it to own needs
Tool base -   Reachable
Approachable
Confides
Similarities – one way
Time limiting. Goal
Participant 4- Date: 11-5-04 Time: 4.00pm
Help get better – care
Pre hostel – long term
One way – help in crisis
Trust you – confidence – realism
See when need help
Intuition – Experience - * Sixth sense
In classroom – heard what should do!
See relationships.
Watching – through the years.
Apprenticeship.
Detached – your problems
Obliged – in position to help
Here for money
Your experiences – keep it one way – opinions
Burden them with your issues
Personal space – touch
Artificial – personality betrayed
Primary nursing – personality clashes
Get to know the client – talk. Observe.
Joking
Basic – perceive – scientific debate
Observational – open – approachable
Authoritative

Non judgemental –
Time – making beds –
Medication
College – languages. Not nursing skills
Shouldn't but do.
Non judgemental – distance
Right in middle
You feel they can come to you
Perception – approachable
Trust – trust – open – dependence – independence
Sharing
Trust
Observation – non-verbal
Openness
Can't learn – Intuitive
Past experience
Participant 5- Date: 9-6-04   Time: 3.30pm
Team – MDT –
On hand – being there
Focal – View liase more contact
In awe
Medium Support –
Skills
Link up – draw somebody out. Better rapport
Rapport – trust. Parent
TR – understanding trust help liase link
Confident – best interests

- Listen to – in the firing line
- Block – research – on wards – other staff

In work frame of mind
Step into different – professional
Personally Involved   Intimacy - Boundary
No No   Time
Duty of care. Vulnerable – advocate
Trained – nurses interest – who are you?
First – introduce – word of comfort
Reassurance
Joke – normalising
Stigma
Trial and error – honesty and trust
First impression – friendly face
Revolving door – frustrating

Joke – humour – straight-laced – need to know
Comfortable in your presence
Advocate -   spending time
Direct contact
Overwhelming. Informative
Contentment – comforting to have a nurse.
Participant 6- Date: 5-7-04 Time: 4.00pm
Liaison – doctor – nurse – level
Education – symptom – services
Catchment – socio economic –
Acutely ill –
Action – no formal diagnosis
TR – student? – both people?
Personal skills – tool -   talk
Listen – action
Experience – skill –
Daily activities – hit – miss
Use of knowledge – similarities Code
Professional distance – boundaries
Differently – emotional
Professional requirements – touch –
Drink – therapeutic setting – objective
Paid
Trust – patient requirement – dementia
Intuition – care plan – broad strokes
Assessments
No
Language – short sentences – simple words
Lead – patient
Empathy – skills – knowledge of illness
Cures
Groups –
Non-threatening open eye contact
Dementia
Hypersensitive
Formal plan – relate
Child – open – job specific – interaction
Opinion – attitudes
Non-judgemental – 2-way process
Interaction – dementia – mood lifts
Information – knowledge

Appendix Eleven

Audit trail

It is vital to make explicit decisions made during research process to enable consistency and transparency in the research process. The decision or audit trail for this study began by identifying the research question.

Questions asked during the research process	Decisions made in relation to the questions
Why choose the research question?	The notion that informs this study and what makes it a significant research endeavour is the questioning of the fundamental role of psychiatric nurses. Namely if psychiatric nurses claim to form therapeutic relationships with patients, are they doing this knowingly, with a complete understanding of why, how and when these relationships are formed?
Questions asked during the research process	Decisions made in relation to the questions
Why review the literature?	The literature review in grounded theory provides context to concepts and an awareness of gaps in the literature. Grounded theorists maintain a second literature review is required to link a priori knowledge and new theory or evidence (Hutchinson and Wilson, 2001).
Why choose the Naturalistic paradigm?	Naturalistic inquiry is the most appropriate approach to use in this study. The research question is what determines the method of research adopted and in this case the research question seeks to ascertain what psychiatric nurses perceive to be the constituents of the therapeutic relationship. Naturalistic inquiry accepts that there are many perceptions of what constitutes reality and the objective of this study is to explore perceptions of psychiatric nurses perceptions of what forms the relationship between nurse and patient and what makes this relationship therapeutic.
How does grounded theory 'fit'?	Strauss and Corbin (1990) describe one the purposes of research is to guide practitioners' practices and to develop a basic knowledge. In this study the objective is to form a theory relating to constituents of the therapeutic relationship to inform professional psychiatric nursing practice. Building theory implies interpreting data that must be conceptualised and the concepts related to a view of reality.

Appendix 11 (Continued)	
What rationale for the chosen sample?	Having located the research question and identified research methods it is incumbent upon the researcher to define and access a sample. The sample for this study was a purposive sample of six psychiatric nurses. The rationale for Purposive sampling as opposed to any other form of sampling lies with the selected methodology. Grounded theory requires information to be obtained from a particular research population this population must how the information required. In this study the information required is located in psychiatric nurses who are post qualification between two and ten years.
Questions asked during the research process	Decisions made in relation to the questions
Rationale for inclusion criteria?	The sample nurses was generic psychiatric nurses with no post registration training in counselling or related courses that could bias the data towards a counselling orientation. The research refers to psychiatric nurses' perceptions of the constituents of the therapeutic relationship that could be biased by extra training in counselling. Psychiatric nurses qualified between two and ten years.
With who was access negotiated?	Access to conduct the research was negotiated with a number of gatekeepers before the commencement of the study. These gatekeepers included the Director of Psychiatric Nursing Services, the Programme Manager, Ward Managers and the Individual nurses involved in the study. The researcher must seek to gain ethical approval to conduct the study from appropriate authorities.
How was the sample selected?	The Assistant Director of Nursing department were requested to furnish me with a list of names of nurses who fulfil the inclusion criteria. Nurses who met the inclusion criteria were selected from the list. The nurses who were selected to participate were requested to on the basis of the research question and the notion that they hold the required
Why use semi-structured depth interviews?	Individual semi-structured interviews were chosen as a method of data collection. This method enabled a flexible approach to data collection and fits with grounded theory methodology (Morse and Field, 1985). More structured data collection methods would not be consistent with a grounded theory approach, as it would not allow the participants the opportunity to expand on their responses to the questions posed in the interview.
Why include an interview guide?	It comprised open questions and was used as a reference to prompt me during the interviews, as I am a novice researcher. It was sufficiently structured to allow me to deviate from the guide to explore the participants' world and to expand on important information that was emerging.
Why topics were included in the guide?	An interview guide was developed informed by the available literature and upon my own experiences as a psychiatric nurse.

Questions asked during the research process	Decisions made in relation to the Questions
	Why devise a GANT chart? A GANT chart outlines the sequence of events through focussed on the issue of time and provi-ded deadlines for various phases of the research.
Why conduct a pilot study?	In this investigation the objective of the pilot study will be to test the interview schedule and to ascert-ain whether the answers given and the data collected are appropriate to answer the research question.
What was learned from the pilot study?	The pilot interview was a useful exercise in this particular study, to identify repetitions in the original interview guide that where altered in subsequent interviews. I also learned that the timing of the interview was good and gave sufficient scope to explore areas as they emerged from the participants.
Why interview in situ?	The presenting phenomena are studied in their own context and are specific to circumstance. Naturalistic inquiry seeks to gain knowledge through understanding how individuals interpret their own circumstances (Treacy and Hyde, 1999). To this end data are collected by interviewing and observing participants in situ.
How was transcribing performed?	When the data was transcribed the tapes were played simultaneously to readings the transcripts to verify the content as correct. These transcripts were copied and stored in a locked draw; the original documents were used for analysis.
Informed consent?	Prior to the interview commencing I sought permission to record the interview and to take notes as required, each participant granted this. I reassured each participant of the commitment to maintain confidentiality and anonymity prior to each interview.
What was the analytical process?	When the interviews were transcribed any names reference to names or places was erased or references were coded to maintain anonymity. The constant comparative method was achieved in this study by constantly returning to the data, moving between open coding and axial coding, comparing codes with categories, categories with sub-categories and constantly cycling between these areas. This constant cycling allowed me to engage fully with the emerging data and to provide concepts to explain phenomenon.
Why include memos?	To induce a grounded theory the analysis of data must be elicited at a theoretical level. Memos were part of this procedure to apply principles of constant comparative analysis, in the form of index cards, journal recordings or on a computer to establish connections between the data.

Appendix 11 (Continued)	
Questions asked during the research process	Decisions made in relation to the questions
How did I arrive at the categories?	The process of amalgamating sub-categories and codes was commenced tentatively at the beginning of the analysis. The process as stated is a constant comparative method and referring to the codes sub-categories and memos, I began to link sub-categories with concepts or ideas that encapsulated the amalgamated sub-categories and codes. The categories that were produced encapsulated the open codes represented more abstract definitions of the sub-categories. Sub-categories were allocated to categories as they emerged and seemed to describe the resultant data.
Is the study rigorous?	Sandelowski (1986) describes four aspects of trustworthiness promoting rigor within the naturalistic paradigm. These four criteria refer to credibility, applicability, consistency and confirmability. These four principles of trustworthiness have been upheld throughout the research process.
What ethical considerations were made?	Confidentiality must be considered in relation to ethical considerations, it is based on the right to anonymity and linked to the ethical principle of the respect of person. Informed consent must be given in the light of the following and may be withdrawn at any stage of the research process. Ethical approval to conduct the study was sought from the Director of Nursing and Regional Manager.
How did I check confirmability?	Confirmability is reinforced in this study by the production of research notes made during each interview and the transparency of the decision trail. Notes were taken during each interview to assist in the data collection process and to assist in the data analysis.

Appendix Twelve

Feedback from psychiatric nurses and participants
regarding the findings of the study
John (pseudonym)- Community Mental Health Nurse- 25 years psychiatric nursing experience.

I clearly identify with the findings of the study, particularly in relation to

- The professional relationship aspect of the findings.
- Individual needs of patient care

It was interesting to identify the issue of temporary admission patients and the difficulties identified in relation to forming relationships. As a CMHN I am a bit removed from that scenario.

What I can relate to when in contact with staff on the wards is how limited numbers of staff and the continuity of staff effects the development of the therapeutic relationship.

One interesting point that I would have been aware of but possibly not the degree emphasised in the study is the effect my practice has on more inexperienced psychiatric nurses.

The final aspect taken from the study was the notion of genuineness; it wasn't there 20 years ago. Nurses today have a far more educative role than when I trained.

Peter (pseudonym)- Community Mental Health Nurse (Psychiatry of the old aged)- 25 years experience as a psychiatric nurse.

I haven't anything to add to your findings, I think it's excellent and a good representation of my practice as a psychiatric nurse.

In: Nursing Issues: Psychiatric Nursing, Geriatric Nursing...   ISBN: 978-1-60741-598-5
Editors: C. D. McLaughlin et al., pp. 83-122   © 2010 Nova Science Publishers, Inc.

Chapter II

Biopsychosocial Vulnerability-Stress Modeling for an Incarcerated Population

Deborah Shelton[*]

University of Connecticut, School of Nursing and Department of Medicine, Division of Public Health and Population Sciences, 231 Glenbrook Rd., Unit 2026, Storrs, CT 06269, 860-486-0509

Abstract

This paper discusses individual constructs that form diathesis-stress models and formulates an adapted model for a corrections population. Diathesis-stress models are familiar within psychiatric nursing, but rarely discussed in the literature in their application to correctional population, or for their potential in guiding nursing practice in correctional settings. Of particular interest to this paper is the coping response of inmates to the stressors of incarceration and the implications for clinical care management.

Introduction

Correctional facilities have become the principal agencies for mental health care, with half of all inmates estimated to have a history of mental illness or to have some symptoms of mental illness (Bureau of Justice Statistics, 2006). In a recent Bureau of Statistics report, recent mental health problems are reported to be 24% in state prisons and 21% in local jails (BJS, 2006). Incarcerated individuals are particularly vulnerable to the daily life stressors of such institutions. State prisoners who had a mental health problem were twice as likely as State prisoners without to have been injured in a fight since admission (20% compared to

---

[*] Corresponding author: E-mail: Deborah.Shelton@uconn.edu

10%) and, jail inmates who had a mental health problem (24%) were three times as likely as jail inmates without (8%) to report being physically or sexually abused in the past (BJS, 2006). Despite the need to address this problem, there are many limitations to corrections-based mental health treatment, such as lack of studies conducted to illustrate evidence-based effectiveness of treatment interventions and strained facility resources. This limitation is even more marked in its translation into nursing practice and measurement of the impact nurses have within correctional facilities.

This paper explores the general principles of vulnerability-stress modeling of psychopathology and to expand these principles with conceptualization of risk and diathesis, or vulnerability specific to the incarcerated population. Such modeling has direct implications and application to corrections nursing. The heavy psychiatric nursing component of the correctional nursing role (Shelton 2009) can make best use of those "teachable moments" in which nurses enhance and reinforce the knowledge and skills that enable clients to adapt in their daily lives and in those relationship elements that are supported by empirics, or, linked to patient outcomes. Development of coping skills and the therapeutic elements that define psychiatric nursing's traditional relationship may not, however, cleanly adapt to correctional settings. In fact these relationship elements do not "belong" to any single professional guild. There is a collaborative team science effort underway to identify the evidence-based practices for the treatment of mental illness within restrictive correctional settings. Multiple diathesis factors and their additive effects are considered to be significant in the lives of incarcerated individuals with mental disorders, calling for models that feature psychosocial factors in addition to polygenic factors. In order to provide a sufficiently complex model, existing interpersonal and cognitive models extended to include vulnerability would need to specify the multiple diathesis factors that fall into their respective cognitive and interpersonal categories and articulate the link between them. Similarly, models that highlight biological and psychological factors would also need to specify the link between various processes and how they would jointly work to produce the disorder when life stress is encountered. This paper then, identifies key concepts, constructs and variables for inclusion in a diathesis-stress framework for translation to a correctional environment.

Vulnerability-Stress Models

Vulnerability-stress models, also referred to as diathesis models, are derived from psychological theory that explains behavior as both a result of both biologic and genetic factors, and of life experiences. The model assumes that a disposition towards a certain disorder (frequently mental disorders like schizophrenia, Zubin & Spring, 1977; or depression, Luecken, Appelhans, Kraft, & Brown, 2006) may result from a combination of one's genetics and early learning. The term diathesis, which is often used interchangeably with vulnerability (Ingram & Luxton, 2005) refers to a predispositional factor or set of factors that make the abnormal or diseased condition possible. In this model, a biological or genetic vulnerability or predisposition (the diathesis) interacts with the environment and life events (the stressors) to trigger behaviors or psychological disorders. The greater the underlying vulnerability, the less stress is needed to trigger the behavior or disorder. Conversely, the smaller the genetic influence, the greater the life stressor or combination of stressors is required to produce the poor health outcome. Therefore, a person with a predisposition towards a disorder does not always develop the disorder as both the diathesis and the stressor(s) are required for this to happen.

Important constructs of these models include vulnerability and stress, and expand to consider moderators and mediators of the effects of these functional processes that lead to disorder. There are many descriptions of stress, which include both major and minor life events that disrupt the stability of an individual's physiology, emotion and cognitive state (Ingram & Luxton, 2005). Selye (1963) described these events as a strain on the adaptive capabilities of the individual, events that interrupt routine and habitual functioning or homeostasis. Stress in turn, reflects those factors that interfere with physiologal and psychological homeostasis. Stress can be conceptualized as having origins from within the individual or can be external to the individual (Kuyken, Peters, Power & Lavender, 1998; Wagner, Lorion & Shipley, 1983). Ingram, Miranda & Segal (1998) suggest that it is possible that vulnerable individuals, or those in a disordered state (such as the inmate population), may play a role in creating their own stresses. A second issue of importance to the discussion of stress is the influence of the appraisal process, or that which an individual perceives to be stressful (Monroe & Simons, 1991). There is variability in the intensity in which a stressor is perceived and experienced as stressful. This variability is influenced by numerous factors, such as mental set, coping style, and coping skills.

A diathesis or vulnerability is typically conceptualized as one or more predisposing factors that contribute to the illness or disordered state. Psychopathology models incorporate genetic and biologic factors, as well as psychosocial, cognitive and interpersonal variables (Luecken et.al., 2006; Alloy, Abramson, Walshaw, Keyser, & Gerstein, 2006; McKirnan & Peterson, 1988). Ingram et al (1998) identify core features of vulnerability: that it is a trait, is stable, can change, is endogenous to individuals, and is usually latent. The discussion of vulnerability as permanent and enduring is tied to the idea of genetic endowment of individuals as has been proposed for many years in the case of schizophrenia (Zubin & Spring, 1977). While change is limited in this case, those disciplines that rely on assumptions of dysfunctional learning as the genesis of vulnerability assume that this trait can change. Stability of the trait refers to a resistance to change, and consideration of vulnerability as endogenous to the individual differentiates the trait as residing with the person as opposed to originating from an external life event. Finally, because diatheses are not often easily recognized, they are considered latent, requiring some activation before psychopathology can occur. As an example, an individual with a problem of impulsive aggressive behavior has trait anger and anxiety related to chronic frustration, which contributes to his individual vulnerabilities generated by negative early life events, such as lack of warmth in the caregiver, that leads to inappropriate aggressive characteristics due to the poor parent-child attachment (Smith, Mullis, Kern & Brack, 1999). Such individuals express much aggression in later relationships, and given the limited intimacy in their lives, the anxiety they experience may be so intense that fear of consequences lacks the power to inhibit aggression as they overcompensate for feelings of inferiority by the use of anger and aggression.

Table 1.

Personality Dimension	Strength of dimension	Emotional state	Coping strategies
Neuroticism (accounts for 40% of the variance in coping style- Watson and Hubbard,1996)	high	Negative emotions-depression, anxiety, or anger and tend to be impulsive and self-conscious (McCrae, 1992; McCrae & Costa, 1987)	poorer outcomes overall (Mattlin, Wethington, & Kessler, 1990; Holahan & Moos, 1987; Vitaliano, Mairuro, Russo, & Becker, 1987) an increase in end-of-day distress (Gunthert, Cohen & Armeli., 1999) increased anger and depression on subsequent days (Bolger & Zuckerman, 1995)
Extraversion	high	Positive emotions-tend to be sociable, warm, cheerful, energetic, and assertive (McCrae, 1992; McCrae & Costa, 1987).	problem-focused coping (Hooker, Frazier & Monahan, 1994; McCrae & Costa, 1986); adaptive forms of emotion-focused coping (Hooker et al., 1994; McCrae & Costa, 1986), such as support seeking (David & Suls, 1999; Watson & Hubbard, 1996; Hooker, Frazier & Monahan, 1994;), positive thinking or reinterpretation (McCrae & Costa, 1986; Watson & Hubbard, 1996), and substitution and restraint (McCrae & Costa,, 1987).
Openness	high	creative, imaginative, curious, flexible in thinking, and psychologically minded (Costa & McCrae, 1992). diversity of emotions, broad interests, preference for variety, unconventional values (McCrae, 1992; McCrae & Costa, 1987).	humor in coping (McCrae & Costa, 1986); positive reappraisal (O'Brien & DeLongis, 1996; Watson & Hubbard, 1996); think about or plan coping (Watson & Hubbard, 1996); less likely to rely on faith (Watson & Hubbard, 1996; McCrae & Costa, 1986); empathic with close family and friends suggesting an openness to their own feelings and to the feelings of others (O'Brien & DeLongis, 1996)
Agreeableness	high	altruistic, acquiescent, trusting and helpful (McCrae, 1992; McCrae & Costa, 1987)	cope in ways that engage or protect social relationships such as seeking support (O'Brien & DeLongis, 1996; Hooker, Frazier & Monahan, 1994; Vickers et al., 1989) positive reappraisal and plans problem solving (Watson & Hubbard, 1996; Vickers , Kolar & Hervig,,1989;)

Conscientiousness (accounts for 29% of the variance in coping styles Watson and Hubbard, 1996)	high	organized, reliable, hard working, determined, and self-disciplined (McCrae, 1992; McCrae & Costa, 1987)	active, problem-focused strategies (Hooker, Frazier & Monahan, 1994), such as planning, problem-solving, positive reappraisal, and suppression of competing activities (Watson & Hubbard, 1996).

Incorporated into the model are concepts of risks, moderators and mediators of stress and vulnerability. Risks refer to those factors that put individuals at increased likelihood of experiencing a disorder, but do not specify what causes the disorder (Rutter, 1987). As an example, female gender is a risk factor for post traumatic stress disorder, but the cause of this disparity remains unclear (Cortina & Kubiak, 2006). Moderators are those variables that influence the strength of the association between the predictor (such as early family environment) and disease or behavior onset (such as the individual's tolerance or sensitivity to distress, or stress reactivity) (Slavik & Croake, 2006; Luecken et. al., 2006). Mediators, or those factors that influence the health outcome, might include variables such as social support, hardiness and coping strategies (Hammond, 1988; Conner-Smith & Compas, 2002).

The Response to Stress

Much has been written on responses to stress, leading to two separate lines of inquiry to explain variations in outcomes. The first focus is on coping techniques (Lazarus & Folkman, 1984) and the second, on personality traits (personal resources such as self-efficacy and perceived control) that influence one's vulnerability to stress (Clark, Watson, & Mineka, 1994). Both coping and personality partially predict adjustment following stressful events, influenced by the appraisal of the stress and the subsequent selection of coping strategies (Conner-Smith & Compas, 2002).

Generally the categorizations of coping responses are described in two ways. There is a distinction between an avoidance or disengagement coping strategy and a straight forward approach or engagement coping strategy (Connor-Smith & Compas, 2002; Holohan & Moos, 1985). Individuals who utilize disengagement coping strategies, such as avoidance and denial, have outcomes that are generally associated with heightened symptoms of depression and anxiety (Fukunishi, 1996; Holmes & Stevenson, 1990; Morrow, Thoreson & Penney, 1995). Engagement coping involves attempts to control the stressor or one's emotions, or involves efforts to adapt to the stressor (Compas, Connor-Smith, Thomsen, Saltzman & Wadsworth, 2001; Weisz, McCabe, & Dennig, 1994). Strategies such as problem solving and seeking emotional support are linked to lower levels of distress (Osowiecki & Compas, 1999; Whatley, Foreman, & Richards, 1998), as are cognitive restructuring and distraction (Epping-Jordan , Compas, Osowiecki, Oppedisano, Gerhardt, Primo, Krag , 1999; Nolen-Hoeksema, Parker & Larson, 1994; Wegner, 1994).

Personality plays an important role in the stress and coping process. It has been linked to the likelihood of experiencing stressful situations (Bolger & Schilling, 1991; Bolger & Zuckerman, 1995), the appraisal of an event as stressful (Gunthert, Cohen & Armeli, 1999), the likelihood of engaging in certain coping strategies (Watson & Hubbard, 1996; David & Suls, 1999; McCrae & Costa, 1986), and even influences the effectiveness of the outcomes of these coping strategies (Bolger & Zuckerman, 1995; Gunthert et al., 1999). Costa and McCrae (1995) suggest a five-factor model of personality that has been found useful in understanding coping as a broadly based taxonomy of personality dimensions that represent the minimum number of traits needed to describe personality. The five dimensions are Neuroticism, Extraversion, Openness, Agreeableness and Conscientiousness. Table 1 summarizes the five dimensions and their respective coping strategies. It is interesting to note that Neuroticism and Conscientiousness account for 69% of the variance in coping style (Watson and Hubbard, 1996).

Lee-Baggley, Preece, and DeLongis (2005) in their discussion of this model note that there is limited research done including all five dimensions within the same study, and they identify a need for additional research examining interactions among these dimensions. In their study with all five factors incorporated into a model of stressors and related coping strategies among stepfamilies, these authors concluded that the stress and coping process is complex and intricate, involving both person and situation factors among their interactions. While the use of these five broad personality traits may be a bit simplified in the overall discussion of taxonomies of psychopathology (Watson, 2003), it serves a useful structure for organizing the discussion of coping strategies.

Evolution of Diathesis-Stress Models

Two concepts that have evolved over time in diathesis-vulnerability models are worth noting: dynamic diathesis-stress relationships and a risk-resilience continuum. The idea that the diathesis-stress relationship can change came in response to the concept of "kindling" (Post, 1992). Kindling suggests that neuronal changes related to disorder result in changes in the level of sensitivity to stress. Therefore, heightened sensitivity means that less stress is required to activate those processes that lead to psychopathology. This indicates that the diathesis-stress relationship is changing (Ingram & Luxton, 2005). The second point has been the incorporation of terms such as invulnerability, competence resilience and protective factors to describe the opposite end of the continuum of vulnerability (Ingram & Price, 2001). Resilience, those factors that make a person resistant to the effect of stressors, can include personality traits such as hardiness, as well as learning skills such as social skills and coping responses. As in the previous discussion, when most vulnerable, one needs little stress to trigger symptoms. At the resilient end of the continuum, one needs a greater amount of stress before symptoms emerge.

The evolution of the diathesis–stress model was reformulated for the field of psychiatric rehabilitation as the stress–vulnerability–protective factors model (Liberman, DeRisi, & Mueser, 1989), and as such has been beneficial for people with severe and persistent mental illnesses. It has stimulated research in particular for common stressors that people with mental disorders experience, as well as suggested treatment to reduce the expression of the diathesis, by developing protective factors. Protective factors in this literature have significance for interventions and include psychopharmacology, problem solving, basic communication and social skill building and the development of support systems for individuals with mental disorders (Gutierrez & Scott, 2004; Jones, Sellwood & McGovern, 2005). This reformulation has significance for translation to the field of correctional health and mental health services.

Thus far, vulnerability-stress models have been defined, and the major constructs of stress, vulnerability, risk and coping responses reviewed. The significance of personality dimensions and their influence upon sensitivity to stress and effective use of coping strategies have been introduced. As diathesis models have evolved, they have broadened to include concepts of resilience and protective factors. These components are critical to understanding the framework as adapted to the corrections population.

Inmates as Vulnerable Populations

Vulnerable populations are those who are at risk of poor physical, psychological and, or social health outcomes (Rogers, 1997). Some groups of people carry a higher risk of poor health outcomes as a result of these risk factors, including the homeless, the poor, or the chronically ill and disabled, people with AIDS, people who live in abusing families, pregnant adolescents and their infants, frail elderly people, immigrants and refugees, and those who are mentally ill (Chin, 2005; Rogers, 1997). There is an overlap in the characteristics of these groups and of the individuals who are incarcerated (Williams, 2007; Hatton, Kleffel, Fisher, 2006; Hammett, 2005; Desai, Lam, & Rosenheck, 2000). Similarities in the populations include the burdens of consequences of frequent generational patterns of poor health, multiple chronic stressors and health disparities.

Nearly 2.2 million men and women are incarcerated in prisons and jails in the United States (Harrison & Beck, 2006); a disproportionate number enter the criminal justice system infected with HIV/AIDS, hepatitis, or tuberculosis. Many live with chronic conditions such as diabetes and hypertension; (Colsher, Wallace, Loeffelholz, Sales, 1992) and many have poor oral health, dental cavities, and gum disease (Walsh, Tickle, Milsom, Buchanan, & Zoitopoulos, 2008). The proportion who suffers from substance abuse problems is many times higher in the prison population than in community samples. In a systematic review of the research Fazel, Bains, and Doll (2006), found that inmates with alcohol abuse and dependence ranged from 18 to 30% for males and 10-24% for females. Drug abuse and dependence were associated with 10-48% of male prisoners and 30-60% of female prisoners. However, fewer than one in four incarcerated adults with psychiatric disorders is identified in routine entry screening (Jordan, Federman, Burns, Schlenger, Fairbank, Caddell, 2002; Parsons, Walker, & Grubin, 2001; Teplin, Abram, & McLelland, 1997), and few jailed individuals with mental illness are likely to receive mental health services (Trestman, Ford, Zhang, Wiesbrock, 2007). Taken as a group, prisoners are more likely to suffer serious illness and premature death (Binswanger, Sterns, Deyo, Heagerty, Cheadle, Elmore, Koepsell, 2007; Kim, Ting, Puisis, Rodriquez, Benson, Mennella, & Davis, 2007).

These risks are compounded by the many systemic barriers to receiving needed health services once they are released (Freudenberg, Daniels, Crum, Perkins, Richie, 2005). Once released, many former prisoners have no access to health insurance and thus no entrée to health services. These individuals often return to the communities that are already poor, overburdened, and with limited health resources (Williams, 2007). The effect is to exacerbate health disparities already present. The inability to secure or maintain a job because of criminal history and health issues may set in motion a sequence of events that leads back to prison. Unable to find employment, get housing, pay for medication, and reestablish family and community relationships, an individual may make poor choices that lead to confinement, thus perpetuating a vicious cycle of incarceration and release.

Vulnerability-Stress Models and Corrections

Limited studies were available for review to examine how the vulnerability-stress model in total might be applied to this population and variables one might select for use in the model. In a study of the first 30 days of incarceration, Harding & Zimmermann (1989) examined cognitive stress and vulnerability factors among 208 male inmates in Britain. Three kinds of vulnerability in this sample were noted: life experiences, personality and medical history. Life experiences included the experience of numerous negative life events, an unhappy childhood, and early separation from parents. The authors included a measure of recidivism, employment preceding incarceration, current education level, and current personal relationships or social supports. Pathology of the personality was evaluated using the Minnesota Multiphasic Personality Inventory (Hathaway & McKinley, 1981) and classified as normal, neurotic traits without character disorder, neurotic traits with character disorder, or severe personality disorder. Self-esteem was also measured. Lastly, medical history was collected through self-report, limited to the presence of prior psychiatric problems, regular use of medication, and drug and alcohol abuse. The authors reported that entry into prison was perceived as a serious stressor, and one that is more problematic for those individuals with psychiatric disorders as well as for those who had a close female relationships before imprisonment (in normal circumstances such relationships would be protective). Stress is not only related to the prison environment but also to the legal process and may be a to the disruption of the inmate's social network. The degree to which incarceration acts as a stressor, or disrupts one's social network must be considered within the context of culture as noted in the "'incarceration as rites of passage" literature (Lichtenstein, 2009; Ogilvie & Van Zyl, 2001; Denny, 1995).

A study by Bonner (2006) examined psychosocial vulnerability among 134 male inmates who were suicidal and the effects of segregation housing, or solitary confinement. Segregation housing has been identified as a major risk factor for prisoner suicide secondary to conditions that are considered highly aversive and stressful, leading to desperation and isolation panic (Toch, 1992) and morbid thinking. For this study, the stressor was segregated housing, both current and anticipated. Inmate vulnerabilities measured included mental health problem history, suicide attempt lethality history, hopelessness, and reasons for living, with suicidal ideation. Because the vulnerability factors were likely correlated with depression, a measure of depression was included to control for mood. As hypothesized, this author found that inmates in segregation had higher levels of depression and suicide ideation than in the general prison population, but that they did not differ on hopelessness, histories of mental health problems or suicide attempt lethality. Supported by a hierarchical regression analysis, those vulnerable inmates with greater mental health problems, higher suicide attempt lethality, higher levels of hopelessness were more likely to report suicide intention than inmates who did not perceive segregation as stressful.

In conceptualizing the corrections population as a clinical population, with chronic health problems and health disparities, we see that they have many overlapping health and social concerns with other vulnerable populations. This knowledge is critical to the translation of the expanded diathesis-stress model in its application to the correctional environment.

Biopsychosocial Vulnerability-Stress Model of Mental Illness in Incarcerated Persons

The development of the biopsychosocial vulnerability-stress model as applied to incarcerated persons is adapted from Wong's (2006) clinical case management work in Hong Kong with the mentally ill. The biologic, psychological and social domains with the respective individual vulnerability factors and environmental stressor categories are presented in Table 2. Literature found supporting these variables, specific to incarcerated populations when possible, is briefly discussed in the following section, and has been added to the framework. A graphic representation has been provided for review in Diagram 1.

Vulnerability Factors

Biological Domain

The body's response to stress, the stress response (Selye, 1976) is an arousal response to any perceived threat regardless of source which results in common physiologic responses. Research has linked emotions to arousal of the neuroendocrine system through release of corticosteroids by the hypothalamic-pituitary-adrenal axis, as well as to the action of the neurotransmitter systems, particularly norepinephrine and serotonin (Cohen, 2000). Impaired feedback regulation of the stress response (for example an immune response) may contribute to stress-related pathology including alterations in behavior (Raison & Miller, 2003). Koenig & Cohen (2002) emphasize the mind-body connection that connects psychological states, the immune system and health. A biological tendency for particular psychophysiological responses may be inherited, underscoring the importance of genetics. The genetic theory suggests that any prolonged stress can cause physiologic changes, which result in a physical disorder. People who are chronically anxious or depressed are thought to have a greater vulnerability to psychophysiologic illnesses (Raison & Miller, 2003).

Table 2. Biopsychosocial Vulnerability-Stress Model of Mental Illness in Corrections Populations.

	Biological Domain	Psychological Domain	Social Domain
Individual Vulnerability Factors	Genetic Bio-chemical dispositions	Cognitive distortions-Cognitive rigidity	Lack of social support
	Assessment data:	Personality Dimension	*Low perceived sense of control*
	Age of onset of s/s, behaviors	Aggression & impulsivity	*(inconsistent/harsh parenting contributes to low perceived control which is hypothesized to contribute to vulnerability to anxiety or an inflated sensitivity/cognitive distortion)*
	Hx of violence	*Buss-Perry aggression*	
	Hx of substance abuse	*OAS-M aggression scores*	Religious Affiliation
	Hx of mental illness		
	Family hx of mental illness	DSM Diagnosis	
	Hx abuse	*Axis 1*	
		Co-occurring disorders	
	DOC Assessment data:	*Personality disorders*	
	Mental health need		
	Medical need	Anxiety sensitivity	
	UR System indicators:	Excessive, inappropriate, lack of expression,, emotions	
	Physical illness, clinic visits		
	(Interpret physical s/s as threatening with stressors)	Emotional reactivity to daily life stress *PANAS score*	

	Biological Domain	Psychological Domain	Social Domain
		Behavior Dysfunction Excessive, inappropriate and lack of behavior performance UR System indicators: *Discipline hx during prior incarcerations* *Criminal behavior* *Offense severity* *Disciplinary tickets* *Risk scores*	Self-stigma (concept of stigma) Social information processing-*exhibit biased attention to and encoding of hostile situation cues* *"weathering hypothesis" – cumulative stress of differential racial or health disparities-poverty-burden*
Environmental Stress Factors		Prizonization-normal adaptation effects *-dependence* *-hyper vigilance* *-emotional over control* *-social withdrawal* *-incorporate exploitive norms* *-diminished sense of self-worth* *-retraumatization secondary to* *incarceration*	Family Stress *Separation due to prolonged incarceration, burn-out support network, inmate employment status,* *Marital status* *Family Characteristics:* *Children* *housing* *Housing density* *Poverty* *Employment status Disability/SSI* *Length of incarceration-* *Number of incarcerations*

Table (Continued)

			Stress from interpersonal relationships *Lack social skills, Hyper-vigilance* *Unable to develop successful relationships*
	Demographic Variables *Age* *Gender* *Race* *Education*	Ineffective personal coping responses Ways of Coping Scale *Problem-focused strategies* *Emotion-focused strategies*	Social stigma *Viewed by society as a"con", as mentally ill, as drug addict* *PTSD upon release from trauma of incarceration* *Effects of health disparities- access to services* UR System indicators : *Vocational need* *Discharge plan* *escape hx*
		Ecological or prison-level vulnerabilities Prison environment *(noise, overcrowding, pollutants, organizational factors/ stressors*	Ecological or community-level vulnerabilities *Poor disorganized communities with limited resources (poor housing, pollutants, alcohol/drugs readily accessible, weapons accessible, little social cohesion)*

Adapted from Wong, D. (2006). Clinical Care Management of People with Mental Illness. Hartworth Press. P.32.

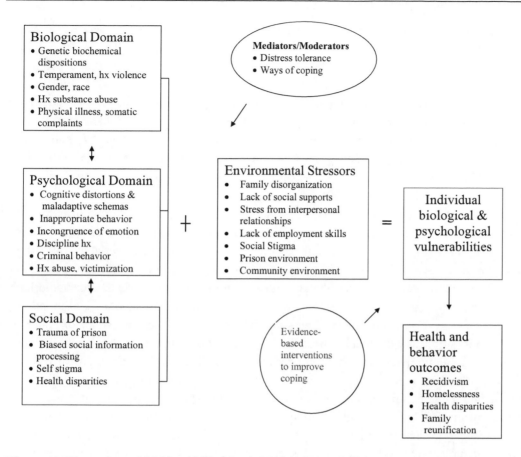

Diagram 1. Biopsychosocial Vulnerability-Stress Model of Mental Illness in Corrections Populations

Although the stress response fulfils an adaptive function, chronic stress for many individuals results in poor physical and psychological health outcomes. McEwen (1998) introduced the concept of allostasis as the adaptive stress response and distinguished allostasis as a state in which individuals meet a given challenge, in contrast to allostatic load which is an overload of their physiological functions due to a continuous activation of their adaptive coping machinery (McEwen & Wingfield, 2003). Function overload appears if allostasis mediators, such as adrenal hormones, neurotransmitters or immunocytokines, among others, are released too often or are used inefficiently, and is more likely to occur when unpredictable social stressors chronically induce physiological and behavioral adjustments that may wear down the underlying physiological functions (Bartolomucci, Palanza, Sacerdote, Panerai, Sgoifo, Dantzer, Parmigiani, 2005; Blanchard, Hebert, Sakai, McKittrick, Henrie, Yudko, McEwen, Blanchard, 1998;).

In the model, a history of or current substance use or abuse is proposed as one of the bio-chemical risk factors. It is possible that selected psychological disorders may play a role in substance and alcohol use (Fishbein & Reuland, 1994). National epidemiologic surveys and clinical studies consistently indicate that substance use disorders and mood and anxiety disorders have strong associations when considered on a lifetime basis (Argawal, Lynskey, Madden, Bucholz & Heath, 2006; Grant, Stinson, Dawson, Chou, Dufour, Compton, Pinkering, Kaplan, 2004; Van Valkenburg & Akiskal, 1999). Cocaine abuse and dependence are associated with increased risk for depression (Rounsaville, 2004), a likelihood that is greatly increased when antisocial personality disorder exists. Aggressiveness and anger directed outward are behaviors that appear to be related to frequent marijuana use (Stoner, 1988), and in studies on opiate users antisocial personality disorder, borderline personality disorder and narcissistic personality are reported as most prevalent (Cohen, Gertmenian-King, Kunik, Weaver, London, & Galynker, 2005; Damen, DeJong, Nass, VanderStaak, Breteler, 2005; Blatt & Berman, 1990).

According to the model (Table 2), under the Biological Domain in the row of Individual Vulnerability Factors are variables for inclusion available from interdisciplinary intake assessments, through system utilization review data and additional variables identified through the literature that would need to be added through targeted research and evaluation studies. These include age of onset of signs and symptoms of psychiatric disorders and high risk behaviors; a history of violence, substance abuse (including alcohol consumption), personal or family history of mental illness and hospitalizations; and a history of abuse or neglect. Information that is obtained from the Department of Correction assessment includes assessment of mental health and medical need, indices utilized in determinations of level of security and housing placements. Variables that are available through the system utilization review would include indicators of service provision such as physical illness and clinic visits. These are of interest as inmates have limited ways in which they can demonstrate control in their environment, and utilization of health care services is one way in which this sense of control is demonstrated. What is not collected regularly is a measure of distress tolerance, which is a common construct in research on affect dysregulation (Simons & Gaher, 2005). Level of distress tolerance has been measured by how long an individual persists in a task that induces physical or psychological discomfort, providing an objectively measured outcome (Lejuez, Kahler, & Brown, 2003; Brown, Lejuez, Kahler, & Strong, 2002). More recently, an effort to develop a self-report measure, the Distress Tolerance Scale (Simons & Gaher, 2005), is in the early stages of development, but has not been tested on clinical samples.

Psychological Domain

The concept of psychopathy has generally been considered a strong predictor of antisocial behavior in adults (Hare, 1991; Harpur, Hare, & Hakstian, 1989). A clinical syndrome marked by profound emotional deficits and pervasive antisocial behavior, psychopathy has been conceptualized in a three factor mode; interpersonal and affective features comprise two separate factors, and impulsive and irresponsible traits comprise the third factor (Hall, Benning & Patrick, 2004). The factor analytic work for this model was validated by Cooke and Michie (2001) using data from the original Psychopathology Checklist-Revised (PCL-R) standardized on a sample of 1,389 incarcerated offenders. These authors labeled factor 1 as an "Arrogant and Deceitful Interpersonal Style" which consisted of a glib and superficial charm, grandiosity, pathological lying and conning, and manipulative behavior style. The second factor, labeled "Deficient Affective Experience", included lack of remorse, shallow affect, lack of empathy, and failure to accept responsibility for one's actions. The third factor, termed "Impulsive and Irresponsible Behavioral Style" included proneness to boredom, impulsivity, irresponsibility, parasitic lifestyle, and lack of realistic goals.

Important to this domain is discussion of cognitive processing, cognitive distortions and emotional response or reactivity and resulting behavior. Among these concepts is the idea of cognitive vulnerability, an idea that is firmly rooted within diathesis-stress perspectives that grew from the studies of depression. This idea suggests that negative cognitive factors emerge during stressful situations. This cognitive reactivity uniquely characterizes individuals who are vulnerable to depression and stimulates processes linked to the onset, relapse, and recurrence of depression (Scher, Ingram & Segal, 2005). Negative moods and negative emotions are mutually reinforcing in depression, facilitating negative cognitive processing, which, in turn, results in negative cognitive interpretations (Beck & Perkins, 2001).

Cognitive processing with anxiety disorders functions a bit differently; there is an appraisal and overestimation of threat represented by environmental or internal bodily stimuli that is in contrast to depression, which centers on ideation relevant to hopelessness and past loss (Riskind, Willimans & Joiner, 2006). In these models, cognitive vulnerability to anxiety disorders hinges on the development of danger schemas that distort information processing (e.g. attention, interpretation, and memory for threat stimuli). As a result, the individual overestimates the magnitude and severity of threat, underestimates coping resources, and overuses compensatory self–protective strategies such as cognitive or behavioral avoidance. A meta-analysis conducted by Beck and Perkins (2001) however, indicates that perceptions of threat and worry are common to both depression and anxiety, an area in need for more extensive research.

Out of the discussion of the stress-vulnerability model of schizophrenia, and again with the application of the model to depression, emerges the importance of emotional reactivity to daily life stressors. Reactivity to life stressors has been defined as the dynamic interplay between daily stressors and mood and involves rapid changes over time (Myin-Germeys & van Os, 2007). The literature has tended to associate early environmental factors with later psychopathic behavior. Attachment theory (Bowlby, 1973) provides a theoretical perspective for understanding an individual's experience of negative mood and interpersonal problems. Generally the theory states that an individuals' emotional experiences with primary caregivers lead to the development of attachment security or insecurity and their ability to relate with others and cope with stress. A poor caregiver experience results in an individual who, as Brennan, Clark, and Shaver (1998) have indicated, as an adult is either attachment anxious or attachment avoidant. Adult attachment anxiety is characterized by fear of rejection and abandonment. Adult attachment avoidance is characterized as the fear of intimacy and dependence, and linked to depression, anxiety and negative affect (Wei, Mallinckrodt, Russell, & Abraham, 2004; Lopez, Mauricio, Gormley, Simko, & Berger, 2001) and pathological narcissism (Wei, Vogel, Ku, Zakalik, 2005). In both situations, these individuals experience difficulties with interpersonal problems, increased feelings of loneliness, and greater hostility toward others. It appears that attachment insecurity contributes to development of maladaptive affect regulation strategies, and the rigid use of maladaptive affect regulation may then contribute to negative mood and interpersonal problems.

Physical aggression, also noted in the proposed vulnerability-stress model of mental illness in incarcerated persons, has been found to be associated with substance use, suggesting that it may be an important antecedent in earlier life pathways to substance use (Fite, Colder, Lochman & Wells, 2007). Subtypes of aggression, proactive and reactive are of particular interest to the discussion of developmental origins and consequences of aggression. Proactive aggression is a goal-oriented and calculated behavior that is motivated by external reward (Dodge, Lochman, Harnish, Bates, Pettit, 1997). In contrast, reactive aggression represents aggressive behavior in response to behavior that is perceived as threatening or intentional. Proactive and reactive aggression has been found to relate differentially to many variables, including peer relations and long term outcomes. Proactively aggressive children are often viewed positively and rated as popular by their peers (Prinstein & Cillessen, 2003) and tend to affiliate with other proactively aggressive children (Poulin & Boivin, 2000). Proactive aggression is also associated with delinquency and violence in adolescence (Brendgen, Vitaro, Tremblay, & Lavoie, 2001) and with high psychopathy scores among adult inmates (Cornell, Warren, Hawk, Stafford, Orem, Pine, 1996). Reactively aggressive children, in contract, are not liked by their peers and are rejected at all ages (Prinstein & Cillessen, 2003). The long-term behavioral outcomes of reactive aggression are mixed, suggesting that proactive aggression is more strongly associated with negative long-term behavioral outcomes.

In a very comprehensive study of personality and violence, Shoham, Askenasy, Rahav, Chard, and Addi (1989) administered eleven different personality assessment instruments among groups of inmates with a range of violent behaviors. These authors found four different groupings of inmates. Group 1 included those who were high in situational-impulsive and premeditated violence and were found to have low levels of emotional stability, poor coping with reality, poor self control and poor interpersonal communication skills. Group 2 included those who were high in premeditated violence only and were found to have low levels of impulsiveness, high in extroversion, low in feelings of social responsibility and high in levels of callousness. Group 3, which included violent inmates high only in situational-impulsive violence, were found to have low emotional stability, weak ego and difficulty remaining in touch with reality. In the last group, inmates low in premeditated and situational-impulsive violence were found to have high levels of anxiety, low in ego strength, self esteem and self-discipline and to have a poor grasp of reality.

Continuing to examine the Psychological Domain in the model, consider the Environmental Stress Factors related to the "incarceration event". The broad psychological effects of incarceration are considered by some as the "retraumatization of incarceration" (Dirks, 2004) given the high number of individuals with traumatic histories. These psychological effects have been termed "prisonization" and refer to the normal adaptation by individuals who are incarcerated (Clemmer, 1940). Behaviors which are seen in the population ass a result of this adaptation are: dependence, hyper vigilance, emotional over control (for fear of exposing a weakness), social withdrawal and isolation (as a survival skill), an incorporation of exploitive norms, diminished sense of self-worth, and symptoms if not the disorder of PTSD (post-traumatic stress disorder) upon release to the community related to the trauma of incarceration. Prisonization originates with the early work of Clemmer (1940, p.270) who studied the inmate social system and suggested that every individual undergoes some degree of prisonization due to the numerous deprivations of confinement. A positive pre-prison socialization and social ties in the community were hypothesized to minimize the negative impact of prison.

From this work, two models: the deprivation and importation models were generated as predictors of prisonization. The deprivation model emphasizes the importance of the pressures and problems caused by the experience of incarceration in creating an inmate subculture. The importation model, on the other hand, emphasizes the effects that pre-prison socialization and experience can have on the inmate social system. It appears in the prison harm literature, studies using both person and situational variables together have achieved greater explanatory strength (Velarde, 2002; Zingraff, 1980). For the inmate with a mental illness, however, the development and retention of adaptations to incarceration is even more problematic. The suffer from stigmatization by other inmates, (Edwards, 2000), incur greater numbers of disciplinary infractions (Toch & Adams, 1986), and may be placed in more restrictive housing units (Lovell, Cloyes, Allen, & Rhodes, 2000). If transferred or released to mental health facilities, their behaviors, such as suspiciousness of others, may hinder their goals in treatment.

Social Domain

Social stress is a recurring factor in most people's lives, and by virtue of its widespread occurrence and the known impact that exposure to chronic social stress has upon many systemic and mental disorders determining the relationships between social factors and individual vulnerability to chronic social stress exposure is important to this discussion of determining individual disease susceptibility. We are reminded that being exposed to social stress does not automatically predict subsequent pathological consequences; not all individuals exposed to social stress will progress to disease or disorder. Within the framework of allostasis and allostatic load briefly mentioned earlier, with chronic stress, the immune response that was stimulated first by the acute stress event becomes depressed resulting in a progressive change in physiology (allostatic load). Studies imply that allostatic overload is more likely to develop when stressors are of a social nature and are unpredictable (Bartolumucci, Palanza, Sacerdote, Panerai, Sgoifo, Dantzer, & Parmigiani, 2005).

Pertinent to the discussion of the Social Domain of our model is the concept of social support and social support networks. Social support is considered important for all people in the promotion of physical health, mental health, stress-coping capability, and community living satisfaction (Bloom, 1990). The behaviors and relationships involved in social support have been conceptualized in various ways: defined as social networks, supportive behaviors, and support appraisals (Vaux, 1988); to be primarily cognitive or psychological characteristics of the individual (Sarason, Sarason, and Pierce, 1990); consist of four components: subjective beliefs, everyday support, potential support, and actual crisis support (Veiel and Baumann, 1992); and specified as listening, task appreciation, task challenge, emotional support, emotional challenge, reality confirmation, tangible assistance, and personal assistance (Richman, Rosenfeld & Hardy, 1993).

In conceptualizing social support, one must appreciate that social supports are probably structured, perceived, and received differently in different populations. The characteristics of social support for seriously mentally ill people and those who have been incarcerated are different from those for the general population. Network structure is an essential support component for re-entry, given that both seriously mentally ill people and persons who have been incarcerated tend to benefit from structure and predictability in their lives (Friestad & Hansen, 2005; Silver & Teasdale, 2005). Hammer (1981) found that is more adaptive for individuals with mental disorders to have involvement with a range of social network clusters each consisting of relatively few people, than fewer clusters each consisting of greater numbers of people. Other studies have found the social networks of people with serious mental illness tend to consist of 10 to 15 people, or half the number found in the networks of the general population (Atkinson, 1986; Cutler, Tatum, & Shore, 1987). The smaller network sizes are thought to be partially the result of social skills deficits, but also to reflect a protective distancing by people with serious mental illness, who function most comfortably with comparatively low levels of stimulation (Gottesman, 1991).

The literature on social stress and crime emphasizes the importance of social support as a key variable because it is considered an important precondition for the provision of effective social controls (Cullen, 1994). Specifically, having a supportive relationship of value may decrease the likelihood that disputes with others will escalate to violence because behaving poorly would risk the loss of valued support (Hirschi, 1969; Hunter, 1985). Individuals involved in supportive relationships are likely to experience a greater degree of social control over their behavior than those who are not involved in such relationships, and individuals with weak attachments to others are expected to experience fewer social controls over their behavior, thereby enabling them to engage in greater amounts of deviance, including violence.

Stigmatization, whether one's personal concept of stigma or a collective social stigma, as a concept or variable, has to be considered in this model. Stigma involves recognition of cues that a person has, resulting in activation of stereotypes, and prejudice or discrimination against that person (Corrigan, 2004). Derived from social identity theory, stigma is a process in which people use social constructs to judge or label someone who is different or disfavored (Overton & Medina, 2008). Not only does the prison inmate treated for mental illness face the stigma of being an ex-convict upon release, but he or she must also live with the stigma of being a mental patient in prison and later when released. In another study of inmates transferred from maximum-security prisons to a state mental hospital, Edwards (1988) suggested that inmates who were in mental hospitals were stigmatized by other inmates.

Two theories of stigma are of particular interest, the first being structural stigma, which describes a process that works to deny people with a mental illness their entitlement to things that people who are considered "normal" take for granted (Johnstone, 2001). The second theory is self-stigma, an internal evaluation process whereby people judge themselves. This judgment could be a result of messages received from societal norms, but ultimately it is the individual who is creating the judgment toward himself or herself. Self-efficacy has an impact on the belief that one can perform; consequently, confidence in one's future is greatly reduced when self-efficacy is poor (Blankertz, 2001; Corrigan, 2004). Individuals may internalize an identity that dehumanizes them, described by Corrigan and Watson (2002) as a private shame that affects ability to live independently.

Lastly, consider the effects of health disparities upon this population. As discussed by Geronimus, Hicken, Keene, Bound (2006), the "weathering hypothesis" suggests that health may decline in early adulthood as a physical consequence of cascading socioeconomic stressors. Allostatic load, as discussed, captures the wear and tear the body experiences as it strives to achieve stability in disruptive environments. Life expectancy (the statistical projection of the length of an individual's life span, based on probabilities and assumptions of living conditions and other affecting factors, described as the best indicator of population health) (PAHO, 2002) needs to be considered to fully understand the how stress-related chronic diseases contribute to excess mortality in marginalized populations, such as those with mental disorders (Dembling, Chen & Vachon, 1999).

In the model (Table 2), under the Psychological Domain column, and in the row for Individual Vulnerability Factors are the variables for inclusion derived from interdisciplinary intake assessments, available through system utilization review data and additional variables identified through the literature that would need to be added through targeted research and evaluation studies. Those variables would reference cognitive measures examining distortions and rigidity and personality dimensions. These would be determined through referral for a more detailed mental health assessment based upon initial intake assessments and mental health risk scores. Psychiatric diagnosis, assessment of co-occurring disorders and presence of personality disorders are to be determined by highly skilled forensic clinicians. The Screening Version of the Psychopathy checklist-Revised (PCL-SV, Hart, Cox & Hare, 1995) designed to complement the Psychopathy Checklist-Revised (Hare, 1991) is commonly used in forensic settings to measure traits of psychopathic personality disorder (Morrissey, Mooney, Hogue, Lindsay & Taylor, 2007; Gray, Snowden, MacCulloch, Phillips, Taylor, MacCulloch, 2004). Of further interest in this model would be an assessment of individual anxiety sensitivity, or emotional reactivity, or lack thereof. The Positive and Negative Affect Scale (PANAS, Watson, Clark & Tellegen, 1988) is a standardized instrument found in research documenting affect in community and psychiatric samples, but was found to have been used in only two studies of prison samples (Crisford, Dare & Evangeli, 2008; Geary, 2003). It may or may not be among the battery of instruments available for psychiatric assessments in correctional settings.

Aggression and impulsivity are of particular interest in this population, and although assessments of these variables are becoming more regular in correctional systems, use of standardized instruments and comparisons with community and mental health populations are not well documented. The Buss-Perry Aggression Scale (Buss & Perry, 1992), a well standardized measure of aggression, has been used the most frequently with inmate populations (Smith, Waterman & Ward, 2006; Diamond, Wang & Buffington-Vollum, 2005; Wang & Diamond, 1999). The Overt Aggression Scale-M (Coccaro, Harvey, Kupsaw-Lawrence & Herbert, 1991) is another standardized aggression scale found in research on aggression in corrections populations (Sevecke, Lemkuhl, Krischer, 2009; Burns, Bird, Leach,Higgins, 2003; Wang, Rogers, Giles, Diamond, Herrington-Wang, Taylor, 1997).

An additional assessment of behavior, to determine excessive, inappropriate and lack of behavior performance would be available from system utilization review indicators such as discipline history during prior incarcerations or prior to incarceration, criminal behavior (severity of offense, pattern and frequency of offending) disciplinary tickets (which are assigned for a wide variety of infractions, and should be examined judiciously), and risk scores (which again are assigned by staff at varying levels in different systems and should be taken into consideration).

Under the Psychological Domain column, in the row for Environmental Stress Factors (Table 2), variables reflecting ineffective personal coping responses would be identified and most likely be obtained through targeted research studies. Standardized instruments found in the literature documenting stress, coping and psychopathology are based upon early work of Lazarus (1966) and include the Ways of Coping Checklist (Aldwin, Folkman, Shaefer, Coyne & Lazarus, 1980), the Coping Strategies Inventory (Tobin, Holroyd ,Reynolds & Wigal, 1989); and the Coping Inventory for Stressful Situations (Endler & Parker, 1990). Examples of studies targeting coping of inmate populations are a study of substance abuse, sex offenders and intimacy deficits (Looman, Abrecen, DiFrazio & Maillett, 2004); coping strategies and attachment in pedophiles (Kear-Colwell & Sawle, 2001); and, mature coping skills of adult and juvenile offenders (Soderstrom, Castellano & Figaro, 2001). An additional assessment, related to coping, would be the Structured Assessment of Correctional Adaptation (SACA) developed by Rotter and collegues (1999, 2005) which assesses the adaptation of mentally ill inmates to the prison environment, but is a fairly new instrument and in need of further reliability and validity testing.

Individual Vulnerability Factors listed under the Social Domain (Table 2) include social supports, or their lack, and stigma. As with community-living persons with mental illness, incarcerated individuals with mental disorders burn-out support networks over time in part due to their maladaptive coping styles and low perceived sense of control. Religious affiliation, as noted in the model, can be a support when utilized, as would a sense of spirituality. These sources of data would be derived from self-report upon intake during the assessment process. The impact of self-stigma, or the internalized experience of mental illness and incarceration, would be assessed by the clinician by determining the inmate's processing of social information to determine if the individual exhibits a biased attention to and encoding of hostile situation cues. Both the Self-stigma of Mental Illness Scale (Corrigan, Watson & Barr, 2006) and the Perceived Devaluation-Discrimination Scale (Link, Cullen, Frank & Wozniak, 1987) have been used with psychiatric samples, but not applied to corrections (Vogel, Wade & Hackler, 2007; Fung, Tsang, Corrigan, Lam, Cheng, 2007). To complete this section of the model, the "weathering hypothesis", which refers to the cumulative effect of stress of differential racial or health disparities such as the burden of poverty, needs be considered here (Geronimus, 1996; Saari,1987).

Environmental Stress Factors

Family Stressors

Regarding family stressors, parallels can be drawn between burdens associated with individuals who suffer mental illnesses and those who are incarcerated, and certainly those individuals who have the experience of both events. Because many prisons are located in rural settings, families and friends of individuals who are incarcerated must cope with the challenge of maintaining a relationship with the incarcerated individual. To maintain a connection with this person is often an additional economic burden, particularly if the incarcerated person is serving a longer sentence, if visits are discouraged (for any number of reasons), or if the economic, physical, and emotional hardships associated with traveling to and from the prison are just too great a burden (Cooke, 2002). Unfortunately, when a parent goes to prison, any cohesion in the family system is disrupted. Burden on the social service system through foster placement for children, for example, is costly as is the additional financial stress to relatives and aging grandparents as they often do not receive similar remuneration as caregivers (Grant, 2000).

In a study of caregivers in Quebec, Provencher, Perreault, St.Onge, and Rousseau (2003) found that caregivers were three times more likely to experience severe psychological distress than reported by those in the general population. This result is consistent with the high prevalence rate of psychological distress in caregivers reported in other studies (Braman, 2004; Saunders, 2003). Uncertainties in caregiving competence as well as conflicts related to multiple roles assumed by caregivers add to the burden of psychological distress felt by caregivers (Provencher et al.,2003). Of critical importance to caregivers are balancing family life and respecting individual needs of family members. In today's managed care environment, caregivers perceive themselves as managers who closely monitor behavioral changes in their ill relatives. In this process, caregivers are left with little time for themselves without assistance and are at risk for experiencing burn-out, poor health and a sense of self-loss.

Only the study by Provencher et al.(2003) examining a stress model of caregiving for mental illness could be found, and no models were found in the literature for caregivers, mental illness and incarceration. However, an examination of the Provencher et al. study is useful to this discussion. These authors propose that primary stressors for caregivers are related to the challenging and problematic behavior of the individual, and secondary stressors are derived from the difficult consequences that emerge from assuming caregiving functions-namely objective and subjective burdens. In their model, moderators referred to resources that help family members to deal with the caregiving stressors, such as informal and formal social supports. These supports were defined as family and friends, access to health care resources, and the number and types of services.

Stress from Interpersonal Relationships

Sociability studies examine inmates' friends and contacts with "outside" relatives, friends, and acquaintances. Similar to community populations, older inmates had smaller and closer social networks (Bond, Thompson & Malloy, 2005). One study found older inmates to have more regular contact with the outside world through visits, letters, and phone calls when contrasted with their younger counterparts (Gallagher, 1990). In a second study, 90% of the older inmates had contact with relatives either by phone or mail, with 43% receiving family visits (Vega & Silverman, 1988).

As mentioned earlier, incarceration has been shown to impose stress upon family relationships, and particularly upon marital and relationship strain (Hairston, 2001). The longer the prison term, the more difficult it becomes for prisoners to maintain relationships and reconnect with their partner upon release (McMurray, 1993). Numerous studies point to the feelings of shame and anger experienced by the non-incarcerated partners placing additional stress on the relationship upon release (Dodge & Pogrebin, 2001; Hairston, 2001). Clearly, incarceration erodes romantic relationships and has potentially devastating consequences for inmates, spouses, and their families. Only one study has investigated the impact of a relationship education intervention with prisoners (Accordino & Guerney, 1998). This was surprising given the documented evidence that for both male and female inmates, maintenance of strong family ties was related to improved coping while in prison, fewer disciplinary problems while incarcerated, and lower recidivism rates (Einhorn, Williams, Stanley, Wunderlin, Markman, Eason, 2008; Dowden and Andrews, 1999; Kemp, Glaser, & Page, 1992).

Social Stigma

The 20th century in the US has been noted by some as the "era of incarceration" because an estimated 7 million or more Americans are under some form of correctional supervision, including probation and parole (Webb, 2007; Rodriguez & Webb, 2007; Walmsley, 2006). The high incarceration rate raises several serious questions that have been posed to a Special Hearing of the Joint Economic Committee of the US Senate in 2007, underscoring the fact that the rate of growth of spending on corrections in state budgets has exceeded that for education, health care, social services, transportation and environmental protection. Hearing witnesses advocated for diversion of individuals who are not threats to public safety into serious and structured community based alternatives to prison (Jacobson, 2007). Prevention strategies, such as increasing high school graduation rates, neighborhood-based law enforcement initiatives and increases in employment and wages to effectively reduce crime are promoted over the greater use of prison (Albert, 2007; Loury & Stoltz, 2007; Western, 2007).

The impact upon the individual is portrayed in a statistic showing that more than half of all inmates released are re-incarcerated within three years (Jacobson, 2007). The strain of trying to adjust in the community after incarceration is not an easy task. After release from prison, offenders face many barriers, often called "invisible punishments" (Nolan, 2007) because they are frequently denied parental rights, driver's licenses, student loans, the right to vote, and they experience the biases that come from having been incarcerated or treated for a mental illness, such as poor public housing, limited employment opportunities (even with skills), and difficulties accessing health care. Transitioning from a world where all decision are made for them, to an environment where these many decisions and choices need be made, They can be overwhelmed by feelings of intense stress and worry.

Ecological or Community-level Vulnerabilities

Gee and Payne-Sturgis (2004) in their discussion of psychosocial environmental concepts, link ethnicity with residential location. These authors note specifically that minorities are often living in communities with differential exposure to health risks. While their discussion is of neighborhood stressors and pollution sources that create adverse health conditions and that are counterbalanced by neighborhood resources, it is reasonable to apply this thinking to correctional settings. Correctional settings, many of which have large minority populations, can be considered "neighborhoods" and as such have their own differential exposures to health risks that create adverse health conditions. Many resources are provided to attend to counterbalancing these stressors. But the opportunity to translate into individual vulnerabilities cannot be ignored, nor the opportunity for structuring health promotion activities. Community stress theory is also derived from research on the stress process among individuals (Lazarus and Folkman 1984; Selye 1976). Community stressors as applied to correctional settings include noise (Ouis 2001), litter, density, and residential crowding (Fleming, Baum & Weiss, 1987; Evans and Lepore, 1993), social disorganization, racial discrimination, fear, and economic deprivation (Krieger and Higgins 2002; Macintyre, Ellaway & Cummings 2002). Chronic activation of the stress system, believed to lead to allostatic load (the "wear and tear" on organ systems) yields way to illness (McEwen 1998).

Living in a group, like other behavioral traits, has costs and benefits. Access to such resources and their distribution are common issues among individuals belonging to social groups. Genetic, experiential and environmental factors interact to determine the position of an individual within a dominance hierarchy and influence the way an individual copes with social and environmental challenges. Archer, Ireland and Power (2007) studied bullying behavior of 1,253 adult offenders (728 men and 525 women) in eleven prisons in the UK. These authors were interested in bullying as a form of displaced aggression in prison samples. In measures of aggression, they used items such as 'Slammed or kicked the door afterwards' to assess displaced physical aggression, and 'Sworn at them after they had gone' for verbal forms to demonstrate ineffective, low-cost, aggression. They found those classed as bullies had higher scores than non-bullies on direct verbal and physical aggression, indirect aggression, verbal and physical displaced aggression, and revenge plans and fantasies; lower values for fear/avoidance; and higher impulsiveness and instrumental and expressive attributions. Those classed as victims showed higher scores than non-victims for fear/avoidance, displaced physical aggression and impulsiveness. Males were clearly more directly physically aggressive and females more fear/avoidant.

The significance of this study lies in understanding the relevance to this model of the effect of overcrowding of the prison environment and its social structure. Archer, Ireland and Power (2007) define displaced aggression as aggression directed towards a target other than the source of the provocation. Miller, Pedersen, Earleywine, and Pollock (2003) highlight that this type of delayed aggressive response can produce a disproportionate aggressive response to a later triggering event secondary to short-term arousal and longer-term rumination over the provoking event. Further, displaced aggression is a low-cost outlet for aggressive impulses in that there is less danger of retaliation, albeit danger from self-injury. Revenge plans and fantasies are also linked to ruminative thoughts about a provoking event. The combination of high provocation and high retaliatory power of the opponent produced a response termed "delayed hostility". This consisted of doing nothing at the time, but feeling frustrated and planning to avenge the provocation later. Sukhodolsky, Golub, and Cromwell (2001) found that men ruminated over anger-inducing events and tended to hold thoughts of revenge longer than women did. This is consistent with findings that men report more homicidal fantasies than women do (Crabb, 2000). The main alternative non-aggressive response to provocation is fear and avoidance. Similar situations can produce either aggression or fear depending on the intensity of the provocation, and internal variables affecting the threshold for fear responses in that individual (Archer, 1976; Berkowitz, 1962). Fear responses to a bullying situation are higher in those who have themselves been victims of bullying than in those who have not, and fewer fear responses in those who are themselves perpetrators than in those who are not perpetrators.

In the model (Table 2), under the Social Domain and in the row of Environmental Stress Factors, the variables for inclusion identify family characteristics (marital status, number of children, relatives living in the home, number of friends and social support network, distance to social units and level of support from social units, employment status, disability) that would be obtained from self-report upon intake assessment or records if available. Disability and vocational need would be determined from a more detailed interdisciplinary assessment. Included under this section of the model would be the length of separation due to prolonged incarceration and the number of incarcerations. Social stigma is viewed from how society views the individual, as a convict, as a mentally ill individual, as a drug addict, certainly influences the outcomes upon re-entry with regard to employment, housing and successful reintegration into the community. Ecological or environmental factors that would impact stress and coping while incarcerated or back in the community include noise, overcrowding, pollutants, and organizational stressors. Gee & Payne-Sturges (2004) provide a discussion of race, community environmental conditions and health that is pertinent to the discussion because it is well documented that, upon re-entry, one of the challenges to success of inmates is that they return to the same environments that encouraged risky behaviors contributing to their incarceration (Petersilia, 2000). Lindquist and Lindquist (1997) and Tataro (2006) discuss the impact of environmental stressors among jail inmates. Many of these variables could be collected from system utilization reviews or from community public health indices.

Discussion

The model as applied to the corrections population provides a framework that can be utilized by an interdisciplinary team of clinicians and researchers collaborating to improve clinical services and patient care outcomes. Use of the biopsychosocial vulnerability stress model as outlined in Table 2 was particularly useful for an examination of the available evidence in the literature, as well as the gaps as it translates to the inmate population. The corrections population is sufficiently similar to community and hospitalized psychiatric samples to provide for translation of the evidence as found in the literature, and, where possible, to include studies that involved inmate populations. What emerged from this discussion were the complexities of such a model, reflective of the complexities of the mentally ill inmate population, and the gaps yet to be demonstrated through research.

The framework provided by this model has begun to capture a picture of the general characteristics of the correctional population. A large number of inmates have mental disorders and co-occurring substance-abuse disorders that bring them into the criminal justice system. A large proportion of the population is male and of minority race. These individuals generally have challenging personality styles, and exhibit impulsive and aggressive behaviors, with a smaller number who are violent. The inmate population appears to have a low tolerance to stress and exhibits poor coping and decision-making skills. Personal resources and supports appear to be inadequate, with issues of poverty, low levels of education, poor vocational skills and poor employment histories. For individuals with extensive lengths of incarceration, or repetitive patterns of incarceration, social networks are even more fragmented and challenged than for the population in general. Reunification with family members is among one of the many emotional demands upon the inmate upon re-entry. Within this framework, interventions can be tailored for individual vulnerabilities, gathering momentum from mediators, moderators, and strengths that can be found in each individual.

Among the next steps would be to begin to apply data to the model to see how it works initially with offender populations, and to see how the model needs to be refined. This research could begin with descriptions or collective case studies of inmate groups by age, race and gender and use of data that are available though record review or utilization review. It would be expected that the younger inmates, particularly males, would have higher levels of aggression and greater difficulty with adjusting to the prison environment, and similarly, have a harder time with re-entry success. Would their utilization of health services be different than that for others of the same gender? We expect a high number of individuals with co-occurring disorders, but what is the significance of the addition of selected medical conditions that might influence behavior and coping? Which individuals are more receptive to clinical interventions and benefit from them? Are there mediators or moderators in the model that we can identify that not only reduce stressors but work to enhance treatment effect? From the model, can we improve matching treatments (such as stress reduction intervention which taps spirituality or teaching recognition of personal stressors and coping strategies) to the individual.

This framework offers yet another systems-based opportunity: to identify standardized measures that could be incorporated into the health care structure of a corrections system that would be useful to both clinicians and researchers. Challenges exist in utilizing technology to reduce burdens to the limited number of clinicians while still meeting the full potential for conducting quality evaluation and research studies. The value of standardized measures has not been missed, since work on the reliability and validity of measures continues. A gap in the literature exists in the publication of standardized instrument scores on corrections populations, or comparisons with mental health and community samples. Further, many corrections systems have endeavored to tailor and standardize instruments for their specific needs, but this makes it difficult to draw comparisons with community samples, particularly when the standard of care in corrections is to be equivalent to that provided in a community setting (Poster, 1992).

The use of the model to support clinical intervention studies to enhance the individual's adaptation (behavioral or medical) while incarcerated and to support re-entry into the community can guide clinical practice. The role of nursing, for example, can be greatly enhanced in corrections to promote this agenda, but the evidence of nursing interventions must be demonstrated in these environments. Nursing roles have the opportunity for many "teachable" moments that can support, enhance and promote inmate health, adherence to medical and mental health regimens as well as behavioral plans. The relationship between nursing interventions and patient outcomes is well documented (Schubert, Glass, Clarke, Aiken, Schaffert-Witviliet, Sloan & De-Geest, 2008). The expectation for nurses to participate in correctional settings in this manner has not always been recognized or desired (Shelton, 2009). As in many other healthcare settings, nurses in correctional settings need to be retooled for the future. There is a large gap in knowledge about evidence-based practices in correctional nursing and evidence-based treatment in correctional settings.

Conclusion

The clinical usefulness of the adapted biopsychosocial vulnerability-stress model is striking in that it is set up as a matrix in which variables can be selected from multiple levels for consideration in development of clinical programming, evaluation of clinical services, or development of a research study. It easily provides for a flexibility to be expanded upon as it is discussed and applied. A framework such as this might guide the development of a quality improvement and informatics system in corrections, or be used to provide a basis of understanding about the shared population between a Department of Corrections and the health care providers.

References

Accordino, M. P. & Guerney, B. (1998). An evaluation of the Relationship Enhancement Program with prisoners and their wives. *International Journal of Offender Therapy and Comparative Criminology.*, *42*, 5-15.

Albert, A. (2007). Testimony to the Special hearing of the Joint Economic Committee of the US Senate on October, 4. *Mass incarceration in the United States: At what cost?*

Retrieved December., *2*, 2008 from http://www.jec.senate.gov/index.cfm?FuseAction= Hearings.HearingsCalendar.

Aldwin, C., Folkman, S. Schaefer, C., Coyne, J. & Lazarus, R. (12980, September). *Ways of Coping Checklist: A process measure.* Paper presented at the annual American Psychological Association meeting, Motreal, Canada.

Alloy, L. B., Abramson, L. Y., Walshaw, P. D., Keyser, J. & Gerstein, R. K. (2006). A cognitive vulnerability–stress perspective on bipolar spectrum disorders in a normative adolescent brain, cognitive, and emotional development context. *Development and Psychopathology.*, *18*, 1055-1103.

Archer J. (1976). Testosterone and fear behavior in male chicks. *Physiology & Behavior.*, *17 (4)*, 561-564.

Archer, J., Ireland, J. L. & Power, C. L. (2007). Differences between bullies and victims, and men and women, on aggression related variables among prisoners. *British Journal of Social Psychology.*, *46*, 299-322

Argawal, A., Lynskey, M. T., Madden, P. A. F., Bucholz, K. K. & Heath, A. C. (2006). A latent class analysis of illicit drug abuse/dependence: results from the National Epidemiological Survey on alcohol and related conditions.*Addiction.*, *102*, 94-104.

Atkinson, D. (1986). Engaging competent others: A study of the support networks of people with mental handicap. *The British Journal of Social Work*, *16*, 83-101.

Bartolomucci, A., Palanza, P., Sacerdote, P., Panerai, A. E., Sgoifo, A., Dantzer, R. & Parmigiani, S. (2005).Social factors and individual vulnerability to chronic stress exposure. *Neuroscience and Biobehavioral Reviews*, *29*, 67-81.

Beck, R. & Perkins, T. S. (2001). Cognitive content-specificity for anxiety and depression: A meta-analysis. *Cognitive Therapy and Research.*, *25*, 651-663.

Beck, A. T., Ward, C. H., Mendelson, M., Mock, J. & Erbaugh, J. (1961). An inventory for measuing depression. *Archives of General Psychiatry.*, *4*, 561-571.

Billings, A. G & Moos, R. H. (1981). The role of coping responses and social resources in attenuating the impact of stressful life events. *Journal of Behavioral Medicine.*, *4*, 139-157.

Binswanger, I. A., Sterns, M. F., Deyo, R. A., Heagerty, P. J., Cheadle, A., Elmore, J. G., Koepsell, T. D. (2007). Release from prison: a high risk of death for former inmates. *New England Journal of Medicine.*, *356(2)*, 157-65.

Blanchard, R. J., Hebert, M., Sakai, R. R. McKittrick, C., Henrie, A., Yudko, E., McEwen, B. S. & Blanchard, D. C. (1998). Chronic social stress changes in behavioral and physiogical indices of emotion. *Aggressive Behavior.*, *24*, 307-321.

Blankertz, L. (2001). Cognitive components of self esteem for individuals with severe mental illness. *American Journal of Orthopsychiatry.*, *77(4)*, 457-465.

Blatt, S. J. & Berman, W. H. (1990). Differentiation of personality types among opiate addicts. *Journal of Personality Assessment.*, *54*, (1&2) 87-104.

Bloom, J. R. (1990). The relationship of social support and health. *Social. Science Medicine*, *30 (5)*, 635-437.

Bolger, N. & Schilling , E. A. (1991). Personality and the problems of everyday life: The role of neuroticism in exposure and reactivity to daily stressors. *Journal of Personality.*, *59(3)*, 322-325.

Bolger, N. & Zuckerman, A. (1995). A framework for studying personality in the stress process. *Journal of Personality and Social Psychology.*, *69(5)*, 890-902.

Bond, G. D., Thompson, L. A. & Malloy, D. M. (2005). Lifespan differences in the social networks of prison inmates. International *Journal of Aging & Human Development.*, *61 (3)*, 161-78.

Bonner, R. L. (2006). Stressful segregation housing and psychosocial vulnerability in prison suicide ideators. *Suicide and Life-Threatening Behavior*, *36(2)*, 250-254.

Bowlby, J. (1973). *Attachment and loss: Vol. 2. Separation: Anxiety and anger.* New York: Basic Books.

Braman, D. (2004). Families and the moral economy of incarceration. *Journal of Religion & Spirituality in Social Work*, *23(1/2)*, 27-50.

Brendgen, M., Vitaro, F., Tremblay, R. E. & Lavoie, F. (2001). Reactive and proactive aggression: Predictions to physical violence in different contexts and moderating effects of parental monitoring and caregiving behavior. *Journal of Abnormal Child Psychology.*, *29*, 293-304.

Brennan, K. A., Clark, C. L. & Shaver, P. R. (1998). Self-report measurement of adult attachment: An integrative overview. In J.A. Simpson & W.S. Rholes (Eds.), *Attachment theory and close relationships* (46-76). NY: Guilford Press.

Brown, R., Lejuez, C. W., Kahler, C. W. & Strong, D. R. (2002). Distress tolerance and duration of past smoking cessation attempts. *Journal of Abnormal Psychology*, *111*, 180-185.

Bureau of Justice Statistics. (2006). Mental health problems of prison and jail inmates. (Pub. # NCJ-213600). Retrieved December 12, 2008 from http://www.ojp.usdoj.gov/bjs/abstract/mhppji.htm.

Burns, M., Bird, D., Leach, C. & Higgins, K. (2003). Anger management training: the effects of a structured programme on the self-reported anger experience of forensic inpatients with learning disability. *Journal of Psychiatric & Mental Health Nursing,10(5)*, 569-578.

Buss, A. H. & Perry, M. (1992). The Aggression Questionnaire. *Journal of Personality and Social Psychology*, *63*, 452-459.

Buss, A. & Perry, M. (1992). The Aggression Questionnaire: Personality Processes and Individual Differences. *Journal of Personality and Social Psychology.*, *63*, 3. 452-459.

Chin, M. H. (2005). Populations at risk: a critical need for research, funding, and action. *Journal of General Internal Medicine.*, *20(5)*, 448-449.

Clark, L. A., Watson, D. & Mineka, S. (1994) .Temperament, personality and the mood and anxiety disorders. Special issue: Personality and psychopathology. *Journal of Abnormal Psychology*, *103(1)*, 103-116.

Clemmer, D. (1940). *The Prison Community.* Boston: The Christopher Publishing House.

Coccaro, E. F., Berman, M. E. & Kavoussi, R. J. (1997). Assessment of life history of aggression: development and a psychometric characteristics. *Psychiatry Research*, *73*, 147-157.

Coccaro, E. F., Harvey, P. D., Kupsaw-Lawrence, E. & Herbert, J. L. (1991). Development of neuropharmacologically based behavioral assessments of impulsive aggressive behavior. *Journal of Neuropsychiatry & Clinical Neurosciences*, *3(2)*, S44-S51.

Coccaro, E. F., Kavoussi, R. J., Sheline, Y. I., Lish, J. D. & Csernansky, J. G. (1996). Impulsive aggression in personality disorder correlates with tritated paroxetine binding in the platelet. *Archives of General Psychiatry*, 53(6)531-536.

Cohen, J. I. (2000). Stress and mental health: A biobehavioral perspective. *Issues in Mental Health Nursing*, 21, 185-202.

Cohen L. J., Gertmenian-King, E., Kunik L., Weaver, C., London, E. D. & Galynker, I. (2005). Personality measures in former heroin users receiving methadone or in protracted abstinence from opiates. *Acta Psychiatric Scandinavica.*, 112, 149-158.

Colsher, P. L., Wallace, R. B., Loeffelholz, P. L. & Sales, M. (1992). Health status of older male prisoners: a comprehensive survey. *American Journal of Public Health.*, 82(6), 881-884.

Cornell, D. G., Warren, J. Hawk, G., Stafford, E., Orem, G. & Pine, D. (1996). Psychopathy in instrumental and reactive violent offenders. *Journal of Consulting and Clinical Psychology*, 64, 783-790.

Cortina, L. M. & Kubiak, S. P. (2006). Gender and posttraumatic stress: Sexual violence as an explanation for women's increased risk. *Journal of Abnormal Psychology.*, 115(4) 753-759.

Compas, B. E., Connor-Smith, J. K., Saltzman, H., Thomsen, A. H. & Wadsworth, M. E. (2001). Coping with stress during childhood and adolescence: problems, progress, and potential in theory and research. *Psychological Bulletin*, 127(1), 87-127.

Conner-Smith, J. K., Compas, B. E. (2002). Vulnerability to social stress: Coping as a mediator or moderator of sociotropy and symptoms of anxiety and depression. *Cognitive Therapy and Research.*, 26(1), 39-55.

Cooke, C. L. (2002). *(Re)presenting African-American men: analyzing discourses on manhood, prison, and relationships.* Unpublished doctoral dissertation, University of Washington, Seattle.

Cooke, D. J. & Michie, C. (2001). Refining the construct of psychopathy: Towards a hierarchical model. *Psychological Assessment.*, 13, 171-188.

Corrigan, P. W. (2004) How stigma interferes with mental health care. *American Psychologist*, 59(7), 614-625.

Corrigan, P. W. & Watson, A. C. (2002). The paradox of self-stigma and mental illness. *Clinical Psychology:Sciences and Practice.*, 9, 35-53.

Corrigan, P. W., Watson, A. C. & Barr, L. (2006). The self-stigma of mental illness: Implications for self-esteem and self-efficacy. *Journal of Social & Clinical Psychology.*, 25(8), 875-884.

Costa, P. T. & McCrae, R. T. (1995). Primary traits of Eysenck's P-E-N system: Three and five factor solutions. *Journal of Personality and Social Psychology*, 69(2), 308-317.

Crabb, P. B. (2001). The material culture of homicidal fantasies. *Aggressive Behavior.*, 26(3), 225-234.

Crisford, H., Dare, H. & Evangeli, M. (2008). Offence-related posttraumatic stress disorder (PTSD) symptomatology and guilt in mentally disordered violent and sexual offenders. *Journal of Forensic Psychiatry & Psychology*, 19(1), 86-107.

Cullen, F. T. (1994). Social support as an organizing concept for criminology: Presidential address to the Academy of Criminal Justice Sciences. *Justice Quarterly.*, 11,527-559.

Cutler, D. L., Tatum, E. & Shore, J. H. (1987). A comparison of schizophrenic patients in different community support treatment approaches. Community Mental Health Journal, 23(2), 103-113.

Damen, K. F. M., DeJong, C. A. J., Nass, G. C. M., VanderStaak, C. P. F., Breteler, M. H. M. (2005). Interpersonal aspects of personality disorders in opioid-dependent patients: The convergence of the ICL-R and the SIDP-IV. *European Addiction Research, 11*, 107-114.

David, J. P. & Sulls, J. (1999). Coping efforts in daily life: Role of big five traits and problem appraisals. *Journal of Personality, 62* (2), 265-294.

Dembling, B. P., Chen, D. T. & Vachon, L. (1999). Life expectancy and causes of death in a population treated for serious mental illness. *Psychiatric Services, 50(8)*, 1036-1042.

Denny, K. (1995). Russian Roulette: A case of questions not asked? *Journal of American Academy of Child and Adolescent Psychiatry, 34(12)*, 682-1683.

Derogistis, L. R., Rickels, K. & Rock, A. (1976). The SCL-90 and the MMPI: A step in the validation of a new self-report scale. *British Journal of Psychiatry., 128*, 280-289.

Desai, R. A., Lam, J. & Rosenheck, R. A. (2000). Childhood risk factors for criminal justice involvement in a sample of homeless people with serious mental illness. *Journal of Nervous and Mental Disease., 88(6)*, 324-332.

Diamond, P. M., Wang, E. W. & Buffington-Vollum, J. (2005). Factor structure of the Buss-Perry Aggression Questionnaire (BPAQ) with mentally ill male prisoners. *Criminal Justice and Behavior., 32(5)*, 546-564.

Dirks, D. (2004). Sexual revictimization and retraumatization of women in prison. *Women's Studies Quarterly, 32*, (3/4)102-115.

Dodge, K. A., Lochman, J. E., Harnish, J. D., Bates, J. E. & Pettit, G. S. (1997). Reactive and proactive aggression in school children and psychiatrically impaired chronically assaultive youth. *Journal of Abnormal Psychology, 106*, 37-51.

Dodge, M. & Pogrebin, M. R. (2001). Collateral costs of imprisonment for women: Complications of reintegration. *The Prison Journal., 81(1)*, 42-54.

Dowden, C. & Andrews, D. A. (1999). What works for female offenders: A meta-analytic review. *Crime and Delinquency., 45*, 438-452.

Edwards, K. A. (1988). Some characteristics of inmates transferred from prison to a state mental hospital.*Behavioral Sciences and the Law., 6(1)*, 131-137.

Einhorn, L., Willimans, T., Stanley, S., Wunderlin, N., Markman, H. & Eason, J. (2008). PREP Inside and Out: Marriage Education for Inmates. *Family Process., 47(3)*, 341-356.

Endler, N. S. & Parker, J. D. A. (1990). The multidimensional assessment of coping: A critical evaluation. *Journal of Personality and Social Psychology., 58*, 844-854.

Engel, G. L. (1977). The need for a new medical model: A challenge for biomedicine. *Science., 196*, 129-136.

Engel, G. L. (1980). The clinical application of the biopsychosocial model. *Am J Psychiatry., 137*, 535-544.

Epping-Jordan, J. E., Compas, B. E., Osowiecki, D. M., Gerri Oppedisano, G., Gerhardt, C., Primo, K. & Krag, D. N. (1999). Psychological adjustment in breast cancer: Processes of emotional distress. *Health Psychology., 18(4)*, 315-326.

Evans, G. W., Lepore S. J. (1993). Household crowding and social support: a quasi-experimental analysis. *J Personal Social Psychology., 65*, 308-316.

Fazel, S., Baines, P. & Doll, H. (2006). Substance abuse and dependence in prisoners: a systematic review. *Addiction.*, *101*, 181-1991.

Fishbein, D. H. & Reuland, M. (1994). Psychological correlates of frequency and type of drug use among jail inmates. *Addictive Behaviors.*, *19(6)*, 583-598.

Fite, P. J., Craig R., Colder, C. R., Lochman, J. E. & Wells, K. C. (2007). Pathways from proactive and reactive aggression to substance use. *Psychology of Addictive Behaviors*, *21(3)*, 355-364.

Fleming, I., Baum, A. & Weiss, L. (1987). Social density and perceived control as mediators of crowding stress in high density residential neighborhoods. *J Personality and Social Psychology.*, *52*, 899-906.

Folkman, S. & Lazarus, R. S. (1980). An analysis of coping in a middle aged community sample. *Journal of Health and Social Behavior.*, *21*, 219-239.

Folkman, S. & Lazarus, R. S. (1988). *Manual for the Ways of Coping Scale.* Palo Alto, CA: Consulting Psychology Press.

Freudenberg, N., Daniels, J., Crum, M., Perkins, T., Rickie, B.E. (2005). Coming home from jail: the social and health consequences of community reentry for women, male adolescents, and their families and communities. *American Journal of Public Health*, *95(10)*, 1725-1736.

Friestad, C. & Hansen, I. L. S. (2005). Mental health Problems among prison inmates: The effect of welfare deficiencies, drug use and self-efficacy. *Journal of Scandinavian Studies in Criminology and Crime Prevention.*, *6*, 183-196.

Fulkunishi, I. (1996). Subclinical depressive symptoms in HIV infection are related to avoidance coping responses: A comparison with end-stage renal failure and breast cancer. Psychological reports, *78(2)*, 483-488.

Fung, K. M. T., Tsang, H. W. H., Corrigan, P. W., Lam, C. S. & Cheng, W. (2007). Measuring self-stigma of mental illness in China and its implications for recovery. *International Journal of Social Psychiatry*, *53(5)*, 408-418.

Gallagher, E. M. (1990). Emotional, social, and physical health characteristics of older men in prison. *International Journal of Aging & Human Development.*, *31(4)*, 251-265.

Geary, The contribution of spirituality to well-being of sex offenders. Dissertation Abstracts International, 64,5-B (UMI# 3090495).

Gee, G. C. & Payne-Sturges, D. C. (2004). Environmental health disparities: A framework integrating psychosocial and environmental concepts. *Environmental Health Perspectives.*, *112(17)*, 1645-1653.

Gerevich, J., Bacskai, E. & Czobor, P. (2007). The generalizability of the Buss-Perry Aggression Questionnaire. *International Journal of Methods in Psychiatric Research*, *16*(3). 124-136.

Geronimus, A. T. (1996). Black/White differences in the relationship of maternal age to birth weight: a population-based test of the weathering hypothesis. Social Science & Medicine, *42(4)*, 589-597.

Geronimus, A. T., Hicken, M., Keene, D. & Bound, J. (2006). "Weathering" and age patterns of allostatic load scores among Blacks and Whites in the United States. *Am J Public Health.*, *96*, 826-833.

Grant, F. (2002). Duty of Care: Implications for teachers/instructors/leaders and other employees working outside the main stream educational arena. *Horizons.*, *20*, 30-35.

Grant, B. F., Stinson, F. S., Dawson, D. A., Chou, S. P. Dufour, M. D., M.C . Compton, W. Pickering, R. P. & Kaplan, K. (2004). Prevalence and co-occurrence of substance use disorders and independent mood and anxiety disorders.

Results from the national epidemiologic survey on alcohol and related conditions. *Archives of General Psychiatry*, *61*, *807*–816.

Gray, N. S., Snowden, R. J., MacCulloch, S., Phillips, H., Taylor, J., MacCulloch, M. J. (2004). Relative efficacy of criminological, clinical, and personality measures of future risk of offending in mentally disordered offenders: A comparative study of HCR-20, PCL:SV, and OGRS. Journal of Consulting and Clinical Psychology, *72(3)*, 523-530.

Gottesman, I. I. (1991). Review of Schizophrenia: Concepts, vulnerability, and intervention. *PsycCRITIQUES*, *36(1)*, 80.

Gunthert, K. C., Cohen, L. H. & Armeli, S. (1999). The role of neuroticism in daily stress and coping, *Journal of Personality and Social Psychology*, *77(5)*, 1087-1100.

Gutierrez, M. J. & Scott, J. (2004). Psychological treatment for bipolar disorders: A review of randomized controlled trials. *European Archives of Psychiatry and Clinical Neuroscience*, *254*, 92-98.

Hairston, C. F. (2001). *Prisoners and families: Parenting issues during incarceration*. Report for the National Policy.

Conference, U. S. Department of Health and Human Services, The Urban Institute, Washington, D. C.

Hall, J. R., Benning, S. D. & Patrick, C. J. (2004). Criterion-related validity of the three-factor model of psychopathy: Personality, behavior, and adaptive functioning. *Assessment.*, *11(1)*, 4-16.

Hart, S. D., Cox, D. N. & Hare, R. D. (1995). *The Hare Psychopathy Checklist: Screening version*. Toronto, ON: Multi-Health Systems.

Hammett, T. M. (1998). Reaching seriously at-risk populations: health interventions in criminal justice settings. *Health Education & Behavior*, *25(1)*, 99-112.

Hammer, M. (1981). Social supports, social networks, and schizophrenia. *Schizophrenia Bulletin*, *7(1)*, 45-57.

Hammond, L. A. (1988, April). *Mediators of stress and role satisfaction in multiple role women.* Paper presented at the annual meeting of the Western Psychological Association, Burlingame, CA.

Harding, T. & Zimmermann, E. (1989). Psychiatric symptoms, cognitive stress and vulnerability factors: A study in a remand prison. *British Journal of Psychiatry*, *155*, 36-43.

Hare, R. D. (1991). *The Hare Psychopathy Checklist–Revised*. Toronto, Ontario: Multi-Health Systems.

Harpur, T. J., Hare, R. D. & Hakstian, A. R. (1989).Two-factor conceptualization of psychopathy: Construct validity and assessment implications. *Psychological Assessment: A Journal of Consulting and Clinical Psychology*, *1*, 6-17.

Hathaway, S. R. & Mckinley, J. C. (1981). Inventaire Multi-phasique de Personnalité (M.M.P.I. et la version MINIMULT). Paris: Les Editions du Centre de Psychologie Appliquée.

Hatton, D. C., Kleffel, D. & Fisher, A. A. (2006). Prisoners' perspectives of health problems and healthcare in a US women's jail. *Women & Health, 44(1)*, 119-136.

Hirschi, T. W (1969). Infraction as action: A study of the antecedents of illegal acts. *Dissertation Abstracts International, 29*(9-A), 69-3614.

Holahan, C. J. & Moos, R. H. (1987). Personal and contextual determinants of coping strategies. *Journal of Personality and Social Psychology, 52(5)*, 946-955.

Holmes, J. A. & Stevenson, C. A. Z. (1990). Differential effects of avoidant and attentional coping strategies on adaptation to chronic and recent-onset pain. *Health Psychology, 9(5)*, 577-584.

Holohan, C. J. & Moos, R. H. (1985). Life stress and health: Personality, coping, and family support in stress resistance. *Journal of Personality and Social Psychology, 49(3)*, 739-747.

Hooker, K., Frazier, L. D. & Monahan, D. J. (1994). Personality and coping among caregivers of spouses with dementia. *The Gerontologist, 34(3)*, 386-92.

Hunter, A. (1985). Private, parochial and public social orders: The problem of crime and incivility in urban communities. In G. D. Suttles & M. N. Zald. (Eds.). *The challenge of social control: Citizenship and institution building in modern society* (230-242). Norwood, NJ: Aldex Publishing..

Ingram, R. E. & Luxton, D. D. (2005). Vulnerability-stress models. In B.J. Hankin & J.R.Z. Abela (Eds.), *Development of psychopathology: a vulnerability-stress perspective.* (32-41). London: Sage Publishers.

Ingram R. E. & Price, J. M. (Eds). (2001). Vulnerability to psychopathology:Risk across the lifespan. NY: Guilford Press.

Ingram, R. E., Miranda, J. & Siegal, Z. (1998). *Cognitive vulnerability to depression.* NY: Guilford Press.

Inez Myin-Germeys, I.,van Os, J. (2007). Stress-reactivity in psychosis: Evidence for an affective pathway to psychosis. *Clinical Psychology Review., 27*, 409-424.

Jacobson, M. (2007). Testimony to a hearing of the Joint Economic Committee entitled *"Mass Incarceration in the United States: At What Cost?"* on October 4, 2007. Special hearing of the Joint Economic Committee of the US Senate. Retrieved December 2, 2008 from http://www.jec.senate.gov/index.cfm?FuseAction=Hearings.HearingsCalendar.

Johnstone, M. J. (2001) Stigma, social justice and the rights of the mentally ill: Challenging the status quo. *Australian and New Zealand Journal of Mental Health Nursing., 10*, 200-209.

Jones, S. H., Sellwood, W. & McGovern, J. (2005). Psychological therapies for bipolar disorder: The role of model-driven approaches to therapy integration. *Bipolar Disorders, 7*, 22-32.

Jordan, B. K., Federman, E. B., Burns, B. J., Schlenger, W. E., Fairbank, J. A., Caddell, J. M. (2002). Lifetime use of mental health and substance abuse treatment services by incarcerated women felons. Psychiatric Services, *53(3)*, 317-325.

Kear-Colwell, J. & Sawle, G. A. (2001). Coping strategies and attachment in pedophiles: Implications for treatment. *International Journal of Offender Therapy and Comparative Criminology.*, *45*, 171-182.

Kemp, G. C., Glaser, B. A. & Page, R. (1992). Influence of family support on men in a minimum security detention center. *Journal of Addictions and Offender Counseling*, *12*, 34-46.

Kim, S., Ting, A., Puisis, M., Rodriquez, S., Benson, R., Mennella, C. & Davis, F. (2007). Deaths in the Cook County jail: 10-year report, 1995-2004. *Journal of Urban Health*, *84(1)*, 70-84.

Koenig, H. G. & Cohen, H. J. (2002). The link between religion and health: Psychoneuroimmunology and the faith factor. NY: Oxford University Press.

Krieger J. & Higgins D. L. (2002). Housing and health: time again for public health action. *American Jouranl of Public Health.*, *92*, 758-768.

Kuyken, W., Peters, E., Power, M. J. & Lavender, T. (2003). Trainee clinical psychologists' adaptation and professional functioning: A longitudinal study. *Clinical Psychology & Psychotherapy.*, *10(1)*, 41-54.

Lazarus, A. A. (1966). Behavior rehearsal vs. non-directive therapy vs. advice in effecting behavior change. *Behavior Research and Therapy*, *4(3)*, 209-212.

Lazarus, R. S. & Folkman, S. (1984). *Stress, Appraisal and Coping*. New York: Springer.

Lee-Baggley, D., Preece, M. & DeLongis, A. (2005). Coping with interpersonal stress: Role of big five traits. *Journal of Personality 73(5)*, 1141-1180.

Lejuez, C. W., Kahler, C. W. & Brown, R. A. (2003). A modified computer version of the paced auditory serial addition task (PASAT) as a laboratory-based stressor. *The Behavior Therapist.*, *26*, 290-293.

Liberman, R. P., DeRisi, W. J. & Mueser, K. T. (1989). *Social skills training for psychiatric patients*. Needham Heights, MA: Allyn & Bacon.

Lichtenstein, B. (2009, February). *Drugs, incarceration, and HIV/AIDS among African American men*. Paper presented at the annual meeting of the American Society of Criminology, Atlanta, Georgia. Retrieved January 2, 2009 from http://www.allacademic. com/meta/p200216_index.html.

Link, B. G., Cullen, F. T., Frank, J. & Wozniak, J. F. (1987). The social rejection of former mental patients: Understanding why labels matter. *American Journal of Sociology.*, *92(6)*, 1461-1500.

Looman, J., Abracen, J., DiFazio, R. & Maillet, G. (2004). Alchol and drug abuse among sexual and nonsexual offenders: relationship to intimacy deficits and coping strategy. *Sexual Abuse. Journal of Research and Treatment*, *16(3)*, 177-189.

Lopez, F. G., Mauricio, A. M., Gormley, B., Simko, T. & Berger, E. (2001). Adult attachment orientations and college student distress: The mediating role of problem coping styles. *Journal of Counseling & Development*, *79*, 459-464.

Loury, G. & Stoltz, M. P. (2007). Mass incarceration and American values. *Testimony to the Special hearing of the Joint Economic Committee of the US Senate on October.*, 4, 2007. *Mass incarceration in the United States: At what cost?* Retrieved December 2, 2008 from http://www.jec.senate.gov/index.cfm?FuseAction=Hearings.HearingsCalendar.

Lovell, D., Cloyes, K., Allen, D. & Rhodes, L. (2000). Who lives in super maximum custody? AWashington State study. *Federal Probation.*, *64*, 33-43.

Luecken, L. J., Appelhans, B. M., Kraft, A. & Brown, A. (2006). Never far from home: A cognitive-affective model of the impact of early-life family relationships on physiological stress responses in adulthood. *Journal of Social and Personal Relationships.*, *2*, 189-203.

Lykke, J, Hesse, M., Austin, S. F. & Oestrich, I. (2008). Validity of the BPRS, the BDI, and the BAI in dual diagnosis patients. *Addictive Behaviors*, *33*, 292-300.

Lindquist, C. H. & Lindquist, C. A. (1997). Gender differences in distress: Mental health consequences of environmental stress among jail inmates. *Behavioral Sciences & the Law.*, *15(4)*, 503-523.

Macintyre, S., Ellaway, A. & Cummins, S. (2002). Place effects on health: how can we conceptualize, operationalize, and measure them? *Social Science Medicine*, *55*,125-139.

Martin, P., Rott, C., Poon, L. W., Courtenay, B. & Lehr, U. (2001). A molecular view of coping behavior in older adults. *Journal of Aging and Health*, *13*, 72-91.

Mattlin, J. A., Wethington, E. & Kessler, R. (1990). Situational determinants of coping and coping effectiveness. *Journal of Health and Social Behavior.*, *31*(1), 103-122.

McCrae, R. R. (1992). Situational determinants of coping. In B.N. Carpenter (Ed.). *Personal coping: Theory, research, and application* (65-76), Westport, CT: Praeger Publishers/Greenwood Publishing Group.

McCrae, R. R. & Costa, P. T. (1986). Personality, coping, and coping effectiveness in an adult sample. *Journal of Personality*, *54 (2)*, 385-405.

McEwing, B. S. (1998). Protective and damaging effects of stress mediators. *New England Journal of Medicine*,*33*, 171-179.

McEwing, B. S. & Wingfield, J. C. (2003). The concept of allostasis in biology and biomedicine. *Hormones and Behavior*, *43* (1), 2-15.

McKirnan, D. J. &. Peterson, P. L. (1988). Stress, expectancies, and vulnerability to substance abuse: A test of a model among homosexual men. Journal of Abnormal Psychology, *97(4)*, 461-466.

McMurray, H. L. (1993). High risk parolees in transition from institution to community life. *Journal of Offender Rehabilitation*, *19(1-2)*, 145-161.

Miller, N., Pedersen, W. C., Earleywine, M. & Pollock, V. E. (2003). A theoretical model of triggered displaced aggression. *Personality & Social Psychology Review*, *7*(1),75-97.

Monroe, S. M. & Simons, A. D. (1991). Diathesis-stress theories in the context of life-stress research: Implications for the depressive disorders. *Psychological Bulletin*, *110*, 406-425.

Morrissey, C., Mooney, P., Hogue, T. E., Lindsay, W. R. & Taylor, J. L. (2007). Predictive validity of the PCL-R for offenders with intellectual disability in a high security hospital: Treatment progress. *Journal of Intellectual & Developmental Disability*, *32(2)*, 125-133.

Morrow, K. A., Thoreson, R. W., Penney, L. L. (1995). Predictors of psychological distress among infertility clinic patients. *Journal of Consulting and Clinical Psychology*, *63(1)*, 163-167.

Mumola, C. & Karberg, J. (2006). Drug use and dependence, state and federal prisoners, 2004 (Bureau of Justice Statistics Special Report, NCJ 213530). Retrieved December 22, 2008 from http://www.ojp.usdoj.gov/bjs/pub/pdf/dudsfp04.pdf.

Nolen, P. (2007). Mass incarceration in the United States: at what cost? Testimony before the Joint Economic Committee on October 4, 2007. Special hearing of the Joint Economic Committee of the US Senate. *Mass incarceration in the United States: At what cost?* Retrieved December., *2*, 2008 from http://www.jec.senate.gov/index.cfm?FuseAction= Hearings.HearingsCalendar.

Nolen-Hoeksema, S., Parker, L. E. & Larson, J. (1994). Ruminative coping with depressed mood following loss. *Journal of Personality and Social Psychology., 67(1)*, 92-104.

O'Brien, T. B. & DeLongis, A. (1996). The interactional context of problem- emotion- and relationship-focused coping: The role of the big five personality factors. *Journal of Personality, 64(4)*, 775-813.

Osowiecki, D. M. & Compas, B. E. (1999). Coping and perceived control in adjustment to breast cancer. *Cognitive Therapy and Research, 23*,169-180.

Ouis D. (2001). Annoyance from road traffic noise: a review. *J Environmental Psychology., 21*, 101-120.

Overall, J. E. & Gorham, D. R. (1962). The Brief Psychiatric Rating Scale. Psychology Rep., *10*, 799-812.

Overton, S. L. & Medina, S. L. (2008). The stigma of mental illness. *Journal of Counseling & Development, 86*, 143-151.

Pan American Health Organization (PAHO). (2002). *Health in the Americas.* Washington, DC: Pan American Health Organization.

Parsons, S.,Walker, L. & Grubin, D. (2001). Prevalence of mental disorder in female remand prisons. *The Journal of Forensic Psychiatry, 12(1)*, 194-202.

Petersilia, J. (2000). Invisible victims. Human Rights: Journal of the Section of Individual *Rights & Responsibilities., 27(1)*, 9-13.

Post, R. M. (1992) Transduction of psychosocial stress into neurobiology of recurrent affective disorder. *American Journal of Psychiatry., 149*, 999-1010.

Poster, M. J. (1992). "The Estelle medical professional judgement standard: The right of those in state custody to receive high-cost medical treatments." *American Journal of Law and Medicine., 18(4)*, 347-368.

Poulin, F. & Boivin, M. (2000). The role of proactive and reactive aggression in the formation and development of boys' friendships. *Developmental Psychology, 36*, 233-240.

Prinstein, M. J. & Cillessen, A. H. N. (2003). Forms and functions of adolescent peer aggression associated with high levels of peer status. *Merrill-Palmer Quarterly., 49*, 310-342.

Provencher, H. L., Perreault, M., St-Onge, M. & Rousseau, M. (2003). Predictors of psychological distress in family caregivers of persons with psychiatric disabilities. *Journal of Psychiatric & Mental Health Nursing., 10 (5)*, 592-607.

Raison, C. L. & Miller, A. H. (2003). When not enough is too much: The role of insufficient glucocorticoid signaling in the pathophysiology of stress related disorders. *American Journal of Psychiatry, 160(9)*, 1554-1565.

Richman, J. M., Rosenfeld, L. B. & Hardy, C. (1993). The social support survey: A validation study of a clinical measure of the social support process. *Research on Social Work Practice, 3*, 288-311.

Riskind, J. H., Williams, N. L. & Joiner, T. E. (2006). The looming cognitive style: A cognitive vulnerability for anxiety disorders. *Journal of Social and Clinical Psychology.*, *25(7)*, 779-801.

Rogers, A. C. (1997). Vulnerability, health and health care. *Journal of Advanced Nursing*, *26*, 65-72.

Rodriguez, N. & Webb, V. J. (2007). Probation violations, revocations, and imprisonment. *Criminal Justice Policy Review*, *18 (1)*, 3-30.

Rotter, M. R., Larkin, S., Schare, M. L., Massaro, J. & Steinbacher, M. (1999). *The clinical impact of doing time: Mental illness and incarceration. Resource manual.* Albany: New York State Department of Labor.

Rotter, M., McQuistion, H. L., Broner, N., Steinbacher, M. & Glazer,W. M. (2005). The impact of "incarceration culture" on re-entry for adults with mental illness: A training and group treatment model. *Psychiatric Services*, *56*, 265-267.

Rutter, M. (1987). Psychosocial resilience and protective mechanisms. *American Journal of Orthopsychiatry*,*57*, 316-331.

Saari, R. C. (1987). The female offender and the criminal justice system. In D.S. Burden & N. Gottlieb (Eds.). The Woman Client: Providing Human Services in a Changing World (pp. 177-194). NY: Travistock Pubs.

Sarason, B., Sarason, I. & Pierce, G. (1990). Traditional views of social support and their impact on measurement. In B., Sarason, I., Sarason, & G. Pierce (Eds.), *Social support: An interactional view* (9-25). New York: John Wiley & Sons.

Saunders, J. C. (2003). Families living with severe mental illness: a literature review. *Issues in Mental Health Nursing*, *24(2)*, 175-198.

Scher, C. D., Ingram, R. E. & Segal, Z. V. (2005). Cognitive reactivity and vulnerability: Empirical evaluation of construct activation and cognitive diatheses in Unipolar Depression. *Clinical Psychology Review*, *25*, 487-510.

Scherer, R. F & Brodzinski, J. D. (1990). An analysis of the Ways of Coping Questionnaire research instrument. *Management Communication Quarterly.*, *3(3)*, 401-418.

Schubert, M., Glass, T. R., Clarke, S. P., Aiken, L.H., Schaffert-Witvliet, B., Sloane, D. M. & De Geest, S. (2008). Rationing of nursing care and its relationship to patient outcomes: The Swiss extension of the international hospital outcomes study. *International Journal of Quality Health Care*, *20(4)*, 227-237.

Selye, H. (1976). *Stress in health and disease.* Reading, Mass.: Butterworths Publishing.

Selye, H. (1963). A syndrome produced by diverse noxious agents. *Nature.*, *138*, 32.

Sevecke, K., Lehmkuhl, G. & Krischer, M. K. (2009). Examining relations between psychopathology and psychopathy dimensions among adolescent female and male offenders.*European Child & Adolescent Psychiatry.*, *18(2)*, 85-95.

Shelton, D. (in press). Forensic nursing in secure environments. *Journal of Forensic Nursing.*

Shoham, S. G., Askenasy, J. J. M., Rahav, G., Chard, F. & Addi, A. (1989). Personality correlates of violent prisoners. *Personality Individual Differences.*, *10(2)*, 137-145.

Silver, E. & Teasdale, B. (2005). Mental disorder and violence: An examination of stressful life events and impaired social support. *Social Problems.*, *52(1)*, 62-78.

Simons, J. S. & Gaher, R. M. (2005). The Distress Tolerance Scale: Development and validation of a self-report measure. *Motivation and Emotion.*, *29(2)*, 83-102.

Slavik, S. & Croake, J. (2006). The individual psychology conception of depression as a stress-diathesis model. *The Journal of Individual Psychology.*, *62*, 4, 417-428.

Smith, S., Mullis, F., Kern, R. M. & Brack, G. (1999). An Adlerian model for the etiology of aggression in adjudicated adolescents. The Family Journal: Counseling and Therapy for Couples and Families., *7(2)*, 135-147.

Smith, P., Waterman, M. & Ward, N. (2006). Driving aggression in forensic and non-forensic populations: Relationships to self-reported levels of aggression, anger and impulsivity. *British Journal of Psychology*, *97*, 387-403.

Soderstrom, I. R., Castellano, T. C. & Figaro, H. R. (2001). Measuring 'mature coping' skills among adult and juvenile offenders. *Criminal Justice and Behavior*, *28(3)*, 300-328.

Spielberger, C. D., Gorsuch, R. L. & Lushene, R. E. (1970). Manual for the State-Traint Anxiety Inventory. Palo Alto, CA: Consulting Psychologists Press.

Stoner, S. B. (1988). Undergraduate marijuana use and anger. *Journal of psychology.*, *122(4)*, 343-347.

Tataro, C. (2006). Watered down: Partial implementation of the new generation jail philosophy. *The Prison Journal*, *86(3)*, 284-300.

Teplin, L. A., Abram, K. M. & McClelland, G. M. (1997). Mentally disordered women in jail: Who receives services? *American Journal of Public Health*, *87(4)*, 604-609.

Sukhodolsky, Denis G., Golub, Arthur; Cromwell, Erin N. (2001). Development and validation of the Anger Rumination Scale. Personality and Individual Differences, 31(5), 689-700.

Tobin, D. L., Holroyd, K. A., Reynolds, R. & Wigal, J. K. (1989). The hierarchical factor structure of the Coping Strategies Inventory. *Cognitive Therapy and Research*, *13*, 343-361.

Trestman, R. L., Ford, J., Zhang, W. & Wiesbrock, V. (2007). Current and lifetime psychiatric illness among inmates not identified as acutely mentally ill at intake in Connecticut's jails. *Journal of the American Academy of Psychiatry and Law*, *35*, 490-500.

Toch, H. (1992). *Mosaic of despair: Human breakdown in prisons*. Washington, DC: The American Psychological Association. H., Toch, & K. Adams, (1986). Pathology and disruptiveness among prison inmates. *Journal of Researchin Crime and Delinquency*, *23*, 7-21.

US Congress. (2007). *Mass incarceration in the United States: At what cost?* Special hearing of the Joint Economic Committee of the US Senate. Retrieved December 2, 2008 from http://www.jec.senate.gov/index.cfm?FuseAction=Hearings.HearingsCalendar.

Van Valkenburg1, C. & Akiskal, H. S. (1999). Which patients presenting with clinical anxiety will abuse benzodiazepines? *Human Psychopharmacology: Clinical & Experimental*, *14*, S45-S51.

Vaux, A. (1988). *Social support: Theory, research, and intervention*. New York: Praeger.

Vega, M. & Silverman, M. (1988). Stress and the elderly convict. *International Journal of Offender Therapy and Comparative Criminology*, *32(2)*, 153-162.

Veiel, H. O. F. & Baumann, U. (1992). *The meaning and measurement of social support.* (pp.xiv, 327). Washington, DC: Hemisphere Publishing.

Velarde, L. D. (2002). Living in prison: Evaluating the deprivation and importation models of inmate adaptation. *Dissertation Abstracts International: Section B: The Sciences and Engineering*, *62*, 4256.

Vickers, R. R., Kolar, D. W. & Hervig, L. K. (1989). *Personality correlates of coping with military basic training.* (Report number: NHRC-89-3), Silver Spring, MD: Naval Health Research Center.

Vitaliano, P. P., Maiuro, R. D., Russo, J. & Becker, J. (1987). Raw versus relative scores in the assessment of coping strategies. *Journal of Behavioral Medicine*, *10(1)*, 1-18.

Vogel, D. L.,Wade, N. G. & Hackler, A. H. (2007). Perceived public stigma and the willingness to seek counseling: The mediating roles of self-stigma and attitudes toward counseling. *Journal of Counseling Psychology*, *54(1)*, 40-50.

Wagner, D. K., Lorion, R. P. & Shipley, T. E. (1983). Insomnia and psychosocial crisis: Two studies of Erikson's developmental theory. *Journal of Consulting and Clinical Psychology*, *51(4)*, 595-603.

Walmsley, R. (2006). U.S. Incarceration rate is largest in the world. *World prison population list.* International Centre for Prison Studies, King's College, London. Retrieved January 15, 2009 from http://www.senate.gov/.

Walsh, T., Tickle, M., Milsom, K, Buchanan, K. & Zoitopoulos, L. (2008). An investigation of the nature of research into dental health in prisons: a systematic review. *British Dental Journal.*, *204(12)*, 683-689.

Wang, E. W. & Diamond, P. M. (1999). Empirically identifying factors related to violence risk in corrections. *Behavioral Sciences & the Law.*, *17(3)*, 377-389.

Wang, E. W., Rogers, R., Giles, C. L., Diamond, P. M., Herrington-Wang, L. E. & Taylor, E. R. (1997). A pilot study of the Personality Assessment Inventory (PAI) in corrections: Assessment of malingering, suicide risk, and aggression in male inmates. *Behavioral Sciences & The Law*, *15(4)*, 469-482.

Watson, D. (2003). Subtypes, specifiers, epicycles and eccentrics: Toward a more parsimonious taxonomy of psychopathology. *Clinical Psychology: Science and Practice*, *10(2)*, 233-238.

Watson, D., Clark L. A. & Tellegen, A. (1988). Development and validation of brief measures of Positive and Negative Affect: The PANAS Scales. *Journal of Personality and Social Psychology*, *54(6)*, 1063-1070.

Watson, D. & Hubbard, B. (1996). Adaptational style and dispositional structure: Coping in the context of the five-factor model. *Journal of Personality.*, *64(4)*, 737-774.

Webb, J. (2007). Mass incarceration in the United States: At what cost? Opening statement before the Joint Economic Committee on October 4, 2007. Special hearing of the Joint Economic Committee of the US Senate. Retrieved December 2, 2008 from http://www.jec.senate.gov/index.cfm?FuseAction=Hearings.HearingsCalendar.

Wegner, W. D. (1994). Support services contributing to patient care. *Nursing Management*, *25(2)*, 64-70.

Wei, M., Mallinckrodt, B., Russell, D. W. & Abraham, W. T. (2004). Maladaptive perfectionism as a mediator and moderator between attachment and negative mood. *Journal of Counseling Psychology.*, *51*, 201-212.

Wei, M., Vogel D. L., Ku, T. Y. & Zakalik, R. A. (2005). Adult attachment, affect regulation, negative mood, and interpersonal problems: The mediating roles of emotional reactivity and emotional cutoff. *Journal of Counseling Psychology, 52(1)*, 14-24.

Weisz, J. R., McCabe, M. A. & Dennig, M. D. (1994). Primary and secondary control among children undergoing medical procedures: Adjustment as a function of coping style. *Journal of Consulting and Clinical Psychology, 62(2)*, 324-332.

Western, B. (2007). Testimony before the Joint Economic Committee on October 4, 2007. Special hearing of the Joint Economic Committee of the US Senate. *Mass incarceration in the United States: At what cost?* Retrieved December 2, 2008 from http://www.jec.senate.gov/index.cfm?FuseAction=Hearings.HearingsCalendar.

Western, B., Lopoo, L. M. & McLanahan, S. (2003). Incarceration and the bonds among parents in fragile families. (Working Paper #02-22-FF). Princeton, NJ: Center for Research on Child Wellbeing. Retrieved January 15, 2009 from http://www.rwjf.org/pr/product.jsp?id=14505.

Whatley, S. L., Foreman, A. C. & Richards, S. (1998). The relationship of coping style to dysphoria, anxiety, and anger. Psychological reports, *83(3)*, 783-791.

Williams, N. H. (2007). Prison health and the health of the public: Ties that bind. *Journal of Correctional Health Care, 13(2).*, 80-92. Retrieved December 31, 2008, from http://jcx.sagepub.com/cgi/content/abstract/13/2/80.

Wong, D. F. K. (2006). *Clinical Case Management for People with Mental Illness: A Biopsychosocial Vulnerability Stress Model*. New York: Haworth Press.

Zingraff, M. T. (1980). Inmate assimilation: A comparison of male and female delinquents. *Criminal Justice and Behavior, 7*, 274-292.

Zubin, J. & Spring, B.(1977). Vulnerability-a new view of schizophrenia. *Journal of Abnormal Psychology, 86(2)*, 103-126.

Chapter III

Risk

Alyson Kettles
University of Aberdeen, Aberdeen, Scotland

Abstract

Risk is discussed and defined in this chapter. Risk assessment and management are introduced along with the terminology, history and some assessment tools. Some tools are described with their associated major references to aid knowledge of this important area of practice. Issues related to the use of risk assessment instruments are discussed as aspects of clinical use, such as education and training, are important to understand.

Introduction

Risk is about people. Risk assessment is about knowing people and being as accurate as you reasonably can be when you conduct a risk assessment and reach a decision. Whether we like it or not risk assessment and management is a regular and daily occurrence in health care. Everyday, people in every capacity will undertake assessments of risk and as a consequence put interventions in place to either manage or reduce those identified risks. For example, a mother will assess the risks in taking a young child to the park and act accordingly by putting on appropriate clothing, checking weather conditions, observing and managing the negotiation of traffic and pedestrians and observe the child as he plays in the park. A nurse will assess and manage the risks to a suicidal patient on an acute care psychiatric ward and a community psychiatric nurse will assess the needs of a patient who has to do his own shopping and then make his own meal in his own residence for the first time since discharge from hospital.

A literature search on risk will provide thousands of results and this confirms both Hayes (1992) assertion that for some time risk has been an important idea in health, the behavioural and social sciences, and criminal justice/legal systems; and Skolbekken's (1995) idea that there is a 'risk epidemic' in medical and healthcare journals.

Woods (1996) states that risk assessment is central to practice and is a requirement by society that we protect those who would need it and those that society needs protecting from. Doyle and Duffy (2006) consider that assessing and managing risk is a key task for mental health clinicians and Doyle (2000) states that "assessing and managing risk is fundamental to the practice of mental health professionals…" Lewis & Webster (2004) argue that risk assessment, and its subsequent management, is one of the highest profile tasks that can be undertaken in mental health and Rose (1998) reports how 'the language of risk now prevails in mental health in the United Kingdom (UK)'. Appleby in the UK Department of Health (2007) document on *Best Practice in Managing Risk* makes it plain that "safety is at the centre of all good healthcare" (p.3).

What is Risk?

Different professionals understand risk in a variety of different ways but in psychiatric and mental health care it means a range of potential adverse events (Kettles, 2004). McClelland (1995) emphasized that a key problem which nurses face in their approach to risk assessment and management, is that it is affected to a considerable degree by who defines that risk and how it is defined. This is in itself problematic in that if we as psychiatric and mental health nurses do not agree what is or is not a risk and to what extent it is a risk then how can we go on to provide care, safety and protection and ultimately, continuity of care across the range of services, and needless to say good risk management? Risk can be considered to be "the probability of harm to self or others or a serious unwanted event; risk assessment as the process of determining this probability; and risk management as the process or intervention through which identified risks are reduced or alleviated" (Kettles and Woods, 2009). So risk can be considered from all points of view to range from the person's deterioration in mental health through to suicide or homicide.

Over the past 50 years psychiatric and mental health practice has changed significantly and specific challenges have developed for the psychiatric and mental health nurses' role in both risk assessment and management. Policy and legal changes internationally have seen an increasing emphasis on community care and recovery rather than institutional and hospital care, where in the latter it was easier to assess and manage risk through the added controls and place of asylum that was provided for the patients, despite the associated loss of personhood and autonomy. Hospital beds are fewer in number and the length of stay in hospital tends to be much reduced. This means that those people finding themselves in hospital are likely to be at a higher risk on admission and so they demand enhanced skills from the psychiatric and mental health nurses that care for them. Conversely this also means that those that are not admitted are more likely to be more risky than in the past, demanding different and higher level skills from those nurses working in community care. With this propulsion towards community care and the related crisis intervention and assertive outreach services that have been and are being developed, risk assessment and management has been taken to a new level of complexity.

In view of the UK Department of Health (2001, p11-13) crisis resolution and home treatment teams provide services for adults with severe mental illness with an acute mental crisis of such severity that, without the participation of this type of team, hospitalization would be essential. Current policy throughout the world has developed, and continues to develop, around the idea that people experiencing mental illness should receive treatment and care in the least restrictive environment, to try to minimize disruption in their lives. Crisis resolution and/or home treatment can usually be provided in a range of settings and offers an alternative to inpatient care. As all of this is a complex process effective risk assessment and management is a crucial and challenging part of the process. The UK Department of Health (2001) also provides unambiguous implementation guidelines for assertive outreach services for those people who have difficulty in maintaining lasting and non-resistant contact with services. Often they can suffer from severe mental health problems with complex needs and multiple pathologies and have difficulty engaging with services, often requiring repeat admissions to hospital. Assertive outreach is viewed as an effective approach to the management of people with these types of problems and both good risk assessment and management are central to these services.

In *From values to action: The Chief Nursing Officer's review of mental health nursing* (Department of Health 2006) key recommendation 10 (in relation to improving outcomes for service users) clearly states "Mental Health Nurses need to be well trained in risk assessment and management. They should work closely with service users and others to develop realistic individual care plans" (p.5). Throughout this review issues of good quality risk assessment and management add force to several of the other recommendations. Similarly *Rights, Relationships and Recovery: The Report of the National Review of Mental Health Nursing in Scotland* (Scottish Executive 2006) highlights one of the visions of mental health services as "Enabling, person-centred recovery and strengths-based focus with a move towards positive management of individual risk" with a mental health nursing response of "Adopting frameworks for practice that promote values-based practice, maximizing therapeutic contact time and the therapeutic management of individual risk" (p.11). Again throughout this key review many of the other practice and care issues discussed are in direct relation to good risk assessment and management. An unambiguous blunt message is therefore being sent by two major reviews of mental health nursing in the UK that risk assessment and management is high on the professional agenda.

The provision of forensic psychiatric services and facilities have grown and more psychiatric and mental health nurses are working within these areas with few specific advanced forensic skills to prepare them for the undertaking. Within these services and facilities there is an increased pressure on mental health nurses to provide formalised assessments of risk and level of risk along with related management strategies in highly stressful patient situations and environments. This challenge has been taken up however using systemic approaches such as the "New to Forensic Programme" in Scotland (http://www.forensicnetwork.scot.nhs.uk/newtoforensic.asp) and the use of the new Risk Management Authority (RMA) (http://www.rmascotland.gov.uk/ home.aspx) to make formal assessments for the courts.

When something goes wrong for a patient in the mental health system, it is a break down in risk assessment and management that is frequently reported. This can and does often result in tragic consequences. The consequence of such breakdowns is often a shift in both public and political opinion about the care given and the way in which the system works. There can also be greater expectations placed upon nurses and other health care professionals as a result. Litigation is a real issue for health professionals in the modern world and society places pressure on nurses, and other health care professionals, to provide accurate assessments of risk, which in themselves are often unrealistic. The end result can be that clinicians err on the side of caution and determine someone to be at higher level of risk than they really are. So it needs to be remembered that risk assessment is an inexact science, but it is one that is developing at a rapid pace.

The History of Risk Assessment and Management

Risk assessment is not new but prior to the mid 1960's the term used was 'dangerousness' and this was used with only a few patients. However, Steadman and Cocozza (1974) and Monaghan (1981) argued that the assessments of dangerousness were unreliable and worse, inaccurate. They set about defining what they considered to be the components of risk in three terms:

1. risk assessment is about executive decision-making rather than legal classification
2. It is about where a person is on a scale of risk
3. It is about the day to day management of the potentially risky person.

However, others argue that risk has other concerns. For example, Mason (1998) argues that risk is about three particular types of risk:

1. risk of violence
2. dangerousness
3. risk of recidivism.

It is these three concerns that he goes on to define rather than the term 'risk' itself. He goes on to show that there are different definitions and major conceptual differences about dangerousness between different disciplines and this is why Steadman and Cocozza (1974) argue that the term 'risk' is a more definable term and has more practical use in clinical areas.

Jacobs (2000) discusses how gambling was the beginning of the idea of risk, with the idea of taking a gamble meaning the probability of an event happening along with the extent of the loss or gain that could result from the throw of a die or the turn of a card. For example, in gambling a player will take risks, often for very high stakes and the term "risk everything on the turn of the dice" refers particularly to when a player can either win or lose an extremely large bet on a single throw of the die. This bet can be a large quantity of money, property or any other life changing momentous item. This is also where the term "losing your shirt" comes from when in the past players have literally lost everything, including the clothes they stand up in (a fictional example of this is shown in the film 'A Knight's Tale'[2001]). As a result risk became a calculable construct in the framework of gambling. Gifford (1986) suggests that risk has always included the idea of danger but that it has not always included ideas of chance. Jacobs shows the derivation of the word 'risk' from the Latin 'resecare' meaning 'to cut back' or 'to cut off short' and the French 'risque' and the Italian including the meaning of 'peril' and the Spanish meaning of 'to venture into danger'.

Risk estimation and epidemiology have developed together since the nineteenth century when epidemiology developed to identify the risk factors of disease and its occurrence through to the prevention of disease through the eradication of the risk factors.

In the 20th century the field of risk analysis grew through its use in nuclear power, as the need for estimating and legitimizing the risks of dealing with nuclear materials and hazardous chemicals became apparent. Risk is also a term that has been used by actuaries in the economics and insurance industries to assess the potentials for events occurring and the gains and losses that can result from particular events. This type of risk involves the use of formal algorithms to calculate complex coefficients and discriminant function equations. This type of approach has been shown to have a greater predictive power than other methods of risk analysis but is very complex to calculate. In the field of mental healthcare few are willing to enter into this type of time consuming and complex activity even if it could be shown to be of benefit to the patient.

Defining Terms in Clinical Risk – Assessment and Management

Confusion surrounds the term 'risk assessment' as people tend not to realise that the idea of risk is simply another word for 'probability'. Risk is a term that has changed from its original meaning in mathematical probability and recently has come to have negative connotations and to represent a combination of probability and something adverse or dangerous.

In psychiatric and mental health services it is the probability (risk) of an event or behaviour (outcome) occurring that we are interested in when we talk about risk assessment. The event or the behaviour is the principal topic of interest because it is usually associated with a degree of severity. This severity can be in relation to illness symptoms and can be referred to as dangerousness. The impact of such severity is exceedingly important because it is possible to have a high risk of an outcome with low impact (such as gesticulating or verbal aggression) or conversely low risk of an outcome with high impact (for example assault).

Common Terminology in use and Some Essential Definitions

In modern day usage 'risk' means different things to different groups of people (Doyle 2000, Jacobs 2000) but for health and social care professionals and for those working in psychiatric and mental health nursing 'risk' is explicitly about the safety of staff, patients and carers (Kettles 2004). Risk is about whether or not an event will occur such as whether or not a patient is likely to abscond or will attempt to commit suicide. In forensic mental health nursing it often means whether or not a patient is likely to become violent.

The insurance industry invests time and money in risk and in order to minimise risk insurers will exclude particular groups from being able to hold their policies. For example, young drivers who have recently passed their driving tests who drive fast sports cars can find it tricky to obtain insurance. They may have to pay more than other drivers to obtain a policy because they are considered to be at a much higher risk than other drivers of being involved in crashes. Other groups include middle aged men with sports cars, and the elderly over the age of 75.

Insurance companies use probability and the statistical tests mentioned above to calculate the possible risks and benefits for individuals and groups seeking policies.

Table 1. An example two-by-two contingency table.

		Outcome	
		Risk event will occur	No risk event will occur
Prediction	Risk event will occur	True Positive	False Positive
	Risk event will not occur	False Negative	True Negative

Table 2. Some Examples of Static risk factors, Stable dynamic factors and Acute dynamic factors.

Static Factors (Hanson *et al.* 1995)	Stable Dynamic Factors (Hanson and Harris 1998)	Acute Dynamic Factors (Hanson and Harris 1998)
•Antisocial personality disorder	•Sees self as no risk	•Victim access
•Prior criminal offences	•Disengaged	•Overall cooperation
•Anger problems	•Number of positive influences	•Disengaged
•Any personality disorder	•Manipulative	•Anger
•Failure to complete treatment	•Low remorse/victim blaming	•Low remorse/victim blaming
•Sexual interest in children	•Victim access	•Substance misuse
•Negative relationship with Mother	•Antisocial lifestyle	•Negative mood
•Early onset of offending	•Number of negative influences	•Sees self as no risk
•Any deviant sexual preference	•Non-attendance/late for treatment	•General hygiene problems
•Victim was a stranger	•Sexual preoccupation	•General social problems
•Offender is <23 years old	•Rape attitudes	•Psychiatric symptoms
•Offender is single	•Substance misuse	•Manipulative
•Victim was a male child	•Hygiene problems	•Non-attendance/late for treatment
•Diverse sex crimes	•Unemployment	•Unemployment

Kettles and Woods (2009) consider that "Probability (The Editors of Chambers 2006) is the chance or the likelihood of something happening and a statistical probability (Hicks 1990, Miller 1989) is the chance or likelihood of an event occurring, often represented on a scale that ranges from 0 to 1: 0 represents no chance of the event occurring; and 1 means that it is certain to occur". When we are conveying the results of research in statistical terms we refer to probability as the *'p'* value and when giving positive results we say that in this circumstance we can reject the likelihood that research results were obtained by chance because the p value is extremely improbable i.e. when p value is less than or equal to 0.05. The smaller the p value the less likely it is that random errors could explain the results (Hicks 1990, Miller 1989, Siegel and Castellan 1988).

Frequently when the results of risk assessment research are described it is done in terms of the correlation coefficient, with researchers highlighting the associated p value as important, when in reality it is the strength of association observed in the correlation that is of particular interest. It is important here to be aware of when the sample size is large the correlation is likely to be significant but small in real terms. The following has been suggested (Cohen and Holliday 1982) as a guide to the specific levels of interest relative to the correlation:

- +0.19 and below can be considered very low
- +0.20 to +0.39 low; +0.40 to +0.69 modest
- +0.70 to +0.89 high; and +0.90 to +1.00 very high.

An **event** is any incidence or occurrence or is 'that which happens' (The Editors of Chambers 2006). So any event or 'outcome' in risk assessment terms is any occurrence of specific assessment items which can be measured in some way. For example, an assessment item might be "Physical aggression following a trigger event" or "Always unable, or refuses, to speak about personal feelings". Morgan (2004, p18) states that in the field of mental health, "event" mostly "refers to behaviours resulting in suicide, self-harm, aggression and violence, and the neglect, abuse and exploitation by self or others". As different assessment instruments use different assessment items and different forms of measurement, this means that any risk assessor needs to know about the tools and instruments of assessment that they are using at any given time and what those tools are aimed at assessing.

A helpful way to think about how events occur is similar to how testing the predictive ability of many risk assessments is worked out by researchers. This is also a useful way to see if outcomes have been successful or not. Two-by-two contingency tables are a superb way to exhibit these results (see Table 1) as it enables correct predictions and error rates to be examined. Two possibilities are likely in this scheme: either the risky event did occur or it did not. This is usually reported as one of the following:

- **true negative** (the patient was predicted to be a risk and risk event did not occur)
- **true positive** (the patient was predicted to be a risk and the risk event did occur)
- **false negative** (the patient was predicted to be not a risk and the risk event did occur)
- **false positive** (the patient was predicted to be a risk and the risk event did not occur).

Behaviour is about the thoughts, cognitions, perceptions, conduct, manners, and emotions that are associated with the behaviour under assessment. Behaviour is about the ways in which a person, in this case the patient, responds to other people and everything they experience (both internally and externally), including nurses and other professionals, other patients, the environment, their symptoms, and the various forms of treatment and intervention that they might receive whilst in either the hospital or the community.

Recurrence of the behaviour at any time and the probability of the risk of recurrence if it is a severe or dangerous behaviour are also issues to be considered.

The severity of any given behaviour is about the level of intensity during the event and can be classified as mild, moderate or severe. Risk to others will usually be termed as 'dangerousness' and this is when injury causing behaviours are present or have been known to be present previously. The negative consequences of dangerousness include serious physical and psychological harm, fear-induction, impulsive destructive and damaging actions, intimidation, feeling unsafe, in peril, at hazard, being and feeling at risk, insecure, the power to hurt, manipulative and destructive (Kemshall 2001, Woods 2001). The preferred term for dangerousness in current common usage is 'risk'.

Being and feeling safe or unsafe is a key concern for staff who conduct risk assessments and so 'safety' or the state of being safe is central to every aspect of psychiatric and mental health nursing including risk assessment and management.

Security is directly related to safety and to the many possible outcomes of risk assessment in psychiatric and mental health nursing (Collins *et al*. 2006). According to Collins (2000) security comes in two kinds

1. Physical security is about the doors, fences and locks (the objects) and the procedures and the use of the materials and items that help procedures to work such as closed circuit television (the systems) that are in position to ensure safety.
2. Relational security is associated very explicitly to risk assessment and management as it involves an in-depth knowledge of each individual patient which develops over time through the nurse-patient relationship. Relational security is only accomplished as an outcome of risk assessment and management through a reliable knowledge and understanding of the risks posed at any given time, as well as the potential risks, and how these might be minimised and the pertinent interventions that are included in the appropriate management for each patient.

The Characteristics of Risk

Risk-taking is a daily occurrence in health and social care and clinicians make decisions to take risks with patients as a matter of course. For example, in acute in-patient mental health services patients who have been placed on high level observation need at some point in their care to have a reduction in the level of observation. At that point in care it becomes a 'risk' to reduce the level of observation, in case the patient is not well enough or has been deceiving the staff, and as a consequence of the reduction the patient harms themselves or others. However, this risk is taken because the clinical staff and relevant others, such as the relatives of the patient, decide that, based on all the available evidence and the risk assessments that have been conducted, the patient is ready for the reduction in the level of observations. This has also been termed positive risk-taking which "is weighing up the potential benefits and harms of exercising one choice of action over another. This means identifying the potential risks involved, and developing plans and actions that reflect the positive potentials and stated priorities of the service user. It involves using available resources and support to achieve desired outcomes, and to minimise potential harmful outcomes. Positive risk-taking is not negligent ignorance of the potential risks. Nobody, especially users or providers of a specific service or activity, will benefit from allowing risks to play out their course through to disaster" (Morgan 2004, p18)

What should be noted here is the use of the terms 'evidence' and 'risk assessments'. Evidence is about both the objective and the subjective evidence that is available. For example, reports from other professionals based upon their health assessments, such as the dieticians and their use of assessment tools such as the Malnutrition Universal Screening Tool (MUST) (Todorovic *et al.* 2003) as well as specific mental health instruments. The term Risk assessment relates to both the possible approaches (clinical judgement, structured clinical judgement, the actuarial approach and the normative approach) (Kettles 2004, MacLean 2000) as well as the numerous and multifaceted instruments (Woods and Kettles, 2009, Kettles *et al.* 2001, 2003, MacCall 2003, MacLean 2000, Risk Management Authority 2007) that are available to attempt to quantify what the risk might be at any given time for individuals to commit some level of harm at any given time. Some of these instruments are about prediction of future behaviour and attempt to say that at any given point in the future the person will offend or re-offend. Other instruments are not designed to be predictive and are for use only as 'snapshot' in time. These tools give a quantification of the existing risk, now and cannot be used to predict future behaviour. Many of these risk assessment instruments are considered by their authors to be suitable for use in research rather than in clinical practice. However, some of these instruments have been taken up for use in clinical practice by practitioners because they need a method to be able to say to other people, such as lawyers, that they have based their decisions on some form of objective assessment. Objective means that it is not simply your own ideas that matter but that there has been a systematic way of collecting the evidence about the person's state of risk that provides a reasonable way of helping the clinician to come to a decision. This systematic method provides items (variables) that have been tested as providing relevant information and which are consistent, valid and reliable, in research terms about providing the information needed to make decisions about the level of risk a person poses at any given time.

What are the Different Types of Risk Assessment?

Variables are the units used to develop risk assessment instruments and they can be classified into the concepts of **actuarial** (or **static**) variables and **clinical** (or **dynamic**) variables.

Variables can be risk factors or personal characteristics, situations, or environmental conditions that contribute to or which predict the onset, continuity, or escalation of behaviour considered to be risky. These variables have been shown to have an empirically-based (scientifically sound) relationship with the risk in question. These are often considered in terms of type of information, and whether the information is static or dynamic in nature.

Static risk variables are considered to be historical in nature and reveal prior life experiences and previous behaviour or behaviours that are associated with a statistically increased likelihood of the risk behaviour occurring. Static risk variables are fixed or inert because they have happened and so they cannot be changed. Whatever degree of risk is implied by these static variables can only change with the introduction of dynamic risk variables. Static risk factors are variables which have been shown to have a relationship with the risk but which are not open to clinical intervention. Typical examples include age, history of violence (physical, psychological or sexual), offending behaviour and previous convictions. These variables affect the probability of a person being either at risk or a risk in the future (for example re-offending) but they cannot be changed by treatment. Static factors, according to Hanson and Bussiere (1998) include variables such as previous sexual offences, deviant sexual preference, previous failure or failures to complete treatment, any personality disorder or (multiple) pathology, anger problems and an elevated Psychopathy Check List-Revised (PCL-R) (Hare 1991) score.

Dynamic Risk Variables, on the other hand, must fulfil a number of conditions. Firstly, a dynamic risk variable must precede and be associated with risk behaviour. Secondly, it must be able to change, and thirdly, changing the variable must change or influence the risk behaviour in some way. Thus, dynamic risk variables must be capable of reducing or exacerbating the risk implied by static variables. Dynamic risk factors have been shown to have a relationship with the risk (using the previous example of re-offending) but these can change as a result of treatment. Examples include symptoms of illness, self-harming behaviours, drug or alcohol use, individual or environmental aspects, deviant sexual interest, sexual fantasy, and negative attitudes to women. Specifically in relation to sex offenders, The National Organisation for the Treatment of Abusers (2007) states that: "the identification of dynamic factors that are associated with reduced recidivism holds particular promise in effectively managing sex offenders because the strengthening of these factors can be encouraged through various supervision and treatment strategies".

Dynamic factors can be categorised into two types of factors: stable and acute factors (Hanson and Harris 1998) and these are shown in Table 1. Stable dynamic factors are characteristics that can change over time, but are still relatively lasting qualities, such as antisocial lifestyle or being manipulative or substance misuse. Hanson and Harris (1998, 2000) suggest that such stable dynamic risk factors also include seeing self as no risk (lack of insight), attitudes (including the attitude of sexual entitlement), negative social influences, being manipulative, sexual preoccupations, rape attitudes, intimacy deficits, sexual/emotional self-regulation as well as general self-regulation.

Hanson and Harris (1998) propose that acute dynamic factors can change over the short term and these variables include victim access, anger, low remorse/victim blaming, substance abuse and the sexual arousal or intoxication that may immediately precede an offence.

The Department of Health (2007, p13-14) categorise risk factors based on the work of Kraemer *et al.* (1997) in a similar but slightly differing way as they consider that *static factors* are those which are unchangeable, for instance, history of violence, offending behaviour. *Dynamic factors* are those that change over time and thus are more amenable to clinical and risk management. For example, individual or environmental aspects such as substance misuse and social networks are amenable to risk management and clinical intervention. *Stable or chronic factors* are those dynamic factors that are fairly stable and which change slowly over time. These could include the examples given for dynamic factors but, it must be remembered, are specific to the individual and so they may take time to change, if at all. Those factors that can be liable to change rapidly are known as *acute factors or triggers* and, as they do change quickly, their influence on the level of risk might be short-lived.

Woods and Kettles (2009) are of the opinion that a full and comprehensive risk assessment will bring together all the different risk assessments that the multidisciplinary team will make. These individualised assessments including those with empirically established acute dynamic risk factors, stable dynamic risk factors, static risk factors, and situational variables will be used to make decisions about care and treatment.

The Major Principles of Conducting Risk Assessment

As has been said earlier, risk assessment is based on actuarial measurement. Actuaries are people who are trained to calculate risks using statistical methods, usually for insurance companies, law firms, or bookmakers. Actuarial scales and instruments are developed and constructed by using statistical analysis of groups with known outcomes (for example, men who have been convicted of a particular violence offence, such as domestic violence, and men who apparently have not re-offended violently). This type of analysis tells us which items or variables do the best job of differentiating between those who re-offended and those who apparently have not re-offended if we use our violence offending example. Since some variables do a better job than others, these types of analyses can tell us how much each variable should be weighted, if at all. These variables are then put together to form a risk assessment scale. This scale is then tested and analysed to see how well it works at making a prediction about those who, again if we use our violence offending example, are likely to re-offend. These types of study, when built up into a body of evidence, provide support for the predictive validity of the scale. The risk assessment scale or instrument is then used on different samples to see how well it works and this establishes cross-validation. When a tool has been used on many different samples, including those that are able to provide normative scores, the scale score can then be used as an estimate of the probability that the individual will or will not have the risk within a specified time. For example, an individual male sex offender with a specific score on a particular risk assessment instrument might have a 40% probability of re-offending within five years; or a particular young woman with borderline personality disorder and is displaying certain behaviours, such as substance misusing, is more at risk from self-harm or abuse.

Actuarial scales seem to work better if variables are weighted. Item weighting views some variables or items as being of more consequence than others in predicting outcome. Item weighting is done using multiple linear regression analysis. This is a statistical method where the result is a "weighted linear prediction". Item weighting, however, is not essential in the development of risk assessment. Some (Schmidt, 1971; Dawes, 1979; Bry et al, 1982;

Kerby, 2003) argue that simple unit item weighting, where each variable is weighted equally, is just as effective. The Psychopathy Check List-Revised (PCL-R) (Hare 1991), for example, is a simple unit item weighting where all items are scored 0, 1, or 2.

Item weighting is a scientific question. In order to conduct item weighting, large samples are required to determine the item weights, and the resulting judgments must be made using empirical science. However, some risk assessment scales use "clinically derived" weightings where clinicians decided the relative importance of each item and weighted each item according to their own clinical judgment. This is not acceptable. Without ample data to intimate otherwise, items should have equal weights.

Until recently, there has been a 'clinical versus actuarial' debate, where people have argued that only actuarial scales gave an accurate risk assessment and that these should be used clinically as opposed to the clinical scales which tried to give an overall picture of an individual's situation. However, this debate has been overtaken by the introduction of structured clinical judgement which uses actuarial assessments as the basis for an complete picture of the patient enabling decision making based on both types of assessment. This is more useful and practical for clinicians, and researchers, as risk assessment is taken to more appropriate levels. For example, comparison of different actuarial assessments can be conducted in clinical practice and structured clinical judgement has enabled the development and use in clinical practice of normative scales such as the BEST-Index (Woods 2008, Ross *et al* 2007). These normative scales are for use over time rather than the traditional single 'snapshot' approach that other actuarial tools such as the HCR-20 employ.

Should the Scores of Risk Scales Ever be "Adjusted" by Clinicians?

Whether or not a clinician (or a researcher) should "adjust" the score from an actuarial scale based upon knowledge or information that the scale does not explain or does not call attention to is a matter of debate. Those recommending adjustment tend to do so because the clinician may be familiar with, possibly, critical information that could affect the risk decision-making process but which is not addressed (or not adequately addressed) by the scale in use in the clinical area. Examples of this type of information might include that the person being assessed could be very depressed due to personal circumstances or is very angry after being thrown out of the house, a partner or girl/boy friend has suddenly ended a relationship, or having a relevant other person die (or be killed). When risk assessment is conducted, these types of acute events need to be taken note of and they need to be included in the overall picture of risk when it comes to decision-making.

However, the score of any empirically-validated risk assessment scale or instrument should never be changed without re-validation of the scale. The reason is that it is very difficult, if not impossible, to provide adequate ground rules for ensuring uniform adjustment in the field or clinical area. How much a score is adjusted and in what circumstances the adjustment is made is up to the individual clinician in the field, and this introduces both error and unreliability in the use of the scale. Changing the score on any validated risk assessment scale based on "new" information is equivalent to changing the score on a standardised personality scale, such as the Minnesota Multi-phasic Personality Inventory (MMPI), after acknowledging that the client's score on the risk scale does not take into consideration the "new" information. It would plainly be extremely unethical to change scores on standardized tests. It is, in this author's view, equally unethical to alter the scores on validated risk assessment scales.

So, how do we take into account information that is obviously important but which is not scored for in a risk assessment scale? Critical, risk-relevant information should be incorporated into a comprehensive multidisciplinary assessment of risk in the way that structured clinical judgement is used. Rather than adjust the numerical score of a scale, it is only proper, and recommended, that all such information be used to "adjust" the conclusions of the inclusive risk assessment. All information is presented, along with the score that most accurately reflects the actuarial scale that has been used. The team would reach a conclusion based on the score, each team member's assessments and any additional information from whatever source, such as the police, and those conclusions might, if appropriate, state something like the following, "We note that the 'risk assessment scale' score is fairly low, however, there are some specific issues at this time that may increase this individual's risk and these include...". Actuarial factors should serve as an secure basis for more dynamic clinical risk assessment. This has been called 'third generation' research and is known as the *structured clinical judgement approach* (Doyle and Dolan 2002).

Can you Improve your Reliability when Scoring on Validated Scales?

If the items on the scale you are using are clear and the criteria for scoring the items are also clearly identified, then the most important factor in unreliability is the ambiguity of the information used to score the items. How ambiguous the information is can vary massively from person to person. There are no known infallible ways of dealing with ambiguous information.

To improve reliability, it is strongly recommended that clinicians (and researchers) use as many sources of information as possible when scoring the scale variables and items. It is recommended that the scale be scored by two independent raters (clinicians or researchers) who will then compare and discuss their scores to minimise error. Agreed scores will then be used. When the information from all accessible sources is limited, unclear, or incomplete, items should be scored "conservatively" (in the direction of lower risk), and it should be noted, that the resulting score could underestimate the risk.

Nurses and clinicians in all disciplines who are using specific scales should study the Training Manual for that particular scale and it is always essential to complete the training, and the associated training on case examples, before using the scale for real in clinical practice. The importance of appropriate and adequate training on practice case examples cannot be overstated.

So in essence, the principles are:

- Use validated scales in preference to 'homemade', cobbled together scales
- Use the validated scales as they have been developed

- Do not 'adjust' validated scales as this makes them unreliable and you cannot then trust the scores
- Only use validated scales when you have the prepared manual for those scales and preferably undertake the associated training to use the scales correctly, if such training is recommended.
- Score conservatively, if there is ambiguous information i.e. in the direction of lower risk
- Use actuarial risk assessment scales and instruments as part of the Structured Clinical Judgement Approach

Which Risk Assessments Should Be Used? Instrumentation is an issue that has developed from the idea fifty years ago that the clinician's own judgement is good enough to base decision making on to the present day where we know that decision making based on clinical judgement is wrong at least one in three times (Monahan, 1981; Steadman et al, 1993) and that assessments of dangerousness were unreliable and inaccurate (Steadman and Cocozza, 1974). So the development of more accurate and reliable assessments based on the idea of risk rather than dangerousness has happened in the last thirty years and is an ongoing phenomenon.

Instruments used to assess (and consequently manage) risk by mental health nurses should have been developed through rigorous research which will have considered the impact these assessments have on health and related behaviour/s. Poorly manufactured instruments or the development of such instruments without the appropriate strategies and resources in place must be discouraged. For example, would you drive a car that had not been tested and was not reliable? Therefore it should be just as important for risk assessments you use to be equally reliable and fit for their purpose?

As will become apparent many valid and reliable instruments already exist to assess risk, so what is the point in developing your own risk assessment when it has already been done and done to a much higher standard than you can do in a clinical area? "Re-inventing the wheel" is a terrible waste of your valuable clinical time when it is so much easier to access those that have undergone, or are currently undergoing, the rigorous process of research and development.

Reliability and Validity

The development of any assessment instrument involves two fundamental elements: reliability and validity. Kerlinger sums the issues up with a seminal quote: "If one does not know the reliability and validity of one's data little faith can be put in the results obtained and conclusions drawn from the results" (1973, p.442). Robson (1993, p.66) point out that this is about establishing 'trustworthiness' from your enquiries.

Bech (1994, p.293) outlines a model for evaluation which includes: the construct validity of a scale; the external validity; and inter-rater reliability. This model takes in to account the representativeness of the items; the extent to which items contribute towards the scale; the way in which the scale corresponds to other variables and the potential for prediction of behaviour; and the extent to which the scale communicates its meaning to the user.

Reliability

To be reliable something needs to be relied on; of sound and consistent character or quality (Oxford University Press 1995). In research the term 'reliability' is used to mean dependability, stability, consistency, predictability, accuracy (Kerlinger 1973); consistency, external and internal (Bryman and Cramer 1997, p.63); and to what extent an empirical scale consistently measures a given phenomenon (Robson 1993, p.220-4). So reliability concerns itself with how accurately and how safe it is to conclude that the measure used has accounted for the error that is inherent in any observation. Polit and Hungler (1993, p.244-8) use three means to do this:

1. **Stability** *is concerned with how suitably the instrument obtains similar results following repeated measures. It is the consistency over time (Bryman and Cramer 1997, p.63) or external reliability that is measured. The method used for examining this is test-retest reliability.*

2. **Equivalence** *is about the extent to which the instrument can determine consistently the same result for the same subject. The most common method for measurining this is inter-rater reliability. Two or, preferably, more raters assess the same subject at the same time. This is a measure of how closely raters agree in their scoring within a scale or in using the same instrument.*

3. **Internal consistency** *is when a scale is thought to measure a single underlying continuum and all its items should be strongly positively related to each other (Oppenheim 1992, p.160). In order to verify this, the scale's homogeneity can be measured using an internal consistency method. There are a few methods for doing this but the method that has come into common use is Cronbach's Alpha.*

Validity

Validity means to be sound or defensible; and well-grounded (Oxford University Press, 1995). In research usage the validity of a measure is involved with how well it measures the concept which it is supposed to be measuring. Conceptual clarity is a necessary antecedent to measurement validity, which can be accomplished through rigorous definitions which in turn enable theoretical understanding and consistency of measurement (Moody 1990, p.250-1).

The relationship between reliability and validity is reciprocal. However, simply because a measure is reliable in itself it does not necessarily follow that it is valid. An instrument can be extremely reliable at 'measuring'; but not at measuring the concept intended.

A number of established approaches to the examination of validity are available:

Face validity is the extent to which the instrument appears to measure the concept and items under examination.

Predictive validity is the strength of the relationship between the concept being measured and an outcome, for example, can measure *a* predict behaviour *b*?

Construct validity is the extent to which the instrument measures a theoretical construct, such as 'risk'.

Internal validity is the extent to which items in the measure present a matching and reasonable description of the items under study.

Criterion-related validity is the competence with which the instrument measures the underlying and related constructs.

Content validity is the expert opinion that the instrument effectively measures the what it purports to measure.

External validity is where a positive correlation exists between the measure and other known measures that purport to measure the same thing.

Predictive validity and internal consistency

Item analysis is a test of predictive validity and the internal consistency of an instrument, carried out by measuring the extent to which each item contributes to the scale as a whole (Oppenheim 1992, p.198-9). The correlation achieved by each item is a direct measure of its predictive validity as an appropriate contributor to the scale as a whole. However, it should be noted that if an item do not correlate significantly with total scores, this does not necessarily mean that the item is invalid. There are a number of reasons why this can happen:

- There may not be data to show a correlation, which may only become evident when more data has been collected and analysed.
- Raters may be inexperienced in the use of an instrument.
- For a variety of reasons, raters may not have the information necessary to conduct an effective assessment. This may mean increased variability and loss of an obvious pattern in the resulting scores.
- Raters may either not have precise operational definitions for items or they may misunderstand the given definitions or they might not use or consult the definitions during the assessment.

Instruments should be developed from rigorous research which concentrates on reliability and validity. This is not easy for any clinical researcher but it is an essential one to ensure that instruments meet standards.

Improper use of Instruments

Inappropriate use of instruments is worse than not using them at all. Incorrect interpretation and infringement of copyright are serious problems which should not occur. Improper use has further implications which can be serious as risk management decisions are taken on the results of the use of these instruments. Litigation becomes a very real possibility if the application of valid risk assessment has been wrong in any way. Abuse and misuse of screening and assessment instruments appears to take place daily in mental health practice.

Some of this can be unwittingly done and at other times seems to be knowingly done. Either way, this can have serious consequences.

Ignoring Copyright

Many risk assessment instruments are subject to copyright for a number of reasons. Primarily, ownership can be clearly established and will usually expect permission for use to be requested. This permission may be required because the owner wants users to have specific training to use it or they may wish to charge you to use the instrument they have invested so much effort in to developing. Some instruments are not registered for copyright but are published as part of an article, a book chapter, or on the internet. In these cases the publisher will have to be asked in order to obtain permission to reproduce the instrument. Where an instrument is published on the internet, the same applies about asking permission to use the instrument from the author. Consequently, it is important that mental health nurses explore any copyright issues for the instruments they intend to use before including them in their practice. Failure to follow copyright procedure can mean mental health nurses leave themselves open to legal penalties.

"Stealing" the Instrument

Using an instrument as if it was your own, or including it in another instrument without permission from the copyright holder or author, or even without reference to the author, is "theft" at worst or plagiarism at best. The message here is that if you want to include an instrument in assessment documentation you need to gain permission to do this. Do not alter the instrument or the format in any way, unless permission is given, and always cite that permission was given, by whom and when. If an instrument's copyright not restricted, or for any reason you cannot make contact with the copyright holder or author, then it may still be possible for you to include it in your documentation (if it is not altered) but you need to check with your legal department at work first or you can check with the Copyright Licensing Agency http://www.cla.co.uk/ in the United Kingdom (UK).

Altering the Scores on Instruments

This was discussed earlier and the reader is directed back to the section to clarify these issues.

Adapting the Content of Instruments

An important issue is when someone decides to adapt an instrument for use locally. They change words or ideas within the instrument and this affects its reliability and validity. There have been cases where valid and reliable assessment instruments have been adapted, then adapted again, then they have been published as another instrument. This has then involved lengthy legal battles to establish their real authorship. As has been seen instruments develop through rigorous data collection and analysis. Risk assessment items go through fastidious scrutiny to be included. Items can be removed from time to time in revised versions of any instrument but this is usually following rigorous statistical analysis of the items and their relationship to the outcome measures. Thus, it is important that mental health nurses do not remove or add items because they think they should without consulting the instrument author(s) BEFORE they make any changes.

Training

Most valid, researched instruments require the user to have specific training, qualifications or background information to enable them to use them. Many have manuals to help with the scoring and interpretation of the results to enable reliable scoring to be obtained. It is important for mental health nurses to be cognisant of the requirements and only to use instruments with the proper skills, knowledge and training. Failure to do this can severely affect the reliability and validity of the results and the resultant decision making.

Using Instruments for Purposes Other Than The Purposes They Were Designed For

Development involves significant work and validation, usually involving years of work by the developers. Numerous assessment instruments are designed for use with specific populations and if they are used in other populations their reliability and validity has been altered and so the results of their use is questionable to say the least.

Risk assessment instruments have been developed in an effort to minimise error, they are not perfect, but then neither are the humans who use them. However, they are the best we currently have and in essence, the principles of use are:

- Always use valid and reliable instruments, where possible
- Do not change or alter the use of the instrument in any way
- Seek appropriate permission to use the instrument
- If you must change or alter the instrument, consult the authors FIRST
- Keep the instrument within the population it was designed for
- Take any training that is recommended for the instrument you intend to use.

Which Instruments are Available?

There are many available instruments that the mental health nurse can use to conduct risk assessments. A sample of instruments follow that are only intended to draw attention to some of those that are available for mental health nurses to use in their clinical practice. It is up to the individual mental health nurse practitioner to decide if and how any assessment meets their needs and whether or not they have the relevant training (and experience) to use them appropriately. None of the instruments that follow are explicitly suggested for use but are merely examples of the many that exist.

Box 1: Short Term Assessment of Risk and Treatability [START]
(Webster *et al.* 2004).

Training

A structured education/training program is supported by the authors for all staff using START. A trainers' manual is also available (see Desmarais *et al*. 2006 reference).

Availability and access

START is available to buy from http://www.bcmhas.ca/Research/Research_START.htm

Email: *start@forensic.bc.ca*

References:

Desmarais, S.L., Webster, C.D., Martin, M.L., Dassinger, C., Brink, J. &Nicholls, T.L. (2006). *Manual for the Short Term Assessment of Risk and Treatability (START): Instructors' Guide and Workbook* (Version 2). St. Joseph's Healthcare, Hamilton, Ontario, Canada, and Forensic Psychiatric Services Commission, Port Coquitlam, British Columbia, Canada.

Webster, C.D., Nicholls, T.L., Martin, M.L., Desmarais, S.L. & Brink, J. (2006). Short-Term Assessment of Risk and Treatability (START): The Case for a New Structured Professional Judgement Scheme. *Behavioral Sciences and the Law*, 24, 747-766.

Nicholls, T.L., Brink, J., Desmarais, S.L., Webster, C.D. & Martin, M.L. (2006). The Short-Term Assessment of Risk and Treatability (START): A Prospective Validation Study in a Forensic Psychiatric Sample. *Assessment*, 13(3), 313-327.

General Risk Assessment

There are many instruments that have been developed to aid in the assessment of risk in those individuals with general mental health problems and those with multiple mental health problems, such as: the Brief Psychiatric Rating Scale [BPRS] (Overall and Gorham 1962); the Symptom Checklist-90-Revised [SCL-90–R] (Derogatis 1992); and the collection of scales available to measure mental health symptoms such as hallucinations, delusions, fear and anxiety. This group also includes those assessments that concentrate on more specific and multiple risks. For example: the Short Term Assessment of Risk and Treatability [START] (Webster *et al.* 2004); and the Behavioural Status Index [BEST-Index] (Reed and Woods 2000).

START (Webster *et al.* 2004) has 20-items based on the following seven risk domains: violence to others, suicide, self-harm, self-neglect, unauthorized absence, substance use, and victimization. It also enables the assessor to include and record case-specific dynamic risk factors. A three point scale (not present, possibly present, present) is used, and key items are highlighted relative to the 20 items and case specific factors.

START is for use by all disciplines and items are assessed using the descriptions in the published manual. START can be used with adults with mental health, personality and substance misuse related disorders, in both inpatient and community psychiatric settings, as well as in forensic, and correctional populations. Research surrounding START is ongoing but preliminary studies indicate respectable psychometric properties. There is extensive interest in the instrument and Box 1 contains details of training requirements, access details and references.

The Behavioural Status Index (BEST-Index) (Reed and Woods, 2000) evaluates life skills, social risk and related daily behaviours. The BEST-Index consists of six subscales: social risk, insight, communication and social skills, work and recreational activities, self and family care, and empathy. These subscales identify essential components of human social behaviour. The social risk sub-scale contains twenty items measuring constructs commonly associated with risk: such as, overt and covert violence to the more generally disruptive behaviours. The insight sub-scale also consists of twenty items and examines an individual's cognitive constructs of reality. The communication and social skills sub-scales each have thirty items. Social skills or adaptive social behaviours are principally examined in these subscales. The work and recreational activities sub-scale consists of twenty items. In this scale, remunerated work is not necessarily an element and the section is concerned with constructive activities individuals can associate with and may participate in. The self and family care sub-scale has thirty items and measures socially important areas and daily functioning, such as, aspects of self-care, cooking skills, care for other family members and family relationships. The empathy sub-scale consists of thirty items and is intended to assess the ability of patients to empathise with others, especially with victims.

All items in the BEST-Index are scored using a stepwise approach from 1 (worst case) through 5 (best case). Functioning is considered within a normative, rather than a sociopathic frame of reference. In scoring the assessment a higher score indicates a more socially adaptive performance that would be viewed as "socially acceptable" by others in the patient's family and social and cultural networks. Lower scores are indicative of poorer functioning or problems and these should be the main concern. There is extensive interest in the instrument. Box 2 contains details of the BEST-Index training requirements, availability and references.

Box 2: Behavioural Status Index [BEST-Index] (Reed and Woods 2000).

Training

An education/ training program has been developed by the authors for those wishing to use it.

Availability

The BEST-Index is available from the authors.

Email: Dr Val Reed vreed52@aol.com or Dr Phil Woods phil.woods@usask.ca

References:

Woods, P., Reed, V. & Robinson, D. (1999) The behavioral Status Index: Therapeutic assessment of risk, insight and social skills. Journal of Psychiatric and Mental Health Nursing, 6(2), 79-90.

Woods, P., Reed, V. & Collins, M. (2005). The Behavioural Status Index: Testing a social risk assessment model in a high security forensic setting. Journal of Forensic Nursing, 1(1), 9-19.

Ross, T., Woods, P., Reed, V., Sookoo, S., Dean, A., Kettles, A.M., Almvik, R., ter Horst, P., Brown, I., Collins, M., Walker, H. & Pfäfflin, F. (2007). Selecting and Monitoring Living Skills in Forensic Mental Health Care: Cross-Border Validation of the BEST-Index. International Journal of Mental Health, 36(4), 3-17.

Violence Risk and Risk to Others

Many instruments have been developed to assess the risk of violence and the risk to others, with many focussing on sexual offending and violence. Some examples of violence to others assessments include:
- The Historical Clinical Risk-20 [HCR-20] (Webster *et al*. 1997)
- The Violence Risk Appraisal Guide [VRAG] (Quinsey *et al*. 1998)
- The Violence Risk Scale [VRS] (Wong and Gordon 2000)
- The Brøset Violence Checklist [BVC] (Almvik and Woods 1998).

For sexual offence risk examples include:
- The Sex Offender Risk Appraisal Guide [SORAG] (Quinsey *et al*. 1998)
- The Rapid Risk Assessment for Sexual Violence [RRASOR] (Hanson 1997)
- The Static-99 (Hanson and Thornton, 1999)

- The Sexual Violence Risk-20 [SVR-20] (Boer *et al.* 1998)
- The Risk Matrix 2000 [RM2000] (Hanson and Thornton 2000)
- The Sex Offender Need Assessment Rating [SONAR] (Hanson and Harris 2000)
- The Violence Risk Scale: Sexual Offenders [VRS:SO] (Wong *et al.* 2003).

Some instruments have developed around domestic abuse and assault on spouses. Examples include

- The Spousal Assault Risk Assessment Guide [SARA] (Kropp *et al.* 1999)
- The Brief Spousal Assault Form for the Evaluation of Risk [B-SAFER] (Kropp and Hart 2004).

Assessment of anger has also developed and the preeminent assessment is probably the State-Trait Anger Expression Inventory-2 [STAXI-2] (Spielberger 1999). The Psychopathy Checklist-Revised [PCL-R], Hare 1991, 2003 is an instrument that was not developed for risk assessment but has served well in the prediction of violence.

Some assessments tools have been developed to measure aggression after incidents have occurred:

- The Overt Aggression Scale [OAS] (Yudofsky *et al.* 1986)
- The Modified Overt Aggression Scale [MOAS] (Kay *et al.* 1988)
- Staff Observation Aggression Scale-Revised [SOAS-R] (Nijman *et al.* 1999a, 1999b)
- Report Form for Aggressive Episodes [REFA] (Bjørkly 1996)
- Rating Scale for Aggression in the Elderly [RAGE] (Patel and Hope 1992)
- Brief Agitation Rating Scale [BARS] (Finkel *et al.* 1993)
- Cohen-Mansfield Agitation Inventory [CMAI] (Cohen-Mansfield 1986)
- The Attempted and Actual Assault Scale [ATTACKS] (Bowers *et al.* 2007).

The SOAS-R (Nijman *et al.* 1999a, 1999b) is widely used in research and clinical practice as an incident reporting and analysis measure. The SOAS-R through many studies has been reported to have adequate psychometric properties and to be clinically useful. Box 4.7 reports details of the SOAS-R items, training requirements, availability and access details and some related references.

Box 3: Historical Clinical Risk – 20 [HCR-20] (Webster *et al.* 1997)

Training

The HCR-20 website states a degree, certificate, or license to practice in a health care profession (this includes nursing) plus appropriate training and experience in the ethical administration, scoring, and interpretation of clinical behavioral assessment instruments is required. It should also be borne in mind that full completion of the assessment requires a PCL-R rating to be taken which need specific in-depth education. Nurses that do use the HCR-20 often omit the rating for psychopathy.

Availability

The HCR-20 is available for purchase from
http://www3.parinc.com/products/product.aspx?Productid=HCR-20

Related References *(note this is merely a sample of some of those available that the chapter authors have found useful. A literature search will result in many more)*:

Belfrage, H. (1998). Implementing the HCR-20 scheme for risk assessment in a forensic psychiatric hospital: Integrating research and clinical practice. *Journal of Forensic Psychiatry*, 9, 328-338.

Belfrage, H., Fransson, R. & Strand, S. (2000). Prediction of violence using the HCR-20: a prospective study in two maximum-security correctional institutions. *Journal of Forensic Psychiatry*, 11, 167-175.

Dolan, M. & Doyle, M. (2000). Violence Risk Prediction. *British Journal of Psychiatry*, 177, 303-311.

Dolan, M. & Khawaja, A. (2004). The HCR-20 and post-discharge outcome in male patients discharged from medium security in the UK. *Aggressive Behaviour*, 30, 469-483.

Watt, W., Topping-Morris, B., Doyle, M. & Mason, T. (2003). Pre-admission nursing assessments in a Welsh medium secure unit (1991-2000): Part 2 comparison of traditional nursing assessment with the HCR-20 risk assessment tool. *International Journal of Nursing Studies*, 40, 657-662.

The HCR-20 (Webster *et al.* 1997) is one of the most widely known and widely used assessments of potential violent behaviour. It has been in the spotlight of extensive research and its psychometric properties are known to be good. The HCR-20 has 20 items divided into 3 groups: historical (10 items), clinical (5 items) and risk management (5 items). HCR-20 items are assessed on a three point scale (absent, possibly present, definitely present). The historical items are the basis for the risk assessment and repeated measures are taken on the other items over set periods of time. There is also an ultimate level of risk decision that is made, either low, moderate or high, and this is based on careful consideration of the ratings given over all the items. The HCR-20 is intended for use by all disciplines to assess both criminal and psychiatric populations. The items are assessed according to in-depth descriptions provided in the published manual. Training requirements, availability details and some references are given in Box 3.

The BVC (Almvik and Woods 1998) is a short-term violence prediction instrument and the six behaviours are scored for their presence (1) or absence (0). For well-known patients an increase in the behaviour described is scored as 1, whereas the habitual behaviour while being non-violent is scored as 0. Clear definitions of behaviours are provided by the authors. Scoring is by summing the scores for each of the behaviours. The risk is identified by the authors as: 0 = the risk of violence is small; 1-2 = the risk of violence is moderate (preventive measures should be taken); and 2 or above the risk of violence is very high (preventive measures should be taken and plans should be developed to manage the potential violence). Research indicates that the BVC has satisfactory psychometric properties and discriminates the violent from not violent in a 24-hour period. Box 4 contains details of the training requirements, availability and some references.

Risk to self

A number of assessment instruments have been developed for suicide, self-harm and self-neglect. For example in relation to suicide:

- The Beck Hopelessness Scale [BHS] (Beck *et* al. 1974a)
- The Scale for Suicide Ideation [SSI] (Beck and Steer 1991)
- The Suicide Intent Scales [SIS] (Beck *et al*. 1974b)
- The revised SIS (Pierce 1977, 1981)
- SAD PERSONS (Patterson *et al*. 1983)
- The Nurses' Global Assessment of Suicide Risk [NGASR] (Cutliffe and Barker 2004).

A few self-injury scales exist see for example, the self-report Self-Injury Motivation Scale [SIMS] (Osuch *et al*. 1999) and the self report Self-Injury Questionnaire [SIQ] (Alexander 1999). Sub-scales from other instruments, such as the Behavioural Status Index [BEST-Index] (Reed and Woods 2000) can help to assess for this risk.

As has been discussed, a number of assessment instruments are readily available for mental health nurses to use in practice and some of these have been briefly discussed here. However, no specific recommendations are given here as to whether or not mental health nurses should be using these in their practice. The instruments discussed have been found to be useful for clinical risk decision making but practitioners in every service need to search for the other available instruments that are specific to the population that they serve. So the principles for use are:

- Practitioners need to access appropriate instruments themselves.
- Mental health nurses need to evaluate which instruments meet their own clinical needs.

- Whatever instruments mental health nurses do use in their practice, it is essential to ensure they have permission to use the instruments (unchanged) and that they have the skills, competence, knowledge, education and ability to use them.

Box 4: Broset Violence Checklist [BVC] (Almvik and Woods 1998)

Training

No specific training is required but some training materials are available from the authors if required.

Availability

The BVC is available from the authors. Email: Dr Roger Almvik roger.almvik@ntnu.no or Dr Phil Woods phil.woods@usask.ca Although the BVC is copyrighted, permission is always provided for use providing the original source is cited. An electronic version is also available for purchase from http://www.igcn.nl/?p=63&PHPSESSID=3ca87ea52b2e8efe161bcff230a1856f

Related References:

Abderhalden, C., Needham, I., Miserez, B., Almvik, R., Dassen, T., Haug, H.J. & Fischer, J.E. (2004). Predicting inpatient violence in acute psychiatric wards using the Brøset-Violence-Checklist: a multicentre prospective cohort study. *Journal of Psychiatric and Mental Health Nursing,* 11(4), 422-427.

Almvik, R., Woods, P. & Rasmussen, K. (2000). The Brøset Violence Checklist (BVC): Sensitivity, specificity and inter-rater reliability. *Journal of Interpersonal Violence,* 15(12), 1284-1296.

Almvik, R., Woods, P. & Rasmussen, K. (2007). Assessing Risk for Imminent Violence in the Elderly: The Broset Violence Checklist. *International Journal of Geriatric Psychiatry, 22*(9), 862-867.

Björkdahl, A., Olsson, D. & Palmstierna, T. (2006). Nurses' short-term prediction of violence in acute psychiatric intensive care. *Acta Psychiatrica Scandinavica,* 113(3), 224-229.

Woods, P., Ashley, C., Kayto, D. & Heusdens, C. (2008). Piloting Violence and Incident Reporting Measures on one Acute Mental Health Inpatient Unit. *Issues in Mental Health Nursing,* 29(5), 455-469.

Risk Management

Nursing management of clinical risk is a process not a one-off occurrence. The process begins with patient contact with services, whether that is in the community or in hospital. Then the need for assessment is identified and instituted through screening or assessment procedures. The accumulation of information is essential to the process, through all means possible and mental health nurses employ a number of means to elicit the information that is required:

- Interview at the time of admission
- Interviews with relevant others

- Direct observation of the patient
- Available records from all possible sources, e.g. General practitioner (GP), police, social work
- Through therapeutic engagement with the patient and their families or relevant others
- Multidisciplinary Team (MDT) assessment
- Liaison with other agencies e.g. voluntary services
- Use of validated tests and scales

Use of a framework to ensure effective delivery of care is also essential, such as the structured clinical judgement approach. Any approach or framework needs to be organised around ways of working, ideas, policies and literature that are understood by everyone using them. Such frameworks need to be systematic in nature and rooted in both evidence and experience, as well as sensitive to the dynamic nature of risk. Monitoring, evaluation and regular review based in the recovery approach is essential and this part of the process cannot be minimised. Unfortunately, the evidence to date (Kettles, Robinson and Moody, 2003; McCall, 2003; Kettles et al, 2004; Kettles and Paterson, 2007; Gass et al, 2009) is that systematic and valid methods and frameworks of risk assessment are not in general use. Not using systematic and valid instruments and methods means that the patient is not receiving the best possible care and this can be said to be unethical and negligent practice.

Conclusion

'Risk is a risky business' (Prins, 2002) is a very well known saying and risk is known to be unavoidable in mental health services. However, it is not totally unpredictable anymore. The tools and instruments discussed, briefly, here show that although we cannot always be one hundred percent correct, we can now be much more prepared to identify and to deal therapeutically with those individuals who are 'at risk'. To be this prepared, we need to be using the types of instruments that are available and to move into the 21st century in risk assessment and management terms.

Risk is not just a risky business, it is a risky people business and we need to do the best we can with the best available tools to care appropriately for our patients.

References

Almvik, R. & Woods, P. (1998). The Brøset Violence Checklist (BVC) and the prediction of inpatient violence: some preliminary results. *Psychiatric Care., 5(6)*, 208-211.

Bech, P. (1994). Measurement by observations of aggressive behaviour and activities in clinical situations. *Criminal Behaviour and Mental Health., 4*, 290-302.

Beck, A. T. & Steer, R. A. (1991).*Manual for the Beck Scale for Suicide Ideation.* Psychological Corporation, San Antonio, Texas.

Beck, A. T., Weissman, A., Lester, D. & Trexler, L. (1974a). The measurement of pessimism: The hopelessness scale. *Journal of Clinical Psychology.*, *42*, 861-865.

Beck, A. T., Schuyler, D. & Herman, J. (1974b). Development of Suicidal Intent Scales. In: *The Prediction of Suicide* (Beck, A. T., Resnick, H. & Lettieri, D., (Eds.), Charles Press, Bowie, MD.

Bjørkly, S. (1996). Report form for aggressive episodes: preliminary report. *Percept Mot Skills.*, *83(3 Pt 2)*, 1139-1152.

Boer, D., Hart, S., Kropp, P. & Webster, C. (1998). *Manual for the Sexual Violence Risk-20: Professional Guidelines for Assessing Risk of Sexual Violence.* Psychological Assessment Resources, Lutz Florida.

Bowers, L., Nijman, H. & Palmstierna, T. (2007). The attempted and actual assault scale (attacks). *International Journal of Methods Psychiatric Research.*, *16(3)*, 171-176.

Bry, Brenna, H., McKeon, P. & Pandina, R. J. (1982). Extent of drug use as a function of number of risk factors. *Journal of Abnormal Psychology.*, volume *9*, pages 273-279.

Bryman, A. & Cramer, D. (1997). Quantitative data analysis with SPSS for Windows: a guide for social scientists. Routledge, London.

Cohen, L. & Holliday, M. (1982). Statistics for Social Scientists: an introductory text with computer programs in basic. Harper and Row, London.

Cohen-Mansfield, J. (1986). Agitated behaviors in the elderly. II. Preliminary results in the cognitively deteriorated. *Journal of the American Geriatrics Society.*, *34(10)*, 722-727.

Collins, M. (2000). The practitioner new to the role of forensic psychiatric nurse in the UK. In: *Forensic Nursing and Multidisciplinary Care of the mentally Disordered Offender* (Robinson, D. K. & Kettles, A. M., eds), 39-50. Jessica Kingsley Publishers, London.

Collins, M., Davies, S. & Ashwell, C. (2006). The assessment of security need. In: *Forensic Mental Health Nursing: Interventions with people with 'personality disorder'* (The National Forensic Nurses' Research and Development Group., eds). Quay Books, MA Healthcare, London.

Cutliffe, J. R. & Barker, P. (2004). The Nurses' Global Assessment of Suicide Risk (NGASR): developing a tool for clinical practice. *Journal of Psychiatric and Mental Health Nursing.*, *11(4)*, 393-400.

Dawes, Robyn, M. (1979). The robust beauty of improper linear models in decision making. *American Psychologist.*, volume *34*, pages 571-582.

Department of Health (2001) Department of Health. (2001). *Mental Health Policy Implementation Guide.* Department of Health, London.

Department of Health. (2006). *From values to action: The Chief Nursing Officer's review of mental health nursing.* Department of Health, London.

Department of Health. (2007). *Best Practice in Managing Risk: Principles and Evidence for Best Practice in the Assessment and Management of Risk to Self and Others in Mental Health Services.* Department of Health, London.

Derogatis, L. R. (1992). *SCL-90–R: Administration, scoring and procedures manual II for the revised version and other instruments of the Psychopathology Rating Scale Series.* Clinical Psychometric Research, Townson, MD.

Doyle and Duffy, Doyle, M. & Duffy, D. (2006) Assessing and managing risk to self and others. In: *Forensic Mental Health Nursing: Interventions with people with 'personality* disorder' (The National Forensic Nurses' Research and Development Group., eds), 135-150. Quay Books, MA Healthcare, London.

Doyle, M. (2000). Risk Assessment and Management. In: *Forensic Mental Health Nursing: Current Approaches* (Chaloner, C. & Coffey, M., eds), 140-170. Blackwell Science, Oxford.

Doyle, M. & Dolan, M. (2002). Violence risk assessment: combining actuarial and clinical information to structure clinical judgments for the formulation and management of risk. *Journal of Psychiatric and Mental Health Nursing., 9,* 649-657.

The Editors of Chambers. (2006). *The Chambers Dictionary,* 10th edn. Chambers Harrap, London.

Finkel, S. I., Lyons, J. S. & Anderson, R. L. (1993). A brief agitation rating scale (BARS) for nursing home elderly. *Journal of the American Geriatrics Society., 41(1),* 50-52.

Gass, J., Kettles, A. M., Addo, M. A., McKie, A. & Gibb, J. (2009) Observation and Engagement: Clinical decision-making. Journal of Psychiatric and Mental Health Nursing (submitted February).

Gifford, S. M. (1986). The meaning of breast lumps: a case study of the ambiguities of risk. In 'Anthropology and Epidemiology: interdisciplinary Approaches to the Study of Health and Disease' (Eds: In C., Janes, R. Stall, & S. M. Gifford,) 213-246. Kluwer Academic press, Boston MA.

Hanson, R. K. (1997). *The development of a brief actuarial risk scale for sexual offense recidivism.* (User Report 97-04). Department of the Solicitor General of Canada, Ottawa, Canada.

Hanson, R. K. & Bussiere, M. T. (1998). Predicting Relapse: A Meta-Analysis of Sexual Offender Recidivism. *Journal of Consulting and Clinical Psychology,* 66(2), 348-362.

Hanson, R. K. & Harris, A. (1998). *Dynamic Predictors of Sexual Recidivism.* Corrections Research Ottawa, Department of the Solicitor General, Canada. [Online]. Available from: www.sgc.gc.ca/epub/corr/el99801b/el99801b.htm (Accessed 18th October, 2007).

Hanson, R. K. & Harris, A. (2000). Where should we intervene? Dynamic predictors of sexual offence recidivism. *Criminal justice and Behavior* S. M., *27(1),* 6-35.

Hanson, R. K. & Thornton, D. (1999). *Static-99: Improving actuarial risk assessments for sex offenders.* User Report 99-02. Department of the Solicitor General of Canada, Ottawa, Canada.

Hanson, R. & Thornton, D. (2000). Improving Risk Assessments for Sex Offenders: A Comparison of Three Actuarial Scales. *Law & Human Behaviour., 24(1),* 119-136.

Hare, R. D. (1991). *The Hare Psychopathy Checklist-Revised.*: Multi-Health Systems, Toronto, Ontario, Canada.

Hayes, M. V. (1992). On the epistemology of risk: Language, logic and social science. *Social Sciences & Medicine, 35(4),* 401-407.

Hicks, C. (1990). *Research and Statistics: A practical introduction for nurses.* Prentice-Hall, Hemel Hempstead.

Jacobs, L. (2000). An analysis of the concept of risk. Cancer Nursing 23, 12-19.

Kay, S.R., Wolkenfeld, F. & Murrill, L.M. (1988). Profiles of aggression among psychiatric patients. II. Covariates and predictors. *Journal of Nervous and Mental Disease, 176(9),* 547-557.

Kerby, Dave S. (2003). CART analysis with unit-weighted regression to predict suicidal ideation from Big Five traits. *Personality and Individual Differences*, volume 35, pages 249-261.

Kemshall, H. (2001). *Risk Assessment and Management of Known Sexual and Violent Offenders: a review of current issues.* RDSD Police Research Series Paper 140. Home Office, London.

Kerlinger, F. N. (1973). *Foundations of Behavioral Research*, 2nd edn. Holt Rinehart and Winston, New York.

Kettles, A. M., Robinson, D. K. & Moody, E. (2001). Brief Report: a review of clinical risk and related assessments in forensic psychiatric units. *Journal of Psychiatric and Mental Health Nursing*, 8, 281-283.

Kettles, A. M., Robinson, D. K. & Moody, E. (2003). A review of clinical risk and related assessments in forensic psychiatric units. *British Journal of Forensic practice*, 5, 3-12.

Kettles, A. M., Moir, E., Woods, P., Porter, S. & Sutherland, E. (2004). Is there a relationship between risk assessment and observation level? *Journal of Psychiatric and Mental Health Nursing*, 11, 156-164

Kettles, A. & Paterson, K. (2007). Flexible observation: guidelines versus reality. *Journal of Psychiatric and Mental Health Nursing.*, 14(4), 373-381.

Kettles and Woods (2009). Risk Assessment and Management in Mental Health Nursing. Blackwell/Wiley.

Kraemer, H., Kazdin, A., Offord, D., Kessler, R., Jensen, P. & Kupfer, D. (1997). Coming to terms with the terms of risk. *Archives of General Psychiatry.*, 54(4), 337-343.

Kropp, P. & Hart, D. (2004). *The Development of the Brief Spousal Assault Form for the Evaluation of Risk (B-SAFER): A Tool for Criminal Justice Professionals.* Department of Justice Canada, Research and Statistics Division, Ottawa, Canada.

Kropp, P. R., Hart, S. D., Webster, C. D. & Eaves, D. (1999). *Manual for the Spousal Assault Risk Assessment Guide*, 3rd edn. Multi-Health Systems, Toronto, Canada.

Lewis, A. H. O. & Webster, C. D. (2004). General instruments for risk assessment. *Current Opinions in Psychiatry.*, 17, 401-405

MacCall, C. (2003). A Review of Approaches to Forensic Risk Assessment in Australia and New Zealand. *Psychiatry, Psychology and Law.*, 10, 221-226.

McClelland, N. (1995). The assessment of dangerousness: a procedure for predicting potentially dangerous behaviour, *Psychiatric Care.*, 2, 17-19.

Mason, T. (1998) Models of risk assessment in mental health practice: a critical examination. *Mental Health Care.*, 1, 405-407.

Miller, S. (1989). *Experimental Design and Statistics*, 2nd edn. Routledge, London.

Monahan, J. (1981). Predicting violent behaviour. Sage Library of Social Research, Beverly Hills.

Moody, L. E. (1990). *Advancing Nursing Science Through Research*, Vol 1. Sage, London.

Morgan, S. (2004). 'Positive risk-taking: an idea whose time has come'. *Health Care Risk Report.*, October, 18-19.

The National Organisation for the Treatment of Abusers. (2007). *Frequently Asked Questions - Section C. Risk Assessment.* [Online]. Available from: http://www.nota.co.uk/index. php?id=faqrisk_c (Accessed 21st February 2008)

Nijman, H. L. I., Muris, P., Merckelbach, H. L. G. J., Palmstierna, T., Wistedt, B., Vos, A. M., van Rixtel, A. & Allertz, W. (1999a). The Staff Observation Aggression Scale-Revised SOAS-R. *Aggressive Behavior., 25(3)*, 197-209.

Oppenheim, A. N. (1992). *Questionnaire Design, Interviewing and Attitude Measurement.* Pinter Publishers, London.

Osuch, E. A., Noll, J. G. & Putnam, F. W. (1999). The motivations for self-injury in psychiatric inpatients. *Psychiatry., 62*, 334-346.

Overall, J. E. & Gorham, D. R. (1962). The Brief Psychiatric Rating Scale. *Psychological Reports., 10*, 799-812.

Oxford University Press. (1995). *The Oxford Dictionary of Current English.* Oxford University Press, Oxford.

Patel, V. & Hope, R. A. (1992). A rating scale for aggressive behaviour in the elderly: the RAGE. *Psychological Medicine., 22(1)*, 211-221.

Patterson, W., Dohn, H., Bird, J. & Patterson, G. (1983). Evaluation of suicidal patients: The SAD PERSONS Scale. *Psychsomatics, 24*, 343-349.

Pierce, D. W. (1977). Suicidal intent in self-injury. *British Journal of Psychiatry., 130*, 377-385.

Polit, D. F. & Hungler, B. P. (1993). *Essentials of nursing research: methods, appraisal, and utilization*, 3rd edn. Lippincott, Philadelphia.

Prins, H. (2002). Risk assessment: still a risky business. *The British Journal of Forensic Practice., 4(1)*, 3-8.

Quinsey, V. L., Harris, G. T., Rice, M. E. & Cormier, C. A. (1998). *Violent offenders: appraising and managing risk.* American Psychological Association, Washington, DC.

Reed, V. & Woods, P. (2000). *The Behavioral Status Index: A life skills assessment for selecting and monitoring therapy in mental health care.* Psychometric Press, Sheffield, United Kingdom.

Risk Management Authority. (2007). *Risk Assessment Tools Evaluation Directory (RATED Version 2).* Risk Management Authority, Paisley, Scotland. [Online]. Available from: http://www.rmascotland.gov.uk/rmapublications.aspx (Accessed 17th October, 2007).

Robson, C. (1993). Real world research: a resource for social scientists and practitioners-researchers. Blackwell, Oxford.

Rose, N. (1998). Living dangerously: risk thinking and risk management in mental health care. *Mental Health Care., 1*, 263-266.

Ross, T., Woods, P., Reed, V., Sookoo, A., Dean, A., Kettles, A. M., Almvik, R., ter Horst, P., Brown, I., Collins, M., Walker, H. & Pfäfflin, F. (2007). Selecting and Monitoring Living Skills in Forensic Mental Health Care: Cross-Border Validation of the BEST-Index. *International Journal of Mental Health., 36(4)*, 3-17.

Schmidt, Frank L. (1971). The relative efficiency of regression and simple unit predictor weights in applied differential psychology. *Educational and Psychological Measurement*, volume 31, pages 699-714.

Scottish Executive. (2006). *Rights, Relationships and Recovery: The Report of the National Review of Mental Health Nursing in Scotland.* Scottish Executive, Edinburgh.

Siegel, S. & Castellan, N. J. (1988). *Nonparametric Statistics for the Behavioural Sciences*, 2nd edn. McGraw-Hill, New York.

Skolbekken, J. A. (1995). The risk epidemic in medical journals. *Social Science and Medicine.*, *40(3)*, 291-305.

Spielberger, C. D. (1999). *State-Trait Anger Expression Inventory – 2 (STAXI-2).* Psychological Assessment Resources Incorporated, Odessa, Florida, USA.

Steadman, H. J. & Cocozza, J. (1974) Careers of the Criminally Insane: Excessive social control of deviance. Health, Lexington, DC.

Steadman, H. J., Monahan, J., Cark Robbins, P., et al (1993) From dangerousness to risk assessment: Implications for appropriate research strategies. In: Mental Disorder and Crime (Ed. Hodgins, S.) 39-62, Sage, Newbury Park CA.

Todorovic, V., Russell, C., Stratton, R., Ward, J. & Elia, M. (2003). *The 'MUST' Explanatory Booklet: A Guide to the 'Malnutrition Universal Screening Tool' (MUST) for Adults.* Malnutrition Advisory Group (MAG) A Standing Committee of the British Association for Parenteral and Enteral Nutrition (BAPEN), Redditch, Worcestershire.

Webster, C. D., Douglas, K. S., Eaves, D. & Hart, S. D. (1997). *HCR- 20: Assessing risk for violence. Version 2.* Mental Health, Law, & Policy Institute, Simon Fraser University, Burnaby, Canada.

Woods, P. (1996). How nurses make assessments of patient dangerousness. *Mental Health Nursing.*, *16(4)*, 20-22

Woods, P. (2001). Risk assessment and management. In: *Forensic Mental Health Care: Issues in practice* (C. Dale, T. Thompson, & P. Woods Eds.), 85-98. Baillière Tindall/Royal College of Nursing, Edinburgh.

Woods, P. (2008). The forensic mental health nurse's role in risk assessment, measurement and management. In: *Forensic Nursing: Roles, Capabilities and Competencies* (National Forensic Nurses' Research & Development Group – A. Kettles, P. Woods, & R. Byrt Eds.), chapter 10. Quay Books, London.

Wong, S. C. P. & Gordon, A. E. (2000). *Violence Risk Scale.* Research Unit, Regional Psychiatric Centre, Saskatoon, Saskatchewan, Canada.

Yudofsky, S. C., Silver, J. M., Jackson, W., Endicott, J. & Williams, D. (1986). The Overt Aggression Scale for the objective rating of verbal and physical aggression. *American Journal of Psychiatry.*, *143*, 35-39.

In: Nursing Issues: Psychiatric Nursing, Geriatric Nursing…   ISBN: 978-1-60741-598-5
Editors: C. D. McLaughlin et al., pp. 155-173   © 2010 Nova Science Publishers, Inc.

Chapter IV

Nurse Burnout: A Review of the Evidence and Implications for Practice and Research

Laureen Hayes*
University of Toronto, Toronto, Ontario, Canada

Abstract

This chapter involves a comprehensive literature review relating to nursing burnout, an issue that is receiving increased interest from researchers and healthcare administrators over the past few decades. Maslach & Jackson (1981) developed the Maslach Burnout Inventory (MBI) to assess three aspects of the burnout syndrome: a feeling of emotional exhaustion; cynical attitudes toward one's clients (depersonalization); and the tendency to negatively evaluate oneself (low personal accomplishments). Certain conditions in the practice environment are shown to affect nurses' work lives by either contributing to or alleviating burnout. Also, individual attributes including demographic characteristics and personality traits can influence the development of nurse burnout; however, findings are inconsistent across studies. Nurse burnout has negative consequences of stress-related illness, absenteeism and turnover, which impacts quality of care, patient satisfaction and organizational cost. Incidence of nurse burnout is minimized in professional work environments that enable and encourage full scope of nursing practice. There is a critical need to create nursing work environments that support professional practice and put in place leadership development programs to ensure that high quality of patient care is provided. Managers should be aware that certain personality traits may predispose employees to workplace burnout. Clearly, as demonstrated by the evidence to date, the issue of burnout is one that requires policy attention from healthcare administrators, and one that warrants ongoing research toward a better understanding so new evidence can become available to inform future practice. Future research should involve more longitudinal studies and elaborated theoretical models to explain the causal mechanisms that link organizational features and

* Corresponding author: Email: laureen.hayes@utoronto.ca.

processes of care, and how these factors affect outcomes relating to nurse performance and well-being, patient health and satisfaction, and how these outcomes then feed back into and impact the system at the organizational level and beyond.

Introduction

It is not unusual for nurses to feel worn-out after a hectic work shift, however, they may be experiencing burnout if they are constantly feeling frustrated, emotionally drained, and unproductive, and are becoming cynical. Research shows that burnout is prevalent in the nursing profession and predisposes nurses to job related stress and illness, decreased productivity, absenteeism and turnover behavior (Greenglass, Burke, & Fiksenbaum, 2001; Aiken, Clarke, Sloane, Sochalski, & Silber, 2002). High incidence of burnout is a serious human resource problem as it may worsen staffing shortages. An understanding of why nurses are prone to burnout is necessary when considering approaches to prevention therefore it would be worthwhile to examine what is known about the issue to inform future practice and research.

This chapter discusses findings from a comprehensive literature review relating to nurse burnout. It begins by highlighting the relevance of studying nurse burnout, followed by an account of the origins of the burnout concept, and its theoretical basis and measurement. An overview is given of key findings from studies that examined predisposing factors and consequences of nurse burnout. The final part of the chapter discusses implications of the evidence for nursing practice and institutional policy, and possible directions for future research. The approach taken was a summary of relevant findings rather than a systematic review or critique of individual study methodologies. Keyword searches were conducted using Medline, CINAHL, PubMed, and PsycARTICLES electronic databases and bibliography lists of journal articles scanned for further sources of information. While this chapter reflects primarily a North American perspective, the literature searches produced several published articles from other parts of the world, which were included given the global nature of the issue.

Relevance of Burnout Research in Nursing

The term "burnout" started as a non-theoretical concept prior to becoming a metaphor for a number of psychosocial problems among persons who do "people work" (Kristensen, Borritz, Villadsen, & Christensen, 2005). While the occupational health psychology research in the 1970s focused mainly on industrial workers, today the concept of burnout is not only well established in psychosocial research (Maslach & Leiter, 1997) but also a well known metaphor among human service workers in many countries. Sahraian, Fazelzadeh, Mehdizadeh, & Toobaee (2008) describe burnout as a phenomenon in which the cumulative effects of a stressful work environment gradually overwhelm the defenses of staff members, forcing them to withdraw psychologically. Based on this description, researchers and decision-makers should be concerned about environmental factors that could result in burnout and implement change accordingly.

Over the past few decades, healthcare researchers and administers have become more aware of and interested in the issue of nurse burnout. Healthcare restructuring in the 1990's resulted in increased responsibilities for nurses and fewer support staff to assist them, increased patient acuity, and mandatory overtime, leading to exhaustion, demoralization and turnover (Aiken et al. 2001; Baumann et al. 2001). In a large study representing five countries and 43,000 nurses, almost one third of the nurses reported dissatisfaction with their jobs with staffing shortages and insufficient time for patient care; these conditions were associated with high levels of burnout, particularly in younger nurses (Aiken et al., 2001). Other studies report forty percent of nurses have burnout levels that exceed the standards for healthcare workers and twenty percent tend to pursue new employment within a year (Braithwaite, 2008; Funderburk, 2008). For new graduate nurses, some statistics indicate that at least fifty percent leave their positions within the first year (McDonald, 2006; Buerhaus, Donelan, Ulrich, Norman, DesRoaches, & Dittus, 2007; Funderburk, 2008). Such findings would imply that nurses are experiencing frustration and disillusionment, and healthcare institutions are burdened with increased recruitment and hiring costs.

Even though healthcare environments have become more chaotic, staff nurses remain committed to providing high-quality patient care. Nurses value work environments that support their ability to provide high quality patient care that is consistent with the standards of their profession. Nurses who report that their work environment is supportive of professional practice have lower levels of burnout, greater job satisfaction, and lower turnover intentions (Aiken et al., 2001). However, if nurses perceive their unit is inefficient or are lacking involvement in decision-making, they may distance themselves from personal involvement with their patients in order to avoid negative feelings about not having more time to devote to each patient. The likelihood of burnout increases, therefore an understanding of work related factors as well as other possible influences is needed to address the issue.

Concept and Manifestations of Nurse Burnout

The concept of burnout was introduced in 1974 by Dr. Freudenberger, a psychiatrist, who noticed that health care personnel often suffered from chronic physical fatigue, emotional exhaustion and increased distancing from their patients (Freudenberger, 1974, 1975). In the early 1970's, Freudenberger had devoted considerable pro bono time helping develop the free clinic movement in the United States, and was himself troubled with exhaustion, headaches, gastrointestinal problems and other symptoms (Canter & Fredenberger, 2001). Freudenberger described those particularly susceptible to burnout as being dedicated and committed to their jobs in clinics, crisis intervention centers and therapeutic communities. He claimed that long work hours, job pressures, job monotony, lack of organizational goals, and minimal social and organizational support can cause burnout.

During the same time period as Freudenberger's early studies on burnout, social psychological researcher Christina Maslach had been conducting research on emotions in the workplace (Maslach, 1976). Maslach & Jackson (1981) described burnout as a syndrome of emotional exhaustion and cynicism that occurs frequently among individuals who do 'people-work'. The Maslach Burnout Inventory (MBI) was developed to assess three aspects of the burnout syndrome: a feeling of emotional exhaustion; cynical attitudes toward one's clients (depersonalization); and the tendency to negatively evaluate oneself (low personal accomplishments) (Maslach & Jackson, 1981). Higher scores on emotional exhaustion and depersonalization coupled with lower scores on personal accomplishment indicated burnout (Maslach & Jackson, 1981). An *average degree of burnout* is reflected in average scores on the three subscales, and a low degree of burnout is reflected in low scores on the emotional exhaustion and depersonalization subscales and a high score on the personal accomplishment subscales (Maslach & Jackson, 1986). A *low degree of burnout* (low burnout) represents a positive psychological condition rather than the negative condition that is associated with the burnout syndrome. Despite ongoing reports of stressful work environments, some studies have reported evidence of low nurse burnout (ex. Lee & Henderson, 1996; Coffey & Coleman, 2001; Allen & Mellor, 2002; Whittington, 2002).

Early accounts depict manifestations of burnout in behavior and role performance, some being readily noticeable and others more covert. Distancing oneself from patients and treating patients inflexibly or "strictly by the book" may be part of dehumanization, a defensive behavior to avoid emotional investment (Lavandero, 1981). On the other hand, the nurse may become so completely involved with patients and their families that professional objectivity vanishes (Wimbush, 1983). One of the earliest signs of this form of burnout is continually working long hours, and the nurse may be easily irritated and frustrated. Another common defensive behavior is an exaggerated labeling of patient care situations, for example, referring to a patient as the "kidney failure in room 510" (Lavandero, 1981). Finally, there may be a form of victimization in that caregivers may believe that patients are in some way personally to blame for their health conditions and admissions to the hospital. The impact of nurse burnout for the patient was being realized, as Lavandero (1981) emphasized that the patient also suffers as a result of nurse burnout because nursing care is "technical" rather than caring and professional.

As described in later accounts, burnout manifests itself in the form of chronic exhaustion, cynical detachment, and feelings of ineffectiveness (Maslach & Leiter, 1997). Espeland (2006) portrayed the burnout process, stating that negative emotions start slowly, enthusiasm for the job decreases, and productivity and quality of work decline. There may be feelings of boredom or a sense of helplessness to change the situation, and work tardiness and absenteeism occurs. To cope with the stress associated with burnout, compulsive activities may result which include working extra long hours, poor eating habits, smoking, drinking excessive alcohol, and inappropriate use of drugs (Espeland, 2006). The nurse may have problems communicating and exhibit symptoms such as outbursts, hostility, paranoia, withdrawing, and loss of empathy for others. A myriad of physical ailments may follow: insomnia, chronic fatigue, dizziness or lightheadedness, headaches, muscle aches, nausea, allergies or difficulty breathing, and digestive problems. Given the deterioration in physical and mental status of the nurse and subsequent absenteeism, burnout disrupts continuity of care on the nursing unit in addition to becoming a health issue for the individual nurse.

Measurement of Burnout

The Maslach Burnout Inventory has become the dominant measurement tool in burnout research. Three recent versions of the MBI have been developed – a variation on the original MBI for use with human service jobs, a version developed for educational occupations, and the MBI-General Services Scale that is intended for occupations without a significant human service component (Halbesleben & Demerouti, 2005). The newer versions of the MBI reflect the evolution of thinking about burnout as the domain expanded to include non-human services occupations (Halbesleben & Demerouti, 2005). Poghosyan, Aiken, & Sloane (2009) recently evaluated the applicability of the MBI in international nursing research using secondary data representing eight countries, and found it to perform similarly across jurisdictions. It was concluded that the MBI can be used with confidence internationally to determine effectiveness of burnout reduction interventions. Most researchers agree that emotional exhaustion is the core component of burnout, some questioning the necessity of using each of the three MBI components particularly personal accomplishment (Bakker, Demerouti, & Verbeke, 2004).

Other tools to measure burnout have not been as dominant as the MBI in burnout research. The Copenhagen Burnout Inventory (CBI) was presented by Kristensen et al. (2005) who argue that burnout primarily consists of fatigue (exhaustion), and that the depersonalization and personal accomplishment dimensions of the MBI are not part of the burnout phenomenon. The CBI is composed of three scales: *personal burnout* pertains to general symptoms of physical or mental exhaustion and applies to everyone; *work-related burnout* pertains to symptoms of exhaustion that are related to the work and applies to everyone in the workforce; and *client-related burnout* pertains to exhaustion related to the subject's work with clients and applies to employees in human service work such as nurses and teachers (Kristensen et al., 2005; Shimizutani et al., 2008).

Also developed as an alternative to the MBI is the Oldenburg Burnout Inventory (OLBI), originally constructed and validated among different German occupational groups (Demerouti, Bakker, Kantas, & Vardakou, 2002). Similar to the MBI-GS with questions that apply to any occupation, the OLBI comprises scales of exhaustion and disengagement, the latter being the counterpart of depersonalization in the MBI (Halbesleben & Demerouti, 2005). Few studies of English-speaking samples used the OLBI, largely because of a lack of evidence that the English translation of the scale is psychometrically acceptable. Halbesleben & Demerouti (2005) described the psychometric properties of the instrument in a study that is the first to assess its characteristics in an English-speaking sample.

Predisposing Factors of Nursing Burnout

Work Environment

Researchers have investigated factors that contribute to burnout, some of which relate to conditions in the work environment and others having to do with individual attributes of the nurse. Burnout can affect nurses working in any clinical area, although practice settings characterized by emotionally laden demands, such as oncology, intensive care, and psychiatry may have more of an influence. Only a few studies were found that compared level of burnout between clinical areas. Nurses in psychiatry wards were shown to have higher levels of emotional exhaustion than other wards (Yousefy & Ghassemi, 2006; Sahraian et al., 2008), and burn wards nurses showed significantly higher levels of personal accomplishment (Sahraian et al., 2008). Gillespie & Melby (2003) found that nurses working in acute medicine experienced higher levels of emotional exhaustion than nurses in Accident & Emergency. In a recent Spanish study, Santana, Hernández, Eugenio, Sánchez-Palacios, Pérez, & Falcón (2009) reported that emotional exhaustion was more severe in nurses' aides working on admission wards than in those working in the ICU. An earlier study showed no significant differences in burn-out scores among nurses working on AIDS special care units (SCUs), oncology SCUs, medical intensive care units (ICUs) (van Servellen & Leake, 1993). It seems that findings are generally inconsistent with respect to type of clinical setting and incidence of high burnout levels.

In any clinical area, conditions of the work environment influence the development of burnout. There is theoretical support to explain the negative impact of having to care for more patients in less time with fewer resources. In the psychosocial literature, the conservation-of-resources (COR) theory and the job demands-resources model (JD-R) describe the processes leading to burnout. Hobfoll's (1989) COR theory states that if there is a perceived lack of resources to meet work demands, the individual responds by conserving resources, investing less energy in job performance and experiencing stress and burnout. The JD-R model defines the role of job demands and resources; job demands require workers to exert effort and are associated with negative psychological reactions like burnout, and resources facilitate accomplishment and decrease the demands of the job (Demerouti, Bakker, Nachreiner, & Schaufeli, 2001; Halbesleben & Buckley, 2004). For example, quality of the relationships with leaders and mentors represents a valuable resource that can help employees cope with job demands and reduce the likelihood of burnout (Thomas & Lankau, 2009).

In a Swedish study, Hansen, Sverke & Näswall (2009) found burnout (both exhaustion and cynicism) to be most explained by job demands, while job resources had less significance. In nursing, job stressors such as poor staffing, mandatory overtime for high census, forced time off for low census, and lack of materials to complete required tasks, have been shown to contribute to burnout. Unrealistic workload has been frequently reported as a casual factor of anxiety, decreased job satisfaction, and decreased retention rate in registered nurses. Aiken, Clarke, Sloane, Sochalski, & Silber (2002) found that each additional patient per nurse was associated with a 23% increase in the odds of burnout and a 15% increase in the odds of job dissatisfaction. Where nurses are being faced with excessive demands such in their patient assignment, appropriate staffing and other resources (ex. equipment, leadership) are needed to prevent negative responses leading to burnout.

While workload is believed to contribute to burnout, certain factors influence workload and how the overall quality of the work environment is perceived by the nurse. The Mediation Model of Burnout was proposed as a way to link six key areas of nurse's worklife – workload, control, reward, community, fairness, and values – to outcomes such as job satisfaction or turnover (Leiter, 2005; Maslach & Leiter, 2009). According to the model, control has consequences for workload, reward, community and fairness; those who have successfully shaped their workload, rewards, social interactions, and institutional justice are more likely to develop an environment consistent with their values. Disparities or incongruities in these six key areas of worklife are predictive of burnout; research on the interrelationships of these areas suggests that there is a consistent and complex pattern that predicts the level of experienced burnout (Maslach & Leiter 1997, Leiter & Maslach 2004). Recent longitudinal research has found that particular patterns of scores on measures of burnout and the six areas of worklife can serve as early predictors of subsequent change to either burnout or engagement and thus inform prevention strategies (Maslach & Leiter 2008).

Another model presented in the literature is based on five practice domains identified by Lake (2002) as being associated with magnet hospital characteristics and nurses' perceptions of professional practice environments. The Nursing Worklife Model explains how organizational and nursing unit factors affect nurses' lives in the workplace by either contributing to or alleviating burnout (Laschinger & Leiter 2006, Leiter & Laschinger 2006). The five practice domains are: staff nurse participation in hospital affairs; use of a nursing model as the basis for care on a nursing unit; nurse manager ability, leadership and support; staffing and resource adequacy; and collegial nurse– physician relations (Lake, 2002; Manojlovich & Laschinger, 2007). Nursing leadership was shown to be a driving force with direct implications for staffing, physician-nurse relations, and policy impact (Leiter & Laschinger, 2006). The connection of staffing with emotional exhaustion clarifies that a shortfall of resources (i.e. time, personnel, supplies, or equipment) relative to demands is a driving force behind facets of burnout, particularly emotional exhaustion. In terms of values, the research also demonstrated that regardless of level of exhaustion or depersonalization, nurses who were aware of a nursing model of care operating within their hospital were able to derive a deeper sense of accomplishment from their work, thereby buffering against full burnout syndrome.

Nurses who have the necessary support and resources in their workplace should feel psychologically empowered with a sense of competence and control that enables them to perform their job effectively. Laschinger, Finegan, Shamian and Wilk (2003) examined whether perceptions of structural empowerment could predict burnout three years later. According to Kanter (1977, 1993), organizational structures necessary for empowerment are access to information, receiving support, having access to resources necessary to do the job and having the opportunity to learn and grow (Kanter, 1977, 1993). In a Canadian nursing study, structural empowerment was measured by the Conditions for Work Effectiveness-II (CWEQ-II) (Laschinger et al. 2001), psychological empowerment was measured by the Psychological Empowerment Scale (PES) (Spreitzer, 1995) and burnout was assessed by the Emotional Exhaustion subscale of the Maslach Burnout Inventory-General Survey (Schaufeli, Leiter, Maslach & Jackson, 1996). The results revealed that perceptions of structural empowerment had a direct effect on psychological empowerment at Time 1 and an indirect effect on burnout through psychological empowerment, and psychological empowerment at Time 1 had a significant effect on perceived emotional exhaustion at Time 2 (Laschinger et al., 2003). These findings are congruent with Hochwälder's (2008) study reporting that higher levels of empowerment are related to lower levels of burnout, when empowerment and burnout are studied at the same point in time. The evidence from these studies emphasizes the critical role of access to information and other resources so nurses have the opportunity to grow and experience psychological empowerment.

Given the large number of nurses currently approaching retirement, studies are being conducted to examine factors that will promote retention of the new nurses entering the workforce. Cho, Laschinger, & Wong (2006) examined relationships among structural empowerment, six areas of work life (conceptualized as antecedents of work engagement), emotional exhaustion and organizational commitment on a sample of new graduate nurses. As predicted, structural empowerment had a direct positive effect on the areas of work life, which in turn had a direct negative effect on emotional exhaustion. Based on Kanter's theory and subsequent research by Laschinger and colleagues, adequate support and resources are critical to enable nurses to grow in their careers and provide good quality care without experiencing chronic exhaustion from the inherent responsibilities of nursing practice.

Having an adequate number of experienced nurses relative to the total number of nurses within the healthcare institution is important to consider as a resource. Nurse inexperience measured at the hospital level may affect burnout and dissatisfaction of nurses and the quality of care at the unit level. In one study, individual nurse burnout and dissatisfaction and poorer quality of care was associated with workplaces that have larger percentages of inexperienced nurses (Kanai-Pak, Aiken, Sloane, Poghosyan, 2008). As the JD-R model asserts, resources facilitate accomplishment and decrease the demands of the job, thereby minimizing negative psychological reactions and likelihood of burnout.

Research shows that role conflict and role ambiguity in the workplace has a role in development of burnout. Role conflict refers to incompatible or mutually competing expectations or demands, and role ambiguity is a lack of clarity and predictability regarding role expectations (Rizzo, House, & Lirtzman, 1970). Based on a sample of healthcare staff in Hungary, Pilo (2006) determined that role conflict was a factor contributing positively to emotional exhaustion and depersonalization scores. In a study of mental health service providers, Acker (2003) found that role conflict and role ambiguity had statistically significant correlations with several of the burnout dimensions. In a study of care-providers of institutionalized elderly patients with dementia, Barber & Iwai (1996) hypothesized that work environment characteristics (role conflict and role ambiguity) collectively would be the best predictors of burnout. The findings showed that work environment characteristics accounted for more than 60% of the explained variance in burnout with the majority of this variance being explained by the factor of role conflict. A critical component of the practice environment (Lake, 2002) is effective leadership to ensure nurses are clear in terms of their responsibilities and expectations, and receive appropriate support to guide them when necessary.

Individual Factors

Researchers have questioned why some nurses are more likely than others to experience burnout symptoms even if working in the same practice setting. In addition to work related factors, individual characteristics influence how the nurse responds to the work environment. For example, level of education is believed to be a contributing factor as burnout is often claimed to affect the young, highly educated, ambitious professionals (Maslach, Schaufeli, & Leiter, 2001). The incongruence between an individual's expectations and ensuing reality is considered a main characteristic of burnout as may be the case when nurses enter their careers anticipating they will always be able to meet the needs of their clients.

Robinson et al. (1991) reported that younger nurses experienced more depersonalization, suggesting that the older nurses remained in professional practice for the very reason of personal involvement with patients. In the same study, older nurses reported less personal accomplishment; perhaps the job itself becomes less personally rewarding as experience makes the work routine. Chen & McMurray (2001) also found younger nurses (20-29 years of age) the most prone to emotional exhaustion, and Patrick & Lavery (2007) found increasing age to be associated with lower levels of emotional exhaustion and depersonalisation. Yousefy & Ghassemi (2006) reported findings which were contrasting in terms of age; there was a significant positive correlation between age and years of experience, and emotional exhaustion, and longer duration of service was accompanied by higher degree of emotional depersonalization. Similarly, Losa Iglesias, Vallejo, & Fuentes (2009) concluded that being older than 30 years was associated with a nurse's vulnerability to burnout syndrome.

A number of studies examine the relationship between burnout components and other variables relating to the individual nurse. Based on a sample of intensive care nurses, separated and divorced nurses and staff who work full time were the most prone to emotional exhaustion (Chen & McMurray, 2001). Sahraian et al. (2008) also found single nurses to be more emotionally exhausted. In another study, Losa Iglesias et al. (2009) concluded that having more than ten years of experience, being single and smoking were associated with a nurse's vulnerability to burnout syndrome.

Personality traits have been studied in an attempt to discover which types of people may be at greater risk for experiencing burnout. Maslach, Schaufeli, & Leiter (2001) identified hardiness, locus of control, coping styles, personality type, and attitude as important factors in potential burnout. Maslach et al. (2001) states burnout is higher among individuals who have an external locus of control (attributing events and achievements to others or to chance) rather than an internal locus of control (attributing to own ability and effort). Nurses with a "hardy" personality have a feeling of control in life, an optimistic outlook and ability to handle change, were less likely to suffer from burnout (Garrosa, Moreno-Jimenez, Liang, & Gonzalez, 2008). Similarly, Simoni and Paterson (1997) found that nurses with greater hardiness who used direct-active coping behaviours (changing the stressor, confronting the stressor, finding positive aspects in the situation) reported lower burnout than did those who were less hardy and used inactive coping responses. In other words, those who are burned out cope with stressful events in a rather passive, defensive way, whereas active and confrontational coping is associated with less burnout. Layman and Guyden (1997) suggested that introverted people were at higher risk of developing burnout than were extroverted people.

Other personality traits may influence likelihood of burnout. The exhaustion dimension of burnout appears to be linked to "type A" personality behavior characterized by competitiveness, time-pressured lifestyle, hostility, and an excessive need for control (Maslach et al., 2001). Nurses vary in the expectations they bring to their job. Expectations might be high resulting in working too hard, exhaustion and eventual cynicism when the high effort does not yield the expected results. In addition, Sherman (2004) identified personality characteristics such as perfectionism and over-involvement with clients as contributing to compassion fatigue or burnout. Nurses who experience high levels of personal stress are also at increased risk for stress at work that can lead to burnout (Meadors & Lamson, 2008). If nurses have difficulty separating work from personal life, they may bring negative feelings from the workplace to their home and family, or they might bring issues from their home into the work environment.

Consequences of Nurse Burnout

Nurse burnout produces negative outcomes for the nurse, the patient and the healthcare organization. As already discussed, burnout is manifested in a number of physical and mental health issues which may lead to increased absenteeism and sick leave (Malach-Pines, 2006; Eriksson, Starrin, & Janson, 2008; Meadors & Lamson, 2008). Research also demonstrates the impact of burnout on job dissatisfaction, nurse turnover and quality of care. Aiken, Clarke, Sloane, Sochalski, & Silber (2002) found that burnout and dissatisfaction predict nurses' intentions to leave their current jobs within a year, which then has implications for patient safety because nurse surveillance, early detection, and timely intervention are critical for positive patient outcomes. Aiken et al. (2001) provided strong evidence that hospitals lacking in nurse staffing and organizational support for nursing have higher levels of nurse job dissatisfaction and burnout and more frequent adverse patient events such as falls with injuries, patient complaints, and poorer nurse-assessed quality of care.

Patient safety and satisfaction with care are major concerns when nurses begin to experience and exhibit signs of burnout. Findings of a recent study indicate that burnout may decrease the ability to recognize errors and influence the likelihood of reporting errors (Halbesleben, Wakefield, Wakefield, & Cooper, 2008). It was suggested that burned-out healthcare workers feel that reporting an error is too time consuming, that it does not have a significant impact on the patient, or that no action will be taken anyway. Nurses were also more likely to take shortcuts as solutions to problems with work process, leading to failures in established safety precautions (Halbesleben et al., 2008) and difficulty expressing empathy due to negative attitudes for patients and families (Meadors & Lamson, 2008). Studies demonstrate a negative correlation between emotional exhaustion in nurses and patient satisfaction with care (Vahey, Aiken, Sloane, Clarke, & Vargas, 2004; Argentero, Dell'Olivo, & Ferretti, 2008).

Research has been conducted to provide a better understanding of the relationship between burnout and various negative responses to the job. The Mediation Model of Burnout proposed by Leiter & Maslach (2009) links nurse's worklife to outcomes such as job satisfaction or turnover and determines whether burnout mediates the impact of workplace stressors on intentions to leave the job. Leiter & Maslach (2009) demonstrated that burnout was indeed predictive of turnover intention, and it mediated the effect of workplace factors on this outcome. Based on the results, the authors indicate that the primary issue for turnover intention is the extent to which nurses are involved in their work, as the psychological withdrawal of cynicism is associated with the social withdrawal of quitting a job (Leiter and Maslach, 2009). They emphasize that workload leading to exhaustion, lack of support for the nursing model of care leading to values conflict, and inadequate reward systems are the primary issues for cynicism which was critical in the case of turnover intention.

Addressing the issue of nurse burnout would also help address the issue of nurse turnover and its cost impact. Jones' (2004, 2005) work to determine turnover costs by using a Nursing Turnover Cost Calculation Methodology divides the costs of nurse turnover into the two major cost categories of pre-hire and post-hire costs. Pre-hire costs include advertising/recruiting costs, vacancy costs, and hiring costs, and post-hire costs include orientation and training costs, newly hired RN productivity losses, pre-turnover productivity losses, and termination costs (Jones, 2004). Vacancy costs were the highest, followed by orientation and training costs, newly hired RN productivity costs, and advertising and recruiting costs. Recent studies show varying costs of nurse turnover, largely due to conceptual and methodological differences (Jones & Gates, 2007). In a recent inflation-adjusted dollar estimation, Jones (2008) calculated per RN turnover cost would range from approximately $82,000 (if turnover vacancies are filled by experienced RNs) to $88,000 (if vacancies are filled by new RNs). In general, turnover costs have been estimated to range between 0.75 to 2.0 times the salary of the departing individual (McConnell, 1999), depending on education, experience, and tenure of the nurse who leaves, and factors internal and external to the organizational (Jones & Gates, 2007).

The discussion thus far has focused on the theoretical and empirical findings relating to burnout within the nursing context. The concept and manifestations of nurse burnout, its measurement, predisposing factors relating to the work environment and the individual, and the consequences for the nurse, patient and organization have been touched upon. Clearly, as demonstrated by the evidence to date, the issue is one that requires policy attention from healthcare administrators, and one that warrants ongoing research toward a better understanding so new evidence can become available to inform future practice.

Implications of Research Findings

Implications for Nursing Policy and Practice

Given the link between the work environment and nurse, patient and organizational outcomes, it is important ensure that nurses feel they are supported in their job duties in order to help prevent burnout. Nurses comprise the largest component of hospital staff and have the most consistent and direct contact with patients. While there are no easy answers for the complex challenges facing healthcare facilities, neglecting staff well-being may result in patient dissatisfaction and decrease in service utilization. Vahey et al. (2004) pointed out that aspects of the work environment that account for nurses' emotional exhaustion and patient dissatisfaction are modifiable, such as staffing adequacy, administrative support for nursing practice, and better relations between nurses and physicians. While emotionally exhausted nurses are more likely to leave their jobs, positive changes in the work environment would help stabilize the nurse workforce and improve quality of care and patient satisfaction.

Aiken et al. (2001) emphasize that nurse leaders must ensure that nurses are enabled to have control over their practice environments and supported to make practice decisions based on their expertise and knowledge. Nursing leadership has a compelling role in that nurses at all levels in the organization can be influential in their work whether they are staff nurses providing direct care or have a formal leadership position. The need for leadership and supervision may become urgent as current nursing managers approach retirement and younger nurses may be reluctant to take on management roles. There is a critical need to create nursing work environments that support professional practice and put in place leadership development programs to ensure succession planning and continued leader roles that assure that high quality of patient care is provided (Leiter & Laschinger, 2006).

Incidence of nurse burnout is minimized in professional work environments that enable and encourage full scope of nursing practice. Even in high stress areas, nurses do not burn out if they have the necessary resources to provide high quality care and have the opportunity to engage in professional development and learning. In fact, nurses working in low opportunity jobs might be more likely to limit their work aspirations, be resistant to change, and more likely to be burned out (Leiter & Laschinger, 2006). In one study, Moore (2001) found that nurses' stress during restructuring was mediated by viewing restructuring changes as a challenge and by social support and communication by their managers and colleagues. Therefore, identifying and modifying possible areas of boredom and frustration is important in counteracting nurse burnout. Where appropriate, introducing fun in the work environment can reduce emotional exhaustion as shown in one study that demonstrated a significant correlation with regard to low levels of burnout in healthcare professionals (Karl & Peluchette, 2006).

Front-line nursing managers can be instrumental in efforts to minimize staff nurse burnout. Laschinger et al. (2003) provided important recommendations emerging from their research on nurse burnout. Providing access to information about organizational events and future plans can instill a sense of control over their work environment and trust in management. Nursing managers can enhance balance between family and work life through employment opportunities, such as job sharing or self-scheduling. Provision of opportunities for staff nurse growth and development of new skills could include job enrichment activities, such as job exchange programs, managing short-term projects, internship programs and secondments to projects that are critical to work accomplishments. Managers must find ways to ensure that structures and supports are in place to enable nurses to be successful in their responsibilities in a way that is consistent with their professional values and standards.

While managers must make every effort to create working conditions that prevent burnout from occurring, the nature of the work environment is not the only influence in the development of nurse burnout. Harris and Artis (2005) suggest that managers should be aware that certain personality traits may predispose employees to workplace burnout. Nurses who are anxious, obsessive, idealistic, or overly enthusiastic or empathic might be especially prone to develop burnout (Burke & Richardsen, 1996). If these nurses are successfully identified, they will be more likely to receive appropriate intervention. However, nurses should also be accountable in that they should take measures to protect their own well-being even before they experience burnout symptoms. Braithwaite (2008) states nurses should take responsibility for recognizing symptoms of fatigue and ensure adequate time for rest and sleep. Nurses can alleviate some of the effects of stress by maintaining a healthy diet, exercise, relaxation and recreation, and expressing feelings with friends.

Implications for Research

Although this chapter does not focus on methodologies of individual studies, it would be worthwhile to highlight a few points that the researchers identified as important directions in the study of nurse burnout. As cross-sectional designs are limited in determining causality or explaining correlations, one recommendation is to conduct more longitudinal studies (Brewer & Shapard, 2004). Longitudinal studies might explain more fully the correlation and between burnout level and age or experience, leading to more appropriate implications for employers depending on the explanation for the positive or negative correlation. Hansen et al. (2009) claim that cross-sectional designs are also limited in terms of stating direction of causality. For example, it could be that a burned-out employee experience higher job demands and fewer resources, rather than heavy demands and inadequate resources lead to nurse burnout. Longitudinal design with several measurements over time would contribute to a better understanding of direction of the relationship.

Longitudinal studies also have common limitations which need to be considered in future research. Laschinger et al. (2003) refer to the possibility of other unmeasured factors or other occurring events that may account for the results. For example, personality characteristics may mitigate the impact of environmental circumstances on subsequent burnout. Another difficulty with longitudinal research is that the final sample is often considerably smaller than the original, raising the possibility that respondents who reply to a second surveys are different than those who only responded to the first survey or to those who did not respond at all. Future research should focus on obtaining larger sample sizes to help strengthen the findings (Harris & Artis, 2005).

Given the argument that burnout is detrimental to individuals' health, more research is needed on factors that contribute to this state, and the interplay between structural factors, psychosocial work environment and consequences for health outcomes (Hansen et al., 2009). Future research should use more elaborated models to explain the causal mechanisms that link organizational features and processes of care, how these factors affect outcomes relating to nurse performance and well-being, patient health and satisfaction, and how these outcomes then feed back into and impact the system at the organizational level and beyond. Application of theoretical models should have a constructive focus to determine what work structures and processes are needed for work challenges to contribute to low burnout and wellness. Indeed, positive research has the potential to give nursing a more optimistic outlook and portray the profession as more appealing for the next generation.

Conclusion

This chapter provided an overview of the relevant literature which included the theoretical foundations of burnout and some key findings relating to the predisposing factors and consequences for the nurse, patient and healthcare institution. Implications of the research evidence were discussed as they relate to nursing practice at the individual, nursing unit and institutional levels, and directions for future research in this important area. As a large cohort of experienced nurses approaches retirement, it is critical to examine factors that will promote personal well-being and career commitment in the newer workforce. While a substantial body of research already exists and gains have been made in understanding the burnout phenomena, further work is needed in the advancement of coherent theoretical frameworks to derive a clearer understanding of its precursors and consequences as it may apply in various nursing settings and circumstances. In addressing the issue of burnout, new findings could be incorporated into the planning of new initiatives and in modifying existing organizational strategies to promote a healthy and sustainable nursing workforce.

References

Acker, G. M. (2003). Role conflict and ambiguity: do they predict burnout among mental health service providers? *Social Work in Mental Health.*, *1(3)*, 63-80.

Aiken, L. H., Clarke, S. P., Sloane, D. M., Sochalski, J. A., Busse, R., Clarke, H., et al. (2001). Nurses' reports on hospital care in five countries. *Health Affairs (Millwood).*, *20*, 43-53.

Aiken, L. H., Clarke, S. P., Sloane, D. M., Sochalski, J. & Silber, J. H. (2002). Hospital nurse staffing and patient mortality, nurse burnout, and job dissatisfaction. *Journal of the American Medical Association.*, *288(16)*, 1987-1993.

Allen, J. & Mellor, D. (2002). Work context, personal control, and burnout amongst nurses. *Western Journal of Nursing Research.*, *24(8)*, 905-917.

Argentero, P., Dell'Olivo, B. & Ferretti, M. S. (2008). Staff burnout and patient satisfaction with the quality of dialysis care. *American Journal of Kidney Diseases.*, *51(1)*, 80-92.

Bakker, A. B., Demerouti, E. & Verbeke, W. (2004). Using the job demands–resources model to predict burnout and performance. *Human Resource Management.*, *43*, 83-104.

Bakker, A. B., van Emmerik, H. & Euwema, M. C. (2006). Crossover of burnout and engagement in work teams. *Work and Occupations.*, *33(4)*, 464-489.

Barber, C. E. & Iwai, M. (1996). Role conflict and role ambiguity as predictors of burnout among staff caring for elderly dementia patients. *Journal of Gerontological Social Work.*, *26(1/2)*, 101-116.

Baumann, A., O'Brien-Pallas, L., Armstrong-Stassen, M., Blythe, J., Bourbonnais, R., Cameron, S., et al. (2001). *Commitment and care: The benefits of a healthy workplace for nurses, their patients and the system.* Report submitted to the Canadian Health Services Research Foundation, Ottawa, ON.

Braithwaite, M. (2008). Professional growth and development. Nurse burnout and stress in the NICU. *Advances in Neonatal Care.*, *8(6)*, 343-347.

Brewer, E. W. & Shapard, L. (2004). *Employee Burnout*: A meta-analysis of the relationship between age or years of experience. *Human Resource Development Review., 3(2)*, 102-123.

Buerhaus, P., Donelan, K., Ulrich, B., Norman, L., DesRoaches, C. & Dittus, R. (2007). Impact of the nurse shortage on hospital patient care: comparative perspectives. *Health Affairs., 26*, 853-862.

Burke, R. J. & Richardsen, A. M. (1996). Stress, burnout, and health. In C. L. Cooper (Ed.), *Stress, medicine, and health* (pp. 101-117). Boca Raton, FL: CRC Press.

Canter, M. B. & Freudenberger, L. (2001). Obituary: Herbert J. Freudenberger (1926-1999). *American Psychologist., 56(12)*, 1171.

Chen, S. M. & McMurray, A. J. (2001). "Burnout" in intensive care nurses. *The Journal of Nursing Research., 9(5)*, 152-164.

Cho, J., Laschinger, H. K. S. & Wong, C. (2006). Nursing leadership, workplace empowerment, work engagement and organizational commitment of new graduate nurses. *Canadian Journal of Nursing Leadership., 19(3)*, 43-60.

Coffey, M. & Coleman, M. (2001). The relationship between support and stress in forensic community health nursing. *Journal of Advanced Nursing., 34(3)*, 397-407.

Demerouti, E., Bakker, A. B., Nachreiner, F. & Schaufeli, W. B. (2001). The job demands-resources model of burnout. *Journal of Applied Psychology., 86*, 499-512.

Demerouti, E., Bakker, A. B., Vardakou, I. & Kantas, A. (2002). The convergent validity of two burnout instruments: a multitrait-multimethod analysis. *European Journal of Psychological Assessment, 18*, 296-307.

Demir, A., Ulusoy, M. & Ulusoy, M. F. (2003). Investigation of factors influencing burnout levels in the professional and private lives of nurses. *International Journal of Nursing Studies., 40*, 807-827.

Eriksson, U. B., Starrin, B. & Janson, S. (2008). Long-term sickness absence due to burnout: absentees' experiences. *Qualitative Health Research., 18*, 620-632.

Espeland, K. (2006). Overcoming burnout: how to revitalize your career. *Journal of Continuing Education in Nursing., 37*, 179-180.

Freudenberger, H. J. (1974), "Staff burnout", *Journal of Social Issues, 30*, 159-165.

Funderburk, A. (2008). Mentoring: the retention factor in the acute care setting. *Journal for Nurses in Staff Development., 24(3)*, E1-E5.

Freudenberger, H. J. (1975). The staff burn-out syndrome in alternative institutions. *Psychotherapy: Theory, Research & Practice., 12(1)*, 73-82.

Garrosa. E., Moreno-Jiménez, B., Liang, Y. & González, J. L. (2008). The relationship between socio-demographic variables, job stressors, burnout, and hardy personality in nurses: an exploratory study. *International Journal of Nursing Studies., 45(3)*, 418-427.

Gillespie, M. & Melby, V. (2003). Burnout among nursing staff in accident and emergency and acute medicine: a comparative study. *Journal of Clinical Nursing., 12(6)*, 842-851.

Greenglass, E., Burke, R. & Fiksenbaum, L. (2001). Workload and burnout in nurses. *Journal of Community & Applied Social Psychology., 11*, 211-215.

Halbesleben, J. R. B. & Buckley, M. R. (2004). Burnout in organizational life. *Journal of Management., 30*, 859-879.

Halbesleben, J. R. B. & Demerouti, E. (2005). The construct validity of an alternative measure of burnout: Investigating the English translation of the Oldenburg Burnout Inventory, *Work & Stress.*, *19(3)*, 208-220.

Halbesleben, J. R. B., Wakefield, B. J., Wakefield, D. S. & Cooper, L. B. (2008). Nurse burnout and patient safety outcomes: nurse safety perception versus reporting behavior. *Western Journal of Nursing Research.*, *30*, 560-577.

Hansen, N., Sverke, M. & Näswall, K. (2009). Predicting nurse burnout from demands and resources in three acute care hospitals under different forms of ownership: a cross-sectional questionnaire survey. *International Journal of Nursing Studies.*, *46(1)*, 96-107

Harris, E. G. & Artis, A. B. (2005). Exploring patient, co-worker, and management *burnout* in health care: An empirical study. *Health Marketing Quarterly.*, *22(3)*, 3-20.

Hobfoll, S. E. (1989). Conservation of resources: A new attempt at conceptualizing stress. *American Psychologist.*, *44*, 513-524.

Hochwälder, J. (2008). A longitudinal study of the relationship between empowerment and burnout among registered and assistant nurses. *Work.*, *30(4)*, 343-352.

Jones, C. B. (2004). The costs of nursing turnover, Part I: an economic perspective. Journal of Nursing Administration, 34*(12)*, 562-570.

Jones, C. B. (2005). The costs of nursing turnover, part 2: Application of the Nursing Turnover Cost Calculation Methodology. *Journal of Nursing Administration.*, *35(1)*, 41-49.

Jones, C. B. (2008). Revisiting nurse turnover costs: adjusting for inflation. *Journal of Nursing Administration.*, *38(1)*, 11-18.

Jones, C. & Gates, M. (2007). Costs and benefits of nurse turnover: A business case for nurse retention. *Online Journal of Issues in Nursing.*, *12(3)*, Manuscript 4. Available: www.nursingworld.org/MainMenuCategories/ANAMarketplace/ANAPeriodicals/OJIN/T ableofContents/Volume122007/No3Sept07/NurseRetention.aspx Accessed July 28, 2009.

Kanai-Pak, M., Aiken, L. H., Sloane, D. M. & Poghosyan, L. (2008). Poor work environments and nurse inexperience are associated with burnout, job dissatisfaction and quality deficits in Japanese hospitals. *Journal of Clinical Nursing.*, *17(24)*, 3324-3329.

Kanter, R. M. (1977). *Men and Women of the Corporation*. Basic Books, New York.

Kanter, R. M. (1993). *Men and Women of the Corporation*, 2nd ed. Basic Books, New York.

Kristensen, T. S., Borritz, M., Villadsen, E. & Christensen, K. B. (2005). The Copenhagen Burnout Inventory: A new tool for the assessment of burnout. *Work & Stress.*, *19(3)*, 192-207.

Lake, E. T. (2002). Development of the Practice Environment Scale of the Nursing Work Index. *Research in Nursing & Health.*, *25*, 176-188.

Laschinger, H. K. S., Finegan, J., Shamian, J. & Wilk., P. (2001). Impact of structural and psychological empowerment on job strain in nursing work settings: Expanding Kanter's model." *Journal of Nursing Administration.*, *31*, 260-272.

Laschinger, H. K. S., Finegan, J., Shamian, J. & Wilk, P. (2003). Workplace empowerment as a predictor of nurse burnout in restructured health care settings. *Longwoods Review.*, *1(3)*, 2-11.

Laschinger, H. K. S. & Leiter, M. P. (2006). The impact of nursing work environments on patient safety outcomes: the mediating role of burnout/engagement. *Journal of Nursing Administration., 36(5)*, 259-267.

Lavandero, R. (1981). Nurse burnout: What can we learn? *Journal of Nursing Administration.*, 17-23.

Layman, E. & Guyden, J. A. (1997). (1997). Reducing your risk of burnout. *The Health care supervisor., 15(3)*, 57-69.

Lee, V. L. & Henderson, M. C. (1996). Occupational stress and organizational commitment in nurse administrators. *Journal of Nursing Administration., 26(5)*, 21-28.

Leiter, M. P. (2005). Perception of risk: An organizational model of occupational risk, burnout, and physical symptoms. *Anxiety, Stress, & Coping., 18*, 131-144.

Leiter, M. P. & Laschinger, H. K. S. (2006). Relationships of work and practice environment to professional burnout: Testing a causal model nursing research. *55(2)*, 137-146.

Leiter, M. P. & Maslach, C. (2004). Areas of worklife: A structured approach to organizational predictors of job burnout. In P. L. Perrewe, & D. C. Ganster (Eds.), *Research in occupational stress and well-being (Vol. 3*, 91-134). Oxford : Elsevier.

Leiter, M. P. & Maslach, C. (2009). Nurse turnover: the mediating role of burnout. *Journal of Nursing Management., 17(3)*, 331-339.

Losa Iglesias, M. E., Vallejo, R. B. & Fuentes, P. S. (2009). The relationship between experiential avoidance and burnout syndrome in critical care nurses: A cross-sectional questionnaire survey. *International Journal of Nursing Studies*, [Epub ahead of print]

Malach-Pines, A. (2006).Nurses' burnout: an existential psychodynamic perspective. *Journal of Psychosocial Nursing & Mental Health Services., 38(2)*, 23-31.

Manojlovich, M. & Laschinger, H. (2007). The Nursing Worklife Model: Extending and refining a new theory. *Journal of Nursing Management., 15*, 256-263.

Maslach, C. (1976). Burned-out. *Human Behaviour., 5*, 16-22.

Maslach, C. M. & Jackson, S. E. (1986). *Maslach Burnout Inventory: Manual* (2nd ed.). Palo Alto, CA: Consulting Psychologists Press.

Maslach, C, & Jackson, S. (1981). The measurement of experienced burnout. *Journal of Occupational Behavior., 2*, 99-113.

Maslach, C. & Leiter, M. P. (2008). Early predictors of *job burnout* and engagement. *Journal of Applied Psychology., 93(3)*, 498-512.

Maslach, C. & Leiter, M. P. (1997). *The Truth about Burnout* (3rd ed.). San Francisco: Jossey-Bass.

Maslach, C., Schaufeli, W. B. & Leiter, M. P. (2001). Job burnout. *Annual Review of Psychology., 52*, 397-422.

McConnell, C. R. (1999). Staff turnover: Occasional friend, frequent foe, and continuing frustration. *Health Care Manager., 8*, 1-13.

McDonald, P. (2006). Workplace stress and the practice nurse. *Practice Nurse., 32(6)*, 28-32.

Meadors, P. & Lamson, A. (2008). Compassion fatigue and secondary traumatization: provider self care on intensive care units for children. *Journal of Pediatric Health Care., 22*, 24-34.

Moore, K. A. (2001). Hospital restructuring: impact on nurses mediated by social support and a perception of challenge. *Journal of Health & Human Services Administration., 23(4)*, 490-517.

Patrick, K. & Lavery, J. F. (2007). Burnout in nursing. *Australian Journal of Advanced Nursing.*, *24(3)*, 43-48.

Peluchette, J. & Karl, K. A. (2005). Attitudes toward incorporating fun into the health care workplace. *Health Care Manager.*, *24(3)*, 268-275.

Pilo, B. F. (2006). Burnout, role conflict, job satisfaction and psychosocial health among Hungarian health care staff: a questionnaire survey *International Journal of Nursing Studies.*, *43(3)*, 311-318.

Poghosyan, L., Aiken, L. H. & Sloane, D. M. (2009). Factor structure of the Maslach burnout inventory: an analysis of data from large scale cross-sectional surveys of nurses from eight countries. *International Journal of Nursing Studies.*, *46(7)*, 894-902.

Rizzo, J. R., House, R. J. & Lirtzman, S. I. (1970). Role conflict and role ambiguity in complex organizations. *Administrative Science Quarterly.*, *15*, 150-163.

Robinson, S. E., Roth, S. L., Keim, J., Levenson, M., Flentje, J. R. & Bashor, K. (1991) Nurse burnout: Work related and demographic factors as culprits. *Research in Nursing and Health.*, *14*, 223-228.

Sahraian, A., Fazelzadeh, A., Mehdizadeh, A. R., Toobaee, S. H. (2008). Burnout in hospital nurses: a comparison of internal, surgery, psychiatry and burns wards. *International Nursing Review.*, *55(1)*, 62-67.

Santana, C. L., Hernández, M. E., Eugenio, R. P., Sánchez-Palacios, M., Pérez, S. R. & Falcón, M. R. (2009). Burnout syndrome among nurses and nurses' aides in an intensive care unit and admission wards. *Enfermería Clínica.*, *19(1)*, 31-34.

Schaufeli, W.B., Leiter, M., Maslach, C. & Jackson, S. E. (1996). *Maslach Burnout Inventory General Survey*. Palo Alto, CA: Consulting Psychologists.

Schaufeli, W. B., Salanova, M., Gonzalez Roma, V. & Bakker, A. B. (2002). The measurement of engagement and burnout: A two sample confirmatory factor analytic approach. *Journal of Happiness Studies*, *3*, 71-92.

Sherman, D. W. (2004). Nurses' stress & burnout: How to care for yourself when caring for patients and their families experiencing life-threatening illness. *American Journal of Nursing.*, *104(5)*, 48-56.

Shimizutani, M., Odagiri, Y., Ohya, Y., Shimomitsu, T., Kristensen, T. S., Maruta, T. & Iimori, M. (2008). Relationship of nurse burnout with personality characteristics and coping behaviors. *Industrial Health.*, *46*, 326-335.

Simoni, P. S. & Paterson, J. J. (1997). Hardiness, coping, and burnout in the nursing workplace. *Journal of Professional Nursing.*, *13(3)*, 178-185.

Spreitzer, G. (1995). Psychological empowerment in the workplace: Dimensions, measurement, and validation. *Academy of Management Journal 38(5)*, 1442-1462.

Thomas, C. H. & Lankau, M. J. (2009). Preventing burnout: The effects of LMX and mentoring on socialization, role stress, and burnout. *Human Resource Management.*, *48(3)*, 417- 432.

Vahey, D., Aiken, L., Sloane, D., Clarke, S. & Vargas, D. (2004). Nurse burnout and patient satisfaction. *Medical Care.*, *42(2)*, 57-66.

van Servellen, G. & Leake, B. (1993). Burn-out in hospital nurses: a comparison of acquired immunodeficiency syndrome, oncology, general medical, and intensive care unit nurse samples. *Journal of Professional Nursing.*, *9(3)*, 169-177.

Whittington, R. (2002). Attitudes toward patient aggression amongst mental health nurses in the 'Zero Tolerance' Era: Associations with burnout and length of experience. *Journal of Clinical Nursing.*, *11(6)*, 819-825.

Wimbush, F. B. (1983). Nurse burnout: its effect on patient care. *Nursing Management.*, *14(1)*, 55-57.

Yousefy, A. R. & Ghassemi, G. R. (2006). Job burnout in psychiatric and medical nurses in Isfahan, Islamic Republic of Iran. *Eastern Mediterranean Health Journal.*, *12(5)*, 662-669.

In: Nursing Issues: Psychiatric Nursing, Geriatric Nursing…   ISBN: 978-1-60741-598-5
Editors: C. D. McLaughlin et al., pp. 175-191   © 2010 Nova Science Publishers, Inc.

Chapter V

Interpreting and Responding to Expressions of Mental Pain: The Inner and Outer Dialogues of the Mental Health Nurse

Briege Casey and Evelyn Gordon
Dublin City University, Dublin, Ireland.

Keywords: Mental pain, discourse, therapeutic impasse, curiosity, dialogic space.

Introduction

The mental pain expressed by people experiencing mental health problems can be understood in different ways by the mental health/ psychiatric nurse, depending on a number of factors. These include, in addition to the unique nature of the person's story being presented, the nurse's own internal beliefs, perceptions and past experiences regarding people with mental health issues and his/her experiences of interacting with this population (England 2007, Munro and Baker 2007). The nurse's understandings and responses are also influenced by her/his external social and professional environments where there are a range of ways of perceiving and treating people who are in mental distress.

Sense making is a process that emerges from the interaction between such personal, social and professional dialogues and narratives (Bakhtin 1981). When these dialogues are congruent the nurse can enter communication with clarity and purpose, however sometimes it is difficult to simultaneously integrate conflicting internal and external perspectives (for example; those of the nurse, the person in care, professional and societal discourses) and the nurse struggles to know how to interpret, in a meaningful way, the stories and expressions of mental distress that are presented. Contending dialogues can lead to a struggle to integrate and move forward in communication. While these internal and external perceptions may sometimes be conflictual, their presence offers each person in the interaction the opportunity for transformation and development of understandings. The nurse needs to configure these multiple perspectives in self and environment so that s/he can make sense of situations and find ways of engaging in therapeutic interaction. It is through the struggle to integrate these dialogues that the nurse enters into meaningful engagement with the person in care.

In this chapter, using case vignettes from teaching and therapeutic research, the authors explore ways in which inner and outer dialogues are at play as the mental health nurse attempts to make sense of the experiences of mental pain narrated by people in her/his care. Through making some of these dialogues visible and audible, we hope to encourage mental health nurses to examine their own constructions regarding the nature of peoples' experiences of mental pain and to explore helpful ways of engaging with people in these situations. Engaging with multiple perspectives, particularly in a context where certain discourses are privileged, can be challenging, however we argue that when internal and external dialogues within the nurse and her environment interact, it is not just productive, but is essential to a therapeutic relationship and that when these voices are silenced, opportunities are missed and therapeutic impasse occurs in the relationship (Rober 1999).

The authors propose two interlinked communication strategies for engaging with the tensions between apparently conflicting dialogues, the use of which can lead to transformative learning and unanticipated communicative opportunities. These approaches include cultivating a disposition of curiosity (Cecchin 1987) and creating dialogic space (Anderson & Goolishian 1992).

Meaning Making through Dialogue

Part of being human involves interaction with a complex social and relational environment. We are embedded in a multi-vocal, pluralistic milieu and through our engagement we encounter experiences that are satisfying, troubling, limiting and enlightening. We constantly strive to make sense of these multi-dimensional experiences in order to create meaningful accounts of our worlds and our places therein (Mishler 2004). It is argued that we organise our experiences into mental stories about ourselves and thus construct narratives of our lives through time (Bruner 1987, Ricoeur 1991). In this process, often confusing impressions and happenings are configured into life episodes that are in keeping with other prevailing themes of an overall narrative thread. This meaning making is dialogical in nature as we look to available cultural and social understandings and beliefs to help us construct our sense of self and our experiences within a given culture Bakhtin (1981). Langellier (1989 p260) asserts that "narratives are jointly produced by tellers and listeners who are 'social actors' whose 'social and cultural matrices' are marked by gender, age race class and professional status." We share stories to know that we are not alone and the ways in which people respond to our stories further shapes our understandings and the next performance of the story. Bakhtin (1981) claims that there is an interplay between the embodied and the social elements of the self, between intimate discourses, inner speaking and bodily practices formed in the past and the discourses and practices to which people are exposed, in their social environments, in the present (Holland et al 2003). Bakhtin (1981) refers to the process of configuring and making sense of these inner and outer dialogues of the self as the "orchestration of voices" or "self authoring."

Mental illness and/or trauma can bring about a break in the narrative thread as the person's personal and social construction of self is challenged by events/experiences that are difficult to incorporate into ones' existing narrative structure Crossley (2000). These experiences fall outside the persons expectations of themselves and represent 'biographical disruption' (Sandelowski 1994) or 'narrative wreckage' (Frank 1995). As a response to the interruption, people attempt to incorporate this new phenomenon into the narrative of self by reconfiguring or re-storying their lives to accommodate it. Invariably, available cultural explanations are called upon to help in this sense making process.

People who experience mental health issues and people who care for them operate within this landscape of dialogical meaning making and identity construction through cultural stories and self stories. In the same way that the experience of altered mental state needs to be configured into a coherent sense of self for the person experiencing this phenomenon, the experience of being a nurse needs to be storied into a meaningful sense of self and purpose as a professional. In these endeavours, many disparate voices, discourses and possible ways of knowing and being resonate from within and around the mental health nurse and the other(s) in the therapeutic encounter. Bakhtin (1981) claims that in the sense making process, individuals engage with varied, often conflicting dialogues simultaneously. As Mishler (2004 p118) argues "each person has multiple perspectives on the same event, and the one that comes into play depends on variations in contexts, audiences and intentions, that is, how one positions oneself within that set of circumstances."

Dialogues and Discourses at Play for Mental Health Nurses

Some publicly declared imperatives suggest that the nurse should be objective, empirical and able to detach from the influences of personal bias and cultural stereotype (Koh 1999, Hawthorne and Yurkovich 2002). However, it is also acknowledged that individuals develop in environments that shape their views and beliefs and that they interpret and process experiences in many different ways. Crowe (1998 p87) suggests that

"The personal and professional values of mental health nurses, their beliefs about human nature, their educational and experiential background, their emotional experiences and modes of expression, and the way they perceive the self in relation to others all influence the fundamental mental health nursing skill – the therapeutic use of self in the nurse patient relationship."

These factors influence the nurse's perception of mental illness/distress and his/her beliefs as to how (or whether) people with mental health issues can be helped. The nurse's personal and cultural experiences and perceptions come into contact with professional belief systems as s/he engages with the professional socialisation process of nursing and healthcare. The nurse looks to this socially sanctioned knowledge as a means of configuring her/his own myriad impressions of what it may mean to have mental health problems and what it may mean to be a nurse (Stickley and Timmons 2007). In this way the nurse incorporates prevailing discourses into her/his own meaning making and narrative of self. According to Crowe (2000 p962); "particular types of knowledge and ways of acting are sanctioned by the nursing culture in order to ensure its continued existence and to reproduce the existing social order." One example of a type of knowledge sanctioned by nursing culture is the biomedical construction of mental distress. Within this framework mental disorder is seen as indicative of disease or mental illness and therefore amenable to medically influenced treatments. Experiences of mental distress are grouped into sets of symptoms which are viewed as characteristic of various types of mental illness (Collier 2008). The acceptance of these classifications of normality and abnormality means that biomedical explanations become a dominant discourse. Dominant discourses function to impose order on diverse phenomena, however the emphasis on homogeneity can mean that individual perceptions and personal knowledge of mental distress are marginalized and subsumed into a monologue that claims to explain and categorise all experiences of mental dis-order. (Sakayls (2000, Walsh et al 2008). Within mental health nursing, privileging of biomedical discourse can dominate therapeutic practice and prescribe how experiences of mental pain are to be constructed and understood (Harper 1994,Crowe 2006).

The literature also highlights how discourses of gender dominate and shape both socialization in nursing and the construction of meanings of mental distress (Evans, 2004). Nurses, as a predominately female profession, are expected to embody "womanly" attributes of caring and subservience within a healthcare system that is patriarchal in nature. (Fealy 2004). In this context, many nurses argue, individual women's voices and ways of knowing both as nurses and people with mental health problems are marginalized. Stoppard (1997). In relation to the influence of gendered discourse in ascribing meaning to women's mental distress, Busfield (1996 p117) states:

"Since gender is such a key feature of social relations and a major dimension of social difference, gender inevitably features in the constructions of mental disorder."

The causes and experiences of mental distress vary for each individual, however women's experiences of mental pain are often categorized using parameters that reflect male dominated (phallocentric) assumptions, reasoning and language (Harden 2000, Warne and McAndrew (2007). For example, Sayce (2000 p110) claims that including pre-menstrual disorder into the criteria in the Diagnostic and Statistical Manual of Mental Disorders (1994) subjugated other experiences and meanings of mental distress among women by creating a "syndrome" that "made half a million more women pathological at a stroke." This privileged set of beliefs has implications in relation to how the nurse positions self as gendered and how s/he hears and interprets the voices and stories of female and male persons in interaction (Munro and Baker 2007)

Similarly, the influences of race, culture and class identities are seen as inherent in the formulation and expression of meaning (Fernando 1991, Sandelowski 1994, Hinton and Levkoff 1999). Just as patriarchal gender relations can constrain female meanings, so Western assumptions about normality can silence alternative dialogues from service users and nurses from other cultures.

The following vignette from an education context in an Irish university, encountered by one of the authors, highlights the difficulties inherent in appropriating dominant discourses as the only means of interpreting experiences. The scenario described occurred among a cohort of undergraduate mental health nursing students who were using role play to evoke and explore possible experiences of mental distress and therapeutic interventions. One group comprised of four African female students who had chosen 'depression' as their exploratory theme. The group improvised a situation where a woman experienced 'deep sadness' following the birth of her baby. Thus a scenario was enacted where the sad woman (student A) was visited in her home by three neighbours (students B, C, and D). The neighbours brought baskets of food, tidied the house and sat with the sad woman conversing about local events and making practical arrangements for sharing the care of her children while she was sad. The woman sometimes joined in these conversations, sometimes not, but the conversations continued regardless. The woman was not the main subject of the conversation, no-one directly focused on her state of depression, however, her plight of sadness was acknowledged in a pragmatically supportive way. There was no 'resolution' to the students' scenario and one felt that they would have continued talking for a lengthy period were it not for time constraints.

This dramatic re-presentation stimulated much debate and discussion. Questions were raised such as: "Where was the mental health intervention? Would these 'friends' not consider referring this woman, who probably had a diagnosis of post-natal depression, to a mental health practitioner?" "Perhaps she needed a full psychiatric assessment, may be suicidal or may harm the baby? Perhaps she required admission to hospital?" The African women explained that such responses would not occur in their culture, but neighbours, family and friends would provide support. This fuelled further questions: "Was that because it was a poor country? Was support provided by well meaning but unskilled networks because there were few statutory mental health services in place?" The students replied that the woman's sadness would not be seen as something that was appropriate for medical treatment, but rather this sadness had a spiritual cause and the woman would go to a spiritual healer. This different perspective lead to further debate, such as: "What about treatment of depression? Don't you have depressed people in psychiatric hospitals?" The African nurses explained further that in their country the term 'depression' is not used, instead the woman's problem is called 'kufungisisa' which means "thinking too much," while psychiatric hospitals "are for mad people; people who are out of control."

The students in this class had studied, practiced and discussed mental health nursing together for two years, yet this was the first time that their very different perspectives and cultural backgrounds regarding mental illness and "appropriate" care had been shared among the group. Why was this? The African students, although a distinct cohort within the larger group, had submerged themselves into Western constructions of mental distress based on biomedical paradigms, classifications and language, a "slipping" also observed by Stickley and Timmons (2007), yet their own experiences, beliefs and understandings were something other. They had never disclosed these perceptions to the wider student group as they felt these understandings were somehow alien, incorrect or would not be useful or appreciated within their current context of learning about mental illness. Many of the western students were unaware of the differing perspectives of their colleagues and had presumed consensus of attitudes and beliefs in the class based largely on biomedical principles. When the facilitator considered this matter she realized that the curriculum and teaching methods supported and indeed fostered this homogeneity, a view echoed by Chevannes (2002) and Purden (2005). The students' presentation stimulated inquiry, challenged taken for granted perceptions and helped other students in the class to articulate and discuss some of their own experiences and beliefs which had hitherto been assigned to a marginal status.

This vignette is offered not to dispute or assert the 'correctness' of any particular understanding of mental distress over another but rather to suggest that when a group of meanings become privileged they are invested with perceptions of truth and knowledge and that alternative perspectives that do not fit with the privileged model must be suppressed. According to Foucault (1995 pxiii); "the language of psychiatry, which is a monologue of reason about madness, has been established only on the basis of such a silence." This process of suppression happens in most areas of life and is often unchallenged, but in mental health nursing where finding meaning in experiences is one of the prime motivations of both mental health nurses and people in care, such unchallenged, one dimensional assumptions can be problematic. The scenario presented here, and many others like it, demonstrates the difficulty for nurses in configuring the inner voices of their personal gendered experiences, beliefs, history and culture and their interactions with people in care with prevailing "explanatory" and prescriptive frameworks.

The Voice(s) of the Person in Care

Many of the issues facing nurses also confront the person who is experiencing mental health problems; the desire to order confusion, alleviate pain and gain personal knowledge and mastery. People in mental pain and distress may be attempting to make sense of unusual overwhelming voices in their heads (England 2007, Leudar and Thomas 2000), their inner voices of negativity and fear, (Jones 1999) and the voices, expectations and sometimes censure of family and society (Sayce 2000). Like nurses, people with mental health problems construct meaning in these experiences incorporating a range of influences and explanatory frameworks, for example, some people with mental health problems find biomedical explanations of their distress useful, they perceive that they are experiencing an illness or disease and take comfort in the ability of mental health trained professionals to help them. (Hinton and Levkoff 1999). Brown at al (1996 p 1578) claim that "clients' descriptions of their problems are already storied along psychiatric lines." For others, the mental dis-order is spiritual in nature; spirits are communicating through them, perhaps punishing them for past deeds or they perceive themselves to be in spiritual crisis and this needs to be resolved through spiritual means (Wilding et al 2006). Carone and Barone (2001 p989) state that "religious beliefs provide order and understanding to an otherwise chaotic and unpredictable world." Other people believe that their distress is a manifestation of personal, familial, cultural crisis and that healing/recovery needs to be achieved at this level (Chanp 1999, Sarason and Duck 2000). Some people who come into mental health services may not believe that they have any mental health issues but rather are being distressed by external forces (Leudar and Thomas 2000). Some of these explanatory frameworks may sustain a positive conception of self and the world and aid recovery while some may be unhelpful to the person in moving beyond distress.

People in mental distress bring their stories and performances to mental health nurses as well as their expectations and hopes for how the nurse can help them. Their expectations of nurses will also be shaped by societal discourses as well as the person's previous experiences of nurses and mental health care. Crowe (2000) argues that there is hierarchical differentiation in many mental health care relationships, the person with mental health issues is positioned as a 'patient', the person asking for help and therefore less powerful than the care-giver. She further claims that nurses and patients are expected to interact in predictable ways with each other, the nurse, as competent practitioner guiding the intervention and the patient amenable to the nurse's interventions. This hierarchical differentiation and appropriation of power through "knowledge" or "expertise" has come under increasing pressure in contemporary mental health care contexts. Information technology, improved mental health awareness among the general public and the rise of service user and recovery movements with their accompanying critique of privileged constructions of mental disorder and mental health practices (Lindlow 1996, Bee et al 2008) have meant that many people experiencing mental health issues are more likely to pursue dialogue around the nature of their distress rather than appropriating dominant discourses to account for their own individual situations (Barker et al 1999). In contemporary mental health nursing, much work has been done to challenge disempowering constructions of mental distress and treatment (Warne and McAndrew 2007 Barry 2007). The philosophies of poststructuralist thinkers such as Foucault (1980, 1995) have helped nurses to recognize and deconstruct some of the discourses of knowledge and power that operate within the constructions of mental illness, "nurse- patient" interactions and health care systems and to develop ways of exploring and interacting with the experiences of people in mental pain in ways that respect and therapeutically integrate the person's perceptions and strengths (Shanley and Jubb-Shanley 2007, Crowe et al 2008) However, the mental health nurse may find her/himself in the presence of service user voices that distrust the 'psychiatric system' and these interactions can be complex and challenging, given that the nurse is positioned as a representative of what is often seen as a repressive dominant discourse. The following vignette exemplifies this situation. The extract presented here is taken from a larger research study conducted by one of the authors (Casey and Long 2002). That study explored the narratives of mental health services users in relation to their understandings of their mental distress. This conversation occurs between David (D), a research participant and mental health service user and the researcher (B) who identified herself to David as a nurse teacher.

D: Well, what happened to me? I believe it came back to teenage years. My recollection is that within the family until the age of about ten or eleven I felt secure and happy

B: O K

D: But then when it came to teenage years there was just a blank wall in front of me. Nobody talked to me about teenage years, nobody used to talk about teenage years, in fact it was the reverse, nobody wished to talk about it at all, and I was really wanting to know about what was happening my body and what was happening me but there was no, including doctors, they never talked about the teenage years at all. And I believe they're critical to my own personal development

B: Right

D: But they were never talked about. Even to this day I asked for talk therapy with a doctor or some social worker and the chance of me getting it are very slim and I read about a survey that was carried out on four thousand six hundred patients or service users who take tablets in England and they said that the worst tablet they take is Haloperidol, that's the worst from the user's point of view…But nobody has talked to me intimately about the drug and its effects on the personality and you're a tutor and I'm sure you tell your nurses the truth about the drug but you don't tell the users that truth, you see I don't think you do, you can correct me on this by saying do you tell the users what the drug does to them by how does it affect them sexually and things like that and it does have a big effect sexually on people

B: Yeah, it does

D: But no-one does talk about it. It's just a blind wall you come up against and I'm not being helped by it and yet I'm still on the drug and if I get a little bit annoyed why I'm on the drug it's taken as symptoms not natural annoyance why I'm still on the drug ….. What would you say are the effects of the drug?

B: Well….

D: On you sexually

B: Well, it's well known that the drug…

D: I don't know it! I don't know it! I mean you can tell me now with that microphone on what are the effects that it has sexually on the person. Can you tell me that?

B: Yeah…well the effects that it can have sexually are that it can dampen down people's sexual responses.

D: Dampen down? It takes them away completely….takes them away completely and that was the area in which my problem was in the first place and nobody had… and look at where I am now, but the doctors didn't do anything to help me, all they did was pump tablets into me and give me injections and to this very day I'm talking to you, a tutor and you're not helping me very much either, you're listening to me for your degree or for your diploma and nothing will come of this tape that will help me but it will help you

B: Well that's fair enough David, if you don't want to….

D: It's not fair enough with me, I'd like something to be done about my.. my predicament and I'd like to get talking. I'd like someone to talk to me about my predicament, not always to be giving me injections and tablets. Talk, they said it in the survey that was done in England about four thousand six hundred users, most of them thought talk therapy was very successful and highly recommend it. I never got it

B:Hmmm

D The doctors were all hoity toity up on their high horses, looking down on me and asking me questions and then shutting up and making me feel nervous, they didn't accommodate me at all. And em I feel myself that I will not get talk therapy at all because I'm afraid of doctors and I don't talk too well to them due to my past experiences of them; that's only natural that I should be afraid of them cause they wielded their authority without bringing me into their confidence

In this interaction, many voices contend with each other. David voices his anger and bitterness as he claims the validity of his personal understandings against the 'authority' of the doctors he encountered. In his story one can also hear his grief at lost opportunities, sadness and isolation as he is excluded, not brought "into their confidence." Perhaps his request for "talk therapy" is also a request for dialogue that is meaningful and acknowledging of him as an intelligent man with sexual needs. David presents his knowledge of service user research to help him articulate his anger and distrust of the system that he believes has not allowed him to speak. He positions the researcher as a representative of that system, part of that secret exclusive club, present with tape recorder gathering information for personal study purposes.

This encounter evoked personal responses in the researcher/nurse such as sadness for David, as well as guilt on behalf of a system that he perceived to have caused him so much damage. She also felt frustrated and hurt that he saw her as part of his oppression; like the doctors getting information, diagnosing and medicating, claiming that things which are not explained are common knowledge. The nurse/researcher might share many of his criticisms but because of her position as representative of the health care system feels "duty bound" not to articulate these opinions and thus is also silenced.

The researcher's response, reflected in her comment "Well that's fair enough David, if you don't want to...." implies her anger at David for bringing these issues into consciousness and positioning her in this way. David's challenges evoked in the researcher/nurse feelings of impotence sometimes experienced in the 'caring' role and often resulting in the nurse adopting an authoritative and defensive voice. Experiences of transference and counter transference, the most primitive and personal voices in our dialogues, abound in interactions such as these and result in participants shifting positions and power balances. According to Hammarström (2008 p169) "power can be seen as something that is created and that shifts between the interviewer and the interviewed." David scathingly counters "It's not fair enough with me..." thus highlighting his perception of the injustice and inequality of the interaction/relationship/ health care system.

In addition to these intrapersonal struggles within the interaction, simultaneously more external dialogues were contending for dominance; for example the authority/knowledge claims made by service user research presented by David and the possible psychiatric or "therapeutic" interpretations of David's narrative and articulation of distress. The nurse researcher felt compelled to tick off "psychiatric symptom boxes;" mentally noting, as David related his experiences and opinions, his "pressure of speech," and possible "paranoid delusions." She could also hear such authoritative labels as "narcissistic personality disorder", "skewed family dynamics" and "repressed sexual disorder." Holland et al (2003 p15) comment on the implications of this dialogical wrestling;

> Dialogic perspectives such as Bakhtin's (1981) explicitly free us from the idea that we as a group or as individuals can hold only one perspective at a time. Humans are both blessed and cursed by their dialogic nature - their tendency to encompass a number of views in virtual simultaneity and tension, regardless of their logical incompatibility.

This vignette is offered as an example of the complexity of the interaction that can occur when multiple competing dialogues come into play for the nurse and the person in care. How can the nurse make sense of interactions such as this? How can these personal reactions and professional discourses be configured with the meanings that David is trying to articulate? It can be tempting to allow professional explanatory discourse to dominate; David's mental illness means that his perceptions and judgments may be 'irrational' and therefore less credible. It can be claimed that he lacks insight into his condition. This approach offers an approved systematic framework of constructing David's story that smoothes over both David's and the researcher's troubling voices. Indeed, David refers to this, perhaps customary, professional response when he claims "if I get a little bit annoyed why I'm on the drug it's taken as symptoms not natural annoyance why I'm still on the drug." David's perceptions are thus less powerful as biomedical "knowledge" invalidates personal knowledge. Roberts (2005 p 33), in an examination of Foucault's writing, observes that "power and knowledge are central to the process by which human beings are 'made subjects' and therefore how 'psychiatric identities' are produced."

When one considers the limitation of such interchange it becomes clear that alternative ways must be found around such an impasse. These ways involve being open to hearing all the voices in the dialogue and sitting with the discomfort that can sometimes occur in these interactions. Through exploring these points of discomfort and the understandings and discourses that rub up against one another we can achieve deeper understanding and empathy.

Integrating/Reconciling Multiple Voices

The mental health nurse, given her/his central place in the multidisciplinary team and opportunities of extended contact with the person experiencing mental pain, is in a prime position to influence mental health care practices in significant ways. Some of the challenges associated with including marginalized discourses and integrating competing monologues have been demonstrated in the case vignettes above. These vignettes also demonstrate how the mental health nurse sometimes closes the self off to alternative ways of perceiving and acting in the world. Many writers have considered how and why this closing off takes place. For example Menzies Lyth in the 1950's (Menzies-Lyth 1988) and others since (Lakeman 2006, Evans et al 2008, Tognazzini et al, 2008) have observed in nurses, defensive reactions and the investment in routinised tasks as a form of protection against the anxiety inherent in the professional and interactional work of nursing. Foucault (1980) posits that the power that is invested in dominant discourses and knowledges means that people working in these systems relinquish some of their own agency and contradictory beliefs. Richardson (2000 p517) claims that we are "homogenized" through professional socialization and that through this process our own personal perceptions and understandings are suppressed. Eventually, according to Bourdieu (1997), adherence to the established order leads to habitus - traditional taken for granted practices which are taken as "common sense" and therefore unquestioned; people may not stop to critique their validity. Jones (2005 p1177) claims that unlike other professional therapeutic groups, nursing does not have a 'culture' of personal therapy, which facilitates personal and professional critique and development, thus nurses "…are potentially denied opportunities to understand aspects of their unresolved struggles and perhaps gain a better understanding of ways in which others experience difficulties in human relationships."

Challenging taken-for-granted discourses and traditions may involve risk taking and can be anxiety provoking as hitherto widely accepted practices and perspectives are contested. Therefore, the nurse needs to be able to call upon her/his personal and professional resources in such challenging situations in order to ensure that communication, which is a central component of the mental health nurse's role, remains as constructive as possible. Two interlinked communication strategies, cultivating a disposition of 'curiosity' (Cecchin 1987), and creating 'dialogic space' (Anderson & Goolishian 1992) are proposed as key elements in managing the tension between contending dialogues. Each of these will be discussed further in the following sections.

A Disposition of curiosity

Within therapeutic practice a tension exists between the desire to explore the lived experiences of the other, and the orientation towards capturing that experience, defining it and making it amenable to therapeutic intervention. Nurses are acutely aware of the importance of collating objective data, such as the psychiatric history and observable signs and symptoms of mental illness / dis-order in order to make accurate assessments and formulate relevant care plans. This impetus is based on the premise that mental distress / illness can be observed, explained, defined and categorized and then treated on the basis of this assessment activity. While this model provides direction for the nurse, the person's perceptions of their lived experiences of mental distress can sometimes be lost to the realm of the incidental, as the preconceived medical / nursing discourse is privileged, which undermines genuine interest in the individual's story. An alternative perspective is to be able to accept and live with a degree of ambiguity and uncertainty, challenging the idea that there exists a single objective reality and absolute truth and accepting that sometimes it will be difficult to grasp meanings of experiences and / or to facilitate this meaning making with others. This positioning has been referred to as 'curiosity', or a kind of open-mindedness regarding the process and outcome of communication and the unique story of the other (Cecchin 1987). According to Cecchin (1987) when this curiosity is suppressed, it can hinder the practitioner from genuine engagement with the person's unique story and from considering the multiple possible ways forward. An attitude of curiosity presupposes preparedness to learn and to be surprised and welcoming in relation to all dialogues encountered. Such a position requires that one does not engage in interaction with preconceived ideas about the process and outcome of engagement, instead remaining open to the emergence of unanticipated views and moves. Stimulating and sustaining curiosity and preventing dominance of predetermined professional monologues at the expense of the individual perspective, involves a heightened level of self awareness in the nurse. It is suggested (Peplau 1952, Jack and Miller (2008) that self awareness is a prerequisite for reflective and ethical practice. Within the nursing profession reflective practice, which promotes self awareness and self insight, has long been recognised as an essential tool in the interactive process (Schon 1983, Fejes, 2008, Crowe and O Malley 2006). The nurse must examine and address her/his own internal voices; assumptions, biases and potential for closing off dialogue. (Hammarström 2008) According to Jones (1999 p826):

"Listening to others requires the ability to listen to one's own inner voices and recognize how they might guide exchanges. By avoiding conducting conversations in ways dictated by our own fears, worries and fantasies we can listen, and in doing so allow shifts in awareness."

As Crowe (1998 p87) puts it: "Nurses need to be able to acknowledge how their experiences have influenced who they are and how they interact before they can use their self and their skills to help others." This process involves the nurse recognising and acknowledging his/her own embedded fixed beliefs that possibly constrain understanding of and engagment with alternative narratives. The nurse develops the ability to critically examine and de-construct the dialogues and discourses in which s/he is enmeshed (Collier 2008) as well as seeking out and engaging with those that offer possible alternative ways of understanding mental pain and helping people in mental distress. (Stickley and Timmons 2007). Some writers argue that not only will this openness and exploration facilitate enriched engagement and dialogue with people in care but it will also foster a heightened level of empowerment within the nurse (Udod 2008) as s/he "adopt(s) a more critical stance to understanding power and empowerment in nursing (Bradbury-Jones et al 2008 p258).

Thus, the reflective process suggests a systematic way of reviewing and critiquing one's practice enabling identification of unforeseen possibilities for re-engagement in dialogue and considered anticipation of potential challenges and barriers to forward movement, enhancing a disposition of curious engagement with self and other. This critical process makes it possible for the practitioner to remain in the tension between opposing monologues in order to create dialogic space.

Creating dialogic space

It has been suggested that one of the central challenges in overcoming therapeutic impasse is to be able to remain in the tension between opposing monologues, thereby unpacking the contribution of different perspectives in addition to accommodating hitherto unforeseen commonalities / common ground in purpose if not perspective (Rober 1999). Such an endeavor is built upon openness to different perspectives and courses of action, a curiosity about the views and experiences of the other, and the courage to not only tolerate and accept diversity but to invite it and celebrate its potential for learning. This position does not suggest that the mental health practitioner is without or abandons her/his expertise, personal and professional, that can usefully contribute to the alleviation of mental distress. Rather it suggests that s/he use this expertise informatively rather that impositionally with the person in care (Anderson & Goolishian 1992). Sharing one's expertise in this way challenges the traditional view of the 'expert' knower, who holds knowledge that is fixed and superior to other knowledges. Instead it suggests that the nurse's knowledge is evolving and held as one knowledge among multiple ways of knowing.

Thus, the expert nurse is an expert in creating and managing dialogic space and the tension within this rather than being a problem solver who must avoid or resolve such inevitable tensions. S/he is aware that integration of different conversational voices may not only be impossible at tines but it may indeed not be desirable for the practitioner to seek a coming together of voices when remaining in the tension between these affords greater opportunity for creativity in interaction. This requires that the nurse develop confidence and trust in the sense making dynamics occurring in the therapeutic encounter. S/he shares this dialogical sense making process with the person in interaction and invites people in care to influence the nurses' and others understandings and knowledge regarding the experience of mental distress (Houghton et al 2006, Shanley and Jubb Shanley 2007, Crowe et al 2008). This creation of dialogical space demands greater attention as to what the person in care construes as meaningful and helpful to them in their personal experiences.

Conclusion

There are times when the multiple voices and dialogues in the mental health domain converge into a rich interchange where negotiation of meanings occur leading to a deeper perspectives that provide new opportunities for action. When this dialogic exchange takes place the contributors experience a sense of both inclusion in terms of their own voice being valued and transposition whereby they can appreciate and understand the positions and contributions of the other. However, mental health nurses and people in care often experience discordance or imbalance of voices within interactions which, if not recognized and addressed by the nurse in the therapeutic encounter, can lead to withdrawal or stagnation within the relationship.

Thus, within mental health practice the importance of developing the ability to critically examine and de-construct the dialogues and discourses in which one is embedded, that are possibly constraining to the development of understandings of and engagement with alternative versions of reality, is deemed essential to therapeutic interaction. For example, seeking out and engaging with varying approaches to understanding mental pain and helping people in mental distress.

Within nursing it has been proposed that reflective processes, enhanced by clinical supervision / consultation, facilitate the nurse in incorporating multiple perspectives and engaging openly and creatively in the interactive process. In assisting the nurse to move to a more liberating place in her interactions with self and other, some possible strategies have been proposed for managing this dialogic tension. Such proposals incorporate two interlinked processes, the nurse cultivating curiosity and the desire to explore the multiple perspectives that surround her/him in daily therapeutic practice (Cecchin, 1987), and creating space for genuine dialogue by reflexively and therapeutically utilising the tension between inner and outer voices (Anderson & Goolishian 1992; Rober, 1999).

References

Anderson, H. & Goolishian, H. (1992) The Client is the Expert: A not-knowing approach to therapy, in S. McNamee and KJ. Gergen (eds) *Therapy as Social Construction.*, London: SAGE.

Bakhtin, M. (1981). *The Dialogic Imagination*. University of Texas Press, Austin Texas.

Barker, P., Campbell, P. & Davidson, B. (1999). *From the Ashes of Experience: Reflections on Madness Survival and Growth.*, Whurr, London.

Barry, K. (2007). Collective inquiry: understanding the essence of best practice construction in mental health. *Journal of Psychiatric & Mental Health Nursing.*, *14 (6),* 558-565,

Bee, P., Playle, J., Lovell, K., Barnes, P., Gray, R. & Keeley, P. (2008). Service user views and expectations of UK-registered mental health nurses: a systematic review of empirical research. *International Journal of Nursing Studies.*, Mar; *45(3),* 442-57

Bradbury-Jones, C., Sambrook, S. & Irvine, F. (2008). Power and empowerment in nursing: a fourth theoretical approach. *Journal of Advanced Nursing.*, Apr; *62(2),* 258-66.

Brown, B., Nolan, P., Crawford, P. & Lewis, A. (1996) Interaction, language and the "narrative turn" in psychotherapy and psychiatry. *Social Science and Medicine., 43(11),* 1569-78.

Bruner, J. (1987) Life as Narrative. *Social Research., 54,* 11-32.

Busfield, J. (1996) *Men, women and madness. Understanding Gender and Mental Disorder.*, Macmillan, London.

Carone, D. A. & Jr. Barone, D. F. (2001). A social cognitive perspective on religious beliefs: their functions and impact on coping and psychotherapy. *Clinical Psychology Review., 21(7),* 989-1003.

Casey, B. & Long, A. (2002).. Reconciling voices. *Journal of Psychiatric & Mental Health Nursing., 9(5),* 603-10

Cecchin, G. (1987). Hypothesising, Circularity & neutrality Revisited: An Invitation to Curiosity. *Family Process., Vol. 26, 4,* 405-412

Cixous, H. (1997). *Rootprints: Memory and life writing.* London Routledge.

Champ, S. (1999). A Most Precious Thread. In: *From the Ashes of Experience: Reflections on madness, Survival and Growth.* (eds Barker P., Campbell P., Davidson B.), pp. 113-126. Whurr, London.

Collier, E. (2008). Historical development of psychiatric classification and mental illness. *British Journal of Nursing.*, Jul 24-Aug *13, 17(14),* 890-4

Chevannes, M. (2002).. Issues in educating health professionals to meet the diverse needs of patients and other service users from ethnic minority groups. *Journal of Advanced Nursing., 39,* 290-298.

Crossley, M. (2000). *Introducing Narrative Psychology. Self, trauma and the construction of meaning.* Open University Press, Buckingham.

Crowe, M. (1998). Developing advanced mental health nursing practice: A process of change, *Australian and New Zealand Journal of Mental Health Nursing., 7,* 86-94

Crowe, M. (2000). The nurse-patient relationship: a consideration of its discursive context *Journal of Advanced Nursing., 31(4),* 962-967

Crowe, M. T. & O'Malley, J. (2006). Teaching critical reflection skills for advanced mental health nursing practice: a deconstructive-reconstructive approach. *Journal of Advanced Nursing,* Oct., *56(1),* 79-87

Crowe, M., Carlyle, D. & Farmar, R. (2008). Clinical formulation for mental health nursing practice. *Journal of Psychiatric & Mental Health Nursing*, Dec., *15(10),* 800-7

England, M. (2007). Accuracy of nurses' perceptions of voice hearing and psychiatric symptoms. *Journal of Advanced Nursing*, Apr., *58(2)*, 130-9

Evans, J. (2004). Men nurses: A historical and feminist perspective. *Journal of Advanced Nursing., 47(3)*, 321-328.

Evans, A. M., Pereira, D. A. & Parker, J. M. (2008). Discourses of anxiety in nursing practice: a psychoanalytic case study of the change-of-shift handover ritual. *Nursing Inquiry*, Mar., *15(1)*, 40-8

Fealy, G. (2004). 'The good nurse': visions and values in images of the nurse. *Journal of Advanced Nursing* 46(6), 649–656

Fernando, S. (1991*). Mental Health, Race and Culture* Mind/ Macmillan, London.

Fejes, A. (2008). Governing nursing through reflection: a discourse analysis of reflective practices. *Journal of Advanced Nursing*, Vol. 64 Issue 3, p243-250,

Harden, J. (2000). Language, discourse and the chronotype: applying literary theory to the narratives in health care. *Journal of Advanced Nursing., 31(3)*, 506-512.

Foucault, M. (1980). *Power/knowledge: Selected interviews and other writings*, 1972-1977 Pantheon: New York,

Foucault, M. (1995). *Madness and Civilization: A history of insanity in the age of reason.* London. Tavistock Publications.

Frank, A. (1995). *The Wounded Storyteller: Body, Illness and Ethics.* University of Chicago Press, Chicago.

Hammarström, A. (2008). Shift in power during an interview situation: methodological reflections inspired by Foucault and Bourdieu. *Nursing Inquiry., 15(2)*, 169-76.,

Jack, K. & Miller, E. (2008). Exploring self-awareness in mental health practice. *Mental Health Practice, 12(3)*, 31-5

Jones, A. C (2005). Transference, counter-transference and repetition: some implications for nursing practice, *Journal of Clinical Nursing., 14*, 1177-1184

Jones, A. (1999). 'Listen, listen trust your own strange voice' (psychoanalytically informed conversations with a woman suffering serious illness). *Journal of Advanced Nursing,* Apr., *29(4)*, 826-31

Harden, J. (2000). Language, discourse and the chronotype: applying literary theory to the narratives in health care. *Journal of Advanced Nursing., 31(3)*, 506-512.

Harper, D. J. (1994). The professional construction of "paranoia" and the discursive use of diagnostic criteria. *British Journal of Medical Psychology., 67*, 131-143.

Hawthorne, D. L. & Yurkovich, N. J. (2002). Nursing as science: a critical question. *Canadian Journal of Nursing Research., 34(2)*, 53-64.

Herman, J. L. (1994). *Trauma and Recovery.* New York, Pandora.

Hinton, W. L. & Levkoff, S. (1999). Constructing Alzheimer's: narratives of lost identities, confusion and loneliness in old age. *Culture Medicine and Psychiatry., 23(4)*, 453-75.

Holland, D., Lachicotte, W., Skinner, D. & Cain, C. (2003). *Identity and Agency in Cultural Worlds.* Cambridge Mass, London Harvard University Press.

Houghton, P., Shaw, B., Hayward, M. & West, S. (2006). Psychosis revisited: taking a collaborative look at psychosis. *Mental Health Practice., 9(6)*, 40-43.

Karp, D. A. (1992). Illness, ambiguity and the search for meaning. *Journal of Contemporary Ethnography., 21*, 139-170.

Koh, A. (1999). Non-judgemental care as a professional obligation. *Nursing Standard., 13 (37)*, 38-41.

Lakeman, R. (2006). An anxious profession in an age of fear. *Journal of Psychiatric & Mental Health Nursing., 13(4)*, 395-400

Langellier, K. M. (1989). Personal narratives Perspectives on theory and research. *Text And Performance Quarterly., 9*, 243-276.

Leudar, I. & Thomas, P. (2000). *Voices of Reason, Voices of Insanity. Studies of Verbal Hallucinations.* Routledge, London.

Lindlow, V. (1996). What We Want from Community Psychiatric Nurses. In: *Speaking Our Minds. An anthology.* (eds Read J. & Reynolds J.), 186-190. Open University Press/Macmillan, Milton Keynes.

Menzies-Lyth, I. (1988). The functioning of social systems as a defence against anxiety. In: *Containing Anxiety in Institutions.Selected Essay*s., Vol. 1 (ed Menzies-Lyth, I.), 43-85. Free Association Books, London.

Mishler, E. G. (2004). Historians of the self: Restorying lives revising identities. *Research in Human development 1: 1&2* 101-121.

Munro, S. & Baker, JA. (2007). Surveying the attitudes of acute mental health nurses. *Journal of Psychiatric & Mental Health Nursing, 14(2)*, 196-202

Peplau, H. (1952). Interpersonal relations in nursing New York Putman

Purden, M. (2005). Cultural considerations in interprofessional education and Practice *Journal of Interprofessional Care, 1*, 224-234

Rober, P. (1999). The Therapist's Inner Conversation in Family Therapy Practice: Some Ideas about the Self of the Therapsit, Therapeutic Impasse, and the Process of Reflection. *Family Process.*, Vol. 37, 2, 209-228

Roberts, M. (2005). The production of the psychiatric subject: power, knowledge and Michel Foucault. *Nursing Philosophy., 6(1)*, 33-42

Richardson, L. (2000). Writing: A method of inquiry. In NK Denzin & YS Lincoln (eds) *Handbook of Qualitative Research* (2nd edn) Thousand Oaks CA Sage.

Ricoeur, P. (1991). The human experience of time and narrative. In: *A Ricoeur Reader: Reflection and Imagination.* (ed Waldes M.), 88-116. Harvester Wheatsheaf, New York.

Sakalys, J. (2000). The political role of illness narratives. *Journal of Advanced Nursing., 31(6)*, 1469-1475.

Sandelowski , M. (1994). We are the stories we tell. Narrative knowing in nursing practice. *Journal of Holistic Nursing., 12(1)*, 23-33.

Sarason, B. & Duck, S. (2000). *Personal relationships: Implications for Clinical and Community Psychology.*, Routledge Keegan Paul, New York.

Sayce, L. (2000). *From Psychiatric Patient to Citizen.* Macmillan, London..

Shanley, E. & Jubb-Shanley, M. (2007). The recovery alliance theory of mental health nursing. *Journal of Psychiatric & Mental Health Nursing., 14(8)*, 734-743,

Stoppard, J. (1997). Women's bodies, women's lives and depression: towards a reconciliation of material and discourse accounts. In: *Body Talk: The material and Discursive Regulation of Sexuality, Madness and Reproduction.* (ed Usher J.), pp. 10-32. Routledge, London.

Stickley, T. & Timmons, S. (2007). Considering alternatives: student nurses slipping directly from lay beliefs to the medical model of mental illness. *Nurse Education Today.*, *27(2)*, 155-61.

Tognazzini, P., Davis, C., Kean, A., Osborne, M. & Wong, K. k. (2008). Reducing the stigma of mental illness. *Canadian Nurse.*, *104(8)*, 30-3

Udod, S. A. (2008). The power behind empowerment for staff nurses: using Foucault's concepts. *Canadian Journal of Nursing Leadership.*, *21(2)*, 77-92.

Walsh, J., Stevenson, C., Cutliffe, J. & Zinck, K. (2008). Creating a space for recovery-focused psychiatric nursing care. *Nursing Inquiry.*, *15*, *3*, 251-259.

Warne, T. & McAndrew, S. (2007). Bordering on insanity: misnomer, reviewing the case of condemned women. *Journal of Psychiatric & Mental Health Nursing.*, *14(2)*, 155-62

Wilding, C., Muir-Cochrane, E. & May, E. (2006). Treading lightly: spirituality issues in mental health nursing. *International Journal of Mental Health Nursing.*, *15(2)*, 144-52

In: Nursing Issues: Psychiatric Nursing, Geriatric Nursing…   ISBN: 978-1-60741-598-5
Editors: C. D. McLaughlin et al., pp. 193-212   © 2010 Nova Science Publishers, Inc.

Chapter VI

Two New Developments in the Treatment of Burnout

Y. Meesters and C. J. M. van Velzen

University Medical Centre Groningen, The Netherlands.

Abstract

In modern societies, work-stress and burnout complaints are increasingly leading to higher levels of absentee rates at work. Although burnout is not a classified psychiatric disorder, there is a large amount of co-morbidity with psychiatric disorders such as affective disorders. Therefore it is hardly surprising that mental health workers have developed treatment modalities for people suffering from these complaints. This chapter will describe two new developments in the treatment of burnout complaints at the Department of Psychiatry of the University Medical Center Groningen in the Netherlands.

1. In a research project, the effects of light in the treatment of the emotional exhaustion of the burnout syndrome were investigated. The preliminary conclusions of this small pilot study are promising: subjective energy levels increased.
2. At the clinic, a multidisciplinary day-care programme was developed to treat the burnout syndrome. Taking the principles of cognitive behaviour therapy and activation as a starting point, patients developed new coping strategies and social skills in order to become less vulnerable in their daily life and work situations. The effects of this programme were assessed during the programme and in a follow-up session a year later. A significant reduction in burnout symptoms was seen with 74.7 % of the participants being at work one year after having finished the programme.

Introduction

Work is known to play an important role in psychological health and wellbeing (Blustein, 2008). Job dissatisfaction may lead to work-related stress and psychological and physical dysfunctioning. In modern society, work stress and burnout cause an increasing amount of absentee rates.

In the Netherlands, for example, absence caused by work-related psychological problems is a serious matter. 35% of all people unable to work have mental problems (Houtman et. al., 2007). Stress and emotional exhaustion do not only lead to impaired functioning on the job (Maslach and Schaufeli, 1993; Taris, 2006), but also to other problems, such as a significant increase of sick leave (Bekker et. al., 2005). In 36 % of cases, work pressure and work-related stress are the initial reasons for being absent from work and in 10% for conflicts with colleagues, the management or both (Bakhuys-Roozeboom et al., 2009).

As mentioned above, the most well-known work-related complaint is burnout, which has become a serious social problem, with about 4 % of the working population in the Netherlands suffering from severe burnout complaints (Bakker et al., 2000).

After having defined the burnout syndrome, we will describe two new developments in the treatment of burnout: light therapy and day treatment.

Burnout

Burnout (BO) is a prolonged response to chronic emotional and interpersonal stressors on the job, and is defined by three dimensions: exhaustion, cynicism and inefficacy (Maslach et al., 2001). The core symptom of burnout is emotional exhaustion (Maslach and Schaufeli, 1993). This symptom in particular leads to impaired functioning on the job (Taris, 2006). Emotional exhaustion is also known to lead to a significant increase of sick leave (Bekker et al., 2005).

The term *burnout* is introduced as a metaphor for a work-related state of being emotionally exhausted and overstressed. By definition, burnout complaints are associated with disfunctioning on the job, with people who have severe burnout complaints being unable to continue their normal work routines.

Although severe burnout complaints constitute an emotional state with serious consequences to the individual, this syndrome has not – so far – been included in any psychiatric classification system. For this reason, mental healthcare institutions are often confused as to accepting and understanding the diagnosis of burnout.

This confusion is increased by the fact that the symptoms of the burnout syndrome overlap with those of a number of psychiatric syndromes, particularly those of depression and emotional exhaustion, as described by Schaufeli and Enzman (1998). In a meta-analysis, Glass and McKnight (1996) concluded that burnout and depressive symptoms were not just two different terms for the same dysphoric state nor that they were redundant, mutually exclusive concepts (also see, Schaufeli and Enzman, 1998; Bakker et al., 2000; Schaufeli et al., 2001,Ahola et al., 2005; Sonnenschein et al., 2007a).

When looking for a diagnosis, healthcare professionals pragmatically select a psychiatric diagnosis from any classification system which has the largest overlap of symptoms with those of burnout complaints. A common definition of burnout is the ICD-10 (WHO, 1994) diagnosis of work-related neurasthenia (Schaufeli and Enzmann, 1998; Schaap et al., 2001; Schaufeli et al., 2001).

Others use the DSM-IV diagnosis of undifferentiated somatoform disorder, because of the major problem of exhaustion (Schaap et al., 2001).

Although there is little empirical evidence of successful treatment of burnout, activation and cognitive behavioural therapy (CBT) are common treatment procedures (Schaufeli and Enzmann, 1998; Schaap et al., 2001; Willert et al., 2009). These treatments are administered in outpatient clinics or in special, protocolised programmes offered by specialised therapists. Some patients have benefited by this type of programmes, others have not benefited at all or only partially.

The most distinct symptom of the burnout syndrome is emotional exhaustion, the lack of energy (Taris, 2006). Individuals suffering from severe burnout experience a continuous, severe fatigue throughout the day; something which is uncommon in healthy persons (Sonnenschein et al., 2007b). Emotional exhaustion or fatigue is one of the central issues of this chapter.

Light Therapy

Light therapy has been the most successful treatment for people with seasonal affective disorder so far. It has also been shown that mood is not the only aspect that can be improved by light treatment, but that the same holds for energy levels (Rosenthal et al., 1984; Meesters et al., 1993; Avery et al., 2001; Wileman et al., 2001; Golden et al., 2005). In a case study we have described a patient with seasonal fatigue (without mood disorder), who underwent successful treatment by exposure to light (Meesters and Lambers, 1990). In healthy people, exposure to bright light has improved energy levels (Rüger et al., 2005). Similarly, in people who are seriously ill, a relationship has been shown between fatigue and exposure to light during chemotherapy or treatments of the same type (Liu et al., 2005).

We assumed that energy deficits make it difficult for people to benefit from therapy. If it were possible to improve energy levels after exposure to bright light. It was hypothesised that energy levels of patients with burnout complaints could also be improved after exposure to bright light.

In a pilot study, we investigated the effects in burnout sufferers of light therapy on emotional exhaustion compared to a waiting list condition (Meesters and Waslander, 2009).

Day Treatment

We developed a day treatment programme for patients with severe work-related psychological complaints, who were not expected to derive adequate benefit from an outpatient programme or who desired a more intensive type of treatment.

The goal of this treatment was to analyse patients' personal qualities and vulnerabilities when functioning on the job and for patients to learn new coping strategies and social skills in order to make them less vulnerable in stressful situations. We assessed the first results of this treatment programme in several ways en presented the results elsewhere (Meesters et al., 2009). Patients with different work-related complaints were included in the programme, not just those suffering from burnout. For this chapter we selected patients from this group who were suffering from burnout and we will present the results of this sub-group here.

The day treatment programme was developed and based on the principles of CBT, combined with non-verbal therapy and activation (Meesters et al., 2009). Patients were included when they had a job to return to. Patients with severe psychiatric disorders were excluded from the study.

The treatment programme was offered to groups of 5-8 participants and consisted of nine 8-hour days for the duration of a 13-week period. The treatment was scheduled in two 4-week periods during which the group came together one whole day once a week. Between these two periods, one or two individual sessions were scheduled in another 4-week period. In these individual sessions the first steps in the reintegration process took place. After this intermezzo, participants were expected to be actively engaged in the reintegration to their jobs and group treatment continued in the second period. The programme finished at the end of the second period. Four weeks after the programme had finished a booster day with cognitive therapy, a reintegration session and psychological assessments completed the programme. A follow-up session was scheduled one year after completion of the programme to assess the effects of the treatment. Patients filled out psychological questionnaires and participated in a group session to report about their functioning on the job.

The days of the programme each consisted of four 90-minute sessions. Between sessions, group members had coffee, tea or lunch together, without the therapists being present, which made the total length of the treatment day 8 hours.

The first period

The programme started with an introduction and psycho-education. Every second session of this 4-day period consisted of psychomotor therapy. This therapy was included in the programme for several reasons. In people with burnout complaints activation is known to be an effective treatment modality (Schaap et al., 2001). A protocol was developed in which different aspects of working situations were practised, such as cooperating with others, coping with limited energy levels, coping with work pressure. The sessions were videotaped for feedback of the highlights in the next session.

Cognitive therapy is an important part of the treatment (Schaap et al., 2001), as is stress management (including time management and life style aspects). In the first period, both strategies were included in the treatment every day. In two additional sessions, the qualities and limitations of the patients' functioning on the job were investigated and discussed. Role playing was frequently used together with videotaped feedback. Also, one reintegration session was scheduled to prepare patients for the reintegration steps that were to follow in the next period.

In between periods

After the first 4-week treatment period, another 4-week period was scheduled without group programme in which participants took the first steps towards the reintegration process. One or two individual therapeutic sessions supported this activity.

The second period

After this intermezzo, the second part of the group programme focussed on aspects of the participants' personality that influence their functioning on the job. In additional sessions, interpersonal strategies related to coping with conflicts were exercised using role plays and videotaped feedback. The cognitive therapy continued during the second period. Art therapy was used as a non-verbal treatment procedure to gain insight into different aspects of functioning in a job (cooperating with others, working with a dominant colleague, protecting your position, etc). Finally, sessions were held concerning the actual reintegration process, and developing a relapse prevention plan, which was designed to protect participants from relapsing in the future. Participants were also stimulated to look for a "job coach" from their own social circle who would be able to support them in their reintegration process during the following months.

Methods

In both studies participants were diagnosed by an experienced clinical psychologist. As a definition for burnout we used the criteria of neurasthenia according to the ICD 10 which had to be work-related. This diagnosis had to be confirmed after a short standardised clinical interview for DSM-IV (APA, 1994) and ICD-10 psychiatric disorders (Mini International Neuropsychiatric Interview (M.I.N.I.), Sheehan et al., 1998), with an extra set of questions about burnout complaints containing the criteria of work-related neurasthenia from the ICD-10.Complaints are work-related if they impair a person's ability to work.

Patients filled out a battery of psychological questionnaires using a computer program.

Participants who were depressed according to the DSM-IV as assessed by means of the M.I.N.I., were excluded in order to minimize the overlap between burnout complaints and depression.

Light therapy

In order to be included in the light therapy study, patients did not just have to have the diagnosis of burnout, but also had to score at least 3 on the emotional exhaustion subscale of the UBOS (Utrechtse BurnOut Schaal, Schaufeli & Van Dierendonck, 2000) in order to be included in the light therapy study.

After they had been included and had given informed consent, participants were assigned to one of the two conditions. In other studies, it has proved impossible, however, to create a real placebo condition for light treatment. For this reason, the effects of light treatment are often compared to those of other treatment modalities or to waiting list conditions. In this pilot study we have compared the results of the treatment condition to those of a waiting list condition.

This trial took 22 days, starting on Fridays. After 3 baseline days, participants in the treatment condition were offered light treatment on 5 workdays, no light treatment during the weekend, and another 5 days of light treatment, after which they were monitored for another 7 days. Participants in the waiting list condition were assessed in the same way as those of the treatment condition, but were not given light treatment. Participants in the waiting list condition received light treatment the week after the investigation period had finished.

Participants of the treatment condition were exposed to artificial bright light (full spectrum, without UV, 10,000 lux) at the clinic for 45 minutes on weekdays from 8.00-8.45 a.m. from December 2005 till September 2006.

This treatment was based on the treatment protocol of our SAD outpatient clinic and on SAD research protocols we had used before (Gordijn et al., 2006).

Participants were assessed by weekly self-rating questionnaires they filled out at the clinic.

This research protocol had been approved by the hospital's medical ethical committee.

Day treatment

In the present day treatment study, a selection was taken from the participants of the day treatment programme (Meesters et al., 2009) based on UBOS- emotional exhaustion (UBOS-EE) scores. According to the UBOS manual, burnout sufferers show high scores on the subscale of emotional exhaustion and either high scores at the depersonalisation subscale or low scores on the lack of personal accomplishment subscale (Schaufeli and Van Dierendonck, 2000). Patients with an emotional exhaustion score of at least 2.2, and a depersonalization score of at least 2 or a lack of personal accomplishment score of 3.66 at the highest, were included. These figures are based on the UBOS manual.

In this natural field study we looked for the answers to the following question: is the treatment programme effective as measured by the self-rating scales at three assessment times, but also reflected in the number of working hours on the job?

Assessment and Instruments

In addition to the standardised interview used to assess a diagnosis according to the DSM-IV (APA, 1994) the following questionnaires were filled out by patients in both studies:

UBOS

The UBOS (Utrecht's Burnout School; Schaufeli & Van Dierendonk, 2000) is a Dutch version of the Maslach Burnout Inventory (MBI, Maslach and Jackson, 1981), which assesses job-related burnout complaints and divides them into three subscales: emotional exhaustion, depersonalization and lack of professional accomplishment. These items all refer to the work situation.

SFQ

The SFQ (Shortened Fatigue Questionnaire; Alberts et al., 1997) is a short, reliable and easily used instrument to determine the intensity of patients' bodily fatigue.

BDI-II-NL

Although patients diagnosed with depression according to the DSM-IV criteria were excluded, some distortion of mood could still be shown. Therefore, the BDI-II-NL, the Dutch version of the Beck Depression Inventory (Beck et al., 1996; 2002) was used to assess the severity of the depressive mood.

Additionally, the following questionnaires were filled out in the day treatment study:

SCL-90-R

The Symptom CheckList-90 Revised version (Derogatis, 1977; Dutch translation and adaptation: Arrindell and Ettema, 2003) is a self-report inventory designed to screen for psychological distress and global psychopathology during the past week. This instrument does not just give an overall score but also contains 8 sub-scales: anxiety, agoraphobia, depression, somatization, obsessive-compulsive symptoms, paranoid ideation, hostility and sleeping problems.

IOA

The IOA (Inventarisatielijst Omgang met Anderen, Van Dam-Baggen and Kraaimaat, 1987) is a self-rating questionnaire used to assess social skills in two ways. Firstly, the frequencies with which social skills are used in different social situations and secondly, tensions experienced by the patient when social skills are used.

UCL

The UCL (Utrechtse Coping Lijst, Schreurs et al., 1993) is a self-report questionnaire which assesses the way people generally react when confronted with problems or unpleasant situations. It contains seven independent subscales measuring: active problem focusing (analyzing problems, acting confidently and in a goal-directed way), palliative reaction pattern (looking for distraction, relaxation, seeking diversions), avoidance (complying in order to avoid problematic situations, adopting a waiting attitude), support-seeking (seeking comfort and sympathy), worrying (being preoccupied with problems, brooding, feeling unable to act), emotional expression (showing frustrations) and comforting cognition (encouraging oneself, creating soothing thoughts).

Light therapy

In the light therapy study, the psychological self-report questionnaires were filled out on a weekly basis. The scores at day 1 and day 22 were used for the comparison in this chapter. The score on the emotional exhaustion subscale of the UBOS was used as an inclusion criterion (score 3 or higher) and outcome measurement.

Table 1. Participants

	Treatment	Waiting list	Day treatment
Male/female	8/8	8/6	24/22
Age **	44.6 ± 10.8 yr	45.9 ± 13.0 yr	43.0 ± 9.0 yr
Sick leave	12	12	25
Partial sick leave	3	2	14
Full at work	1		7
Education			
Low	1		8
Middle	6	8	14
High	9	6	24
Hours at work*	13 (n=4)	14 (n=2)	9.3 (n=21)
Winter/summer	6/10	4/10	--

* Average working hours per week of participants who are still (partial) at work
** Mean score ± standard deviation

Day treatment

In the day treatment programme, patients filled out the questionnaires at the start and at the end of the programme and one year later.

The actual hours participants went to work were registered at the three assessment moments.

Statistics

The proportional improvement scores and effect sizes (Cohen, 1988) were calculated and ANOVA with repeated measures was used to calculate levels of significance.

Results

Participants in the light therapy study

The light treatment condition had 16 participants, the waiting list condition 14. Six participants were still at work, with 5 working part-time because of their complaints. The others reported they were unable to continue their jobs due to their burnout complaints (see Table 1). The two conditions did not differ in age, gender, level of education, timing in the season of participation in the design (winter or summer), and hours at work or sick leave. Neither did the two conditions differ in mood and energy levels before the start of the programme as indicated by the scores on the different self-rating scales.

Participants in the day treatment study

Patients suffering from burnout and not suffering from a depression according to the DSM-IV and who filled out questionnaires at the three assessment times were selected from our day treatment programme for patients with severe work-related complaints (Meesters, et al., 2009). 46 patients were included (see table 1). Duration of sick leave varied from 0-110 weeks with a mean of 32.3 weeks (± 31.6) and a median of 21 weeks. Other patient characteristics were: married 54.3 %, divorced 8.7%, living alone 23.9 %; living with partner 30.4%; living with partner and child(ren) 41.3 %; living with child(ren) 2.2%; living with others not mentioned before 2.2 %.

Light Therapy

The improvement after light treatment as compared to that of the waiting list condition is statistically significant according to the scores on the SFQ (F (1, 3) = 3.66, p = 0,03; see Figure 1). The scores on the UBOS emotional exhaustion subscale (F (1, 3) = 2.45, p = 0.09)) show a trend in the same direction. Although the UBOS emotional exhaustion scores also show some improvement in the treatment condition when comparing it to the waiting list condition, this difference is not significant.

Day Treatment

Day treatment yields a statistically significant reduction of complaints over time. The effect sizes of the mood and energy scores on the questionnaires are particularly large (see table 2 and figure 1). Social skills and behaviour also showed improvement over time. Coping strategies only improved very slightly to moderately. Reintegration of participants in their jobs measured a year after the programme had finished amounted to 74.7 % of the original contract hours (see Figure 3).

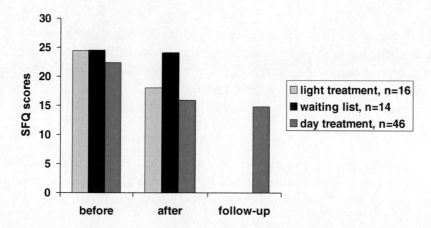

Figure 1. Fatigue scores of the SFQ in the two studies. Before in the light therapy study was the assessment at day 1, after the assessment at day 22 (a week after treatment). Before in the day treatment study was the assessment at the start of the programme, after at the end of the programme, and follow up one year after finishing the programme. The scores in the light treatment condition and the day treatment programme improved significantly (p<0.05).

Participants whose sick leave does not exceed the duration of 21 weeks (median score) show significantly better results in reintegration hours after a year, than those whose sick leave lasts for more than 21 weeks (see Figure 2).

Short vs Long sickness leave

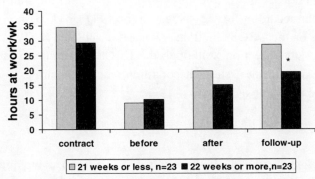

* significant p<0.05

Figure 2. Weekly hours at work at the start and end of the programme and one year later. Contract = weekly hours patients should work according to the contracts with their employers, n=46; 21 weeks or less = a maximum duration of sick leave of 21 weeks; 22 weeks or more = a minimum sick leave duration of 22 weeks.

Emotional exhaustion or fatigue is the most important symptom of the burnout syndrome. Patients with higher levels of fatigue complaints at the start of the programme worked fewer hours than patients with less higher levels of fatigue. The median score on the SFQ was 22.5. If we use this figure to divide the group on the basis of their fatigue, the subgroup with higher levels of fatigue complaints showed higher levels of sick leave of longer duration (see Figure 3).

In the light therapy study, patients were included if they suffered from a certain level of emotional exhaustion as measured by the UBOS. When we apply the same criterion to the day treatment group, this shows that only 6 patients (13%) scored lower than 3 on the UBOS-EE.

The more exhausted patients worked fewer hours at the start of the programme, but also at the other assessments times (Figure 4).They also had longer periods of sick leave before the start of the programme.

Table 2. Results of the day treatment programme

	Range	Before n=46		After, n=46		Follow-up, n=46		% improvement	F	df	p	Effect size
SCL anxiety	10–50	18.9	5.8	15.4	4.9	14.1	4.4	53.9	19.0	1,2	0.00	0.93
SCL agoraphobia	7–35	9.4	2.8	7.9	1.7	7.9	1.6	62.5	7.8	1,2	0.01	0.66
SCL depression	16–80	33.6	9.4	26.0	7.2	24.0	8.5	54.5	22.7	1,2	0.00	1.07
SCL somatzation	12–60	23.9	7.4	19.3	5.9	18.5	6.1	45.4	18.1	1,2	0.00	0.80
SCL obsessive compulsive	9–45	21.9	6.7	17.0	5.4	15.3	5.2	51.2	24.9	1,2	0.00	1.10
SCL paranoid ideation	18–90	29.8	7.3	26.3	7.4	24.6	7.7	44.1	10.7	1,2	0.00	0.69
SCL hostility	6–30	8.6	2.4	7.6	1.8	7.1	1.4	57.7	10.9	1,2	0.00	0.76
SCL sleep problems	3–15	7.4	2.9	6.0	2.5	5.4	2.5	45.5	11.3	1,2	0.00	0.74
SCL–90 total	90–450	167.5	34.4	137.1	30.1	128.5	32.4	50.3	27.6	1,2	0.00	1.17
BDI-II-NL	0–63	18.9	7.1	11.6	7.5	8.2	7.2	56.6	51.4	1,2	0.00	1.50
UBOS exhaustion	0–6	4.5	1.1	2.9	1.3	2.5	1.5	44.4	33.2	1,2	0.00	1.52
UBOS depersonalization	0–6	2.9	1.2	2.4	1.4	1.6	1.2	44.8	20.3	1,2	0.00	1.08
UBOS lack of professional accomplishment	0–6	3.3	1.1	3.7	1.2	4.2	1.0	27.3	15.0	1,2	0.00	0.86

Table 2. (Continued)

	Range	Before n=46		After, n=46		Follow-up, n=46		% improvement	F	df	p	Effect size
SFQ	4-28	22.4	4.5	15.9	6.8	14.8	7.8	41.3	27.3	1,2	0.00	1.19
IOA-frequency	35-175	103.7	11.4	113.6	16.8	118.4	20.4	21.4	12.9	1,2	0.00	0.89
IOA-tension	35-175	71.4	18.4	60.7	14.0	57.4	16.8	38.4	14.7	1,2	0.00	0.79
UCL active problem focussing	7-28	16.8	3.8	18.4	3.5	18.7	3.2	19.4	9.4	1,2	0.00	0.54
UCL palliative reaction pattern	8-32	17.2	3.2	18.2	3.4	17.5	2.6	3.3	2.2	1,2	0.13	0.10
UCL avoidance	8-32	17.8	3.8	16.8	2.9	16.1	3.8	17.3	6.4	1,2	0.04	0.45
UCL support seeking	6-24	11.5	3.3	13.3	3.3	13.5	3.3	36.4	10.5	1,2	0.00	0.61
UCL worrying	7-28	14.3	3.2	12.8	2.8	11.7	3.4	35.6	12.9	1,2	0.00	0.79
UCL emotional expression	3-12	5.7	1.3	6.2	1.2	6.1	1.3	14.8	3.0	1,2	0.06	0.31
UCL comforting cognition	5-20	11.5	2.5	12.2	2.3	12.2	2.3	10.8	3.1	1,2	0.06	0.29
Hours at work/wk		9.3	13.2	17.2	12.1	23.9	14.9	156	16.1	1,2	0.00	1.03
Contract hours at work		32.0	9.5									
Job abstinence period in weeks		32.3	31.6									

More or less fatigue in relation to hours at work (1)

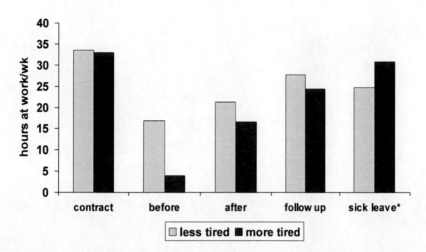

Figure 3. The median score on the SFQ in the day treatment study is 22.5. Less tired is an SFQ score of at most 22.5; more tired is an SFQ score above 22.5; * Sick leave duration in weeks before the start of the programme

More or less fatigue in relation to hours at work (2)

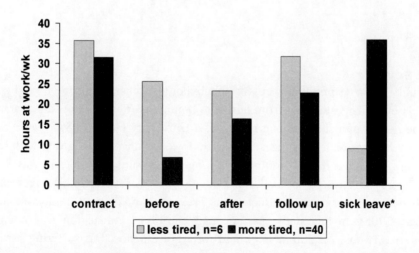

Figure 4. The inclusion score in the light therapy study on UBOS/EE is 3. The patients of the day treatment study have been divided according this criterion. Less tired have an UBOS-EE score of less than 3, more tired have an UBOS-EE score of at least 3 at the start of the programme; * Duration of sick leave in weeks before the start of the programme

Improvement of fatigue in relation to hours at work

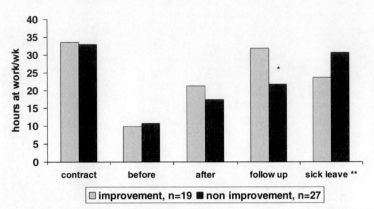

* significant improvement (p <0.05). ** Duration of sick leave in weeks before the start of the
  programme

Figure 5. Improvement is an improvement of at least 50 % on the SFQ at follow-up compared to the
start;

Patients who showed an improvement of 50 % or more on SFQ scores during the
research project, are seen to work significantly longer at the follow-up moment than those
who showed an improvement of less than 50 % (F14.6,df = 1,2, p=0.00; Figure 5). They also
had longer periods of sick leave before the start of the programme.

Discussion

Light therapy

This study shows some evidence for the hypothesis that exposure to light improves
energy levels of patients suffering from burnout complaints. These results are more or less in
line with the results of a study among nurses of a University Hospital, who were exposed to
at least 3 h of daylight on a daily basis. This group was compared to a group with less than 3
h of exposure to light. In the group with longer exposure to light, it was found that
participants were less stressed and had higher levels of work satisfaction. Longer exposure to
light also had an indirect positive effect in the prevention of burnout complaints (Alimoglu
and Donmez, 2005). In this study, participants' emotional exhaustion was equal in both
groups of nurses, who were still at work and were not diagnosed as suffering form burnout
complaints.

Improvement after light treatment was assessed on a weekly basis with instruments that
contained questions about fatigue levels (SFQ). A trend towards improvement was seen after
light treatment based on the UBOS-EE subscale. The UBOS assesses a subject's experience
of complaints at work during the previous week (Schaufeli and Van Dierendonck, 2000).
Most participants did not go to work during the weeks prior to the assessment, but stayed at
home because of their complaints. Therefore, the UBOS may not be the questionnaire best

suited to these participants, which might explain why the results based on this questionnaire are weaker than those based on the other instruments.

When comparing the participants of this study to those of other studies (Ahola et al., 2005) more depressive symptoms were reported. We excluded patients with a DSM-IV diagnosis of depression from the study. Nevertheless, participants in both conditions had elevated scores on a depression questionnaire (BDI-II). The trend towards improvement after light treatment, based on the BDI-II scores can be explained by the items about fatigue and energy. The item about depressed mood remained the same after light treatment. The scores on this item were low from the beginning.

Apart from the small sample size, another limitation of this study is its lack of a placebo control condition. A waiting list condition followed by light treatment was used instead. When we look at the results of the treatment that was offered after the waiting list period, there was no difference in results after this type of light treatment as compared to the light treatment of the protocol: the participants of the waiting list condition showed the same degree of improvement. Some effects of patients' expectations about the result of the treatment cannot be ruled out, however, the effects of the daily visits, and contact with the clinic staff might also account for some of the observed improvements, although the staff were instructed not to talk about the participants' complaints. In the control condition, there were no daily visits to the clinic.

In spite of these shortcomings, the preliminary results of light treatment are promising when treating the emotional exhaustion of the burnout syndrome.

Notwithstanding the small sample size, the effect sizes of light treatment according to the self-rating questionnaires seem promising.

Day treatment

A short, but intensive day treatment programme and its outcomes for patients suffering from severe burnout were described in this chapter. This treatment was protocolised and had as main objective to reduce the complaints, and to teach patients new and more effective coping strategies and social skills in order to make them less vulnerable in future stressful situations. Emotional exhaustion as part of burnout complaints was often seen to be present. The programme contained different approaches, such as cognitive behavioural therapy, non-verbal therapeutic interventions and activation which, when used together, led to a relapse prevention plan at the end and stimulated patients to reintegrate in their jobs. CBT and related interventions were major parts of the programme. In a recent study, De Vente et al. (2008) came to the conclusion that CBT-based interventions were not successful in the treatment of patients with clinical levels of work-related stress. These findings are in line with those of Blonk et al. (2006) who compared an extensive CBT-therapy, a treatment with brief CBT-derived interventions combined with individual-focussed and workplace interventions and a control group of persons with severe work-related psychological complaints. The combination treatment was found to be superior to both the extensive CBT and the control group in shortening the duration of the sick leave. This last finding is probably in line with our own results, in that in our programme, it is not possible to discriminate between the effects of the different elements. In our programme, the total package of interventions might be responsible for the therapeutic outcome. It is not possible to point out a single ingredient of the programme which is responsible for the effect.

When looking at the figures of the follow-up assessment, which was held a year after the programme had been completed, and comparing them to those of the beginning of the programme, a significant reduction of symptoms was found and patients' performance at their jobs amounted to 74.7 % of their contract hours. Before the start of the programme patients had been absent from their jobs for approximately 30 weeks on average. We therefore conclude that the effects of this programme seem promising.

Coping strategies hardly improved at all or very slightly at most. Van Rhenen et al., (2008) showed that active coping strategies are related to the duration of the sick leave. We were unable to confirm these findings; however, there are some differences between the studies. In our study, participants suffer from burnout complaints, whereas in the Van Rhenen study the whole population of a major company was investigated.

In our study, the initial mean scores of coping strategies did not differ from the mean scores of a normal population according to the UCL manual (Schreurs et. al, 1993). Therefore, a major improvement of coping strategies is not very realistic. Nevertheless, improvements, if any, are in the desired direction.

There are, however, some limitations to this study. It is a natural field study with a lack of homogeneity in the psychopathology and without a single intervention technique being responsible for the effects. Since we did not use a placebo condition, it is still possible that the therapeutic results are not superior to any effects over time without treatment. It is therefore impossible to draw conclusions about the working mechanism of the programme.

This programme was developed for and studied with patients in a regular mental healthcare setting, instead of in a randomised controlled scientific laboratory situation. This might increase its chance of being implemented in everyday mental healthcare practice.

Conclusions

Both studies make it clear that the interventions (light therapy and day treatment) improve emotional exhaustion or fatigue levels. If sick leave is relatively short, patients have a better perspective of improvement and reintegration into their jobs. Patients with higher levels of fatigue at the start of the programme worked less at that time. If fatigue complaints decrease, patients may be able to reintegrate into their jobs. Decreasing fatigue levels may lead to a significantly greater amount of hours of reintegration into the job. The conclusion can be that improving emotional exhaustion or fatigue levels should be one of the core goals in the treatment of burnout.

If light treatment indeed has a positive effect on emotional exhaustion or fatigue, it may be assumed that patients can benefit more readily from this treatment if it is administered prior to any other treatment.

Acknowledgment

The authors are grateful to Josie Borger for the improvement of the English of the manuscript.

References

Ahola, K., Honkonen, T., Isometsä, E., Kalimo, R., Nykyri, E., Aromaa, A. & Lönnqvist, J. (2005). The relationship between job-related burnout and depressive disorders – results from the Finnish 2000 Study. *Journal of Affective Disorders.*, *88*, 55-62.

Alberts, M., Smets, E. M. A., Vercoulen, J. H. M. M., Garssen, B. & Bleijenberg, G. (1997). Verkorte vemoeidheidsvragenlijst: een praktisch hulpmiddel bij het scoren van vermoeidheid. *Nederlands Tijdschrift voor de Geneeskunde.*, *141*, 1526-1530.

Alimoglu, M. K., Donmez, (2005). Daylight exposure and the other predictors of burnout among nurses in a University Hospital. *International Journal of Nursing Studies.*, *42*, 549-555

American Psychiatric Association (APA) (1994). Diagnostic and Statistical Manual of Mental Disorders. Fourth Edition.Washington DC: American Psychiatric Association.

Arrindel, W. A., Ettema, J. H. M. (2003). Symptom Checklist SCL-90.Manual.Lisse: Swts & Zeitlinger B. V.

Avery, D. H., Kizer, D., Bolte, M. A. & Hellekson, C. (2001). Bright light therapy of subsyndromal seasonal affective disorder in the workplace: morning versus afternoon exposure. *Acta Psychiatrica Scandinavica.*, *103*, 267-274.

Bakker, A. B., Schaufeli, W. B., Demerouti, E., Janssen, P. P. M., Van der Hulst, R. & Brouwer, J. (2000). Using equity theory to examine the difference between burnout and depression. Anxiety, *Stress and Coping.*, *13*, 247-268

Bakker, A. B., Schaufeli, W. B., Demerouti, E., Janssen, P. P. M., Van der Hulst, R. & Brouwer, J. (2000). Using equity theory to examine the difference between burnout and depression. *Anxiety, Stress and Coping.*, *13,* 247-268.

Bakker, A., Schaufeli, W. & Van Dierendonk, D. (2000). Burnout: prevalentie, risicogroepen en risicofactoren. In: I. D., Houtman, W. B., Schaufeli, T. Taris (Eds.), Psychische vermoeidheid en werk. Alphen a/d Rijn: Samsom

Bakhuys-Roozeboom, M., Gouw, P., Hooftman, W., Houtman, I. & Klein Hesselink, J. (2009).

Arbobalans, 2007/2008. Kwaliteit van de arbeid, effecten en maatregelen in Nederland. Hoofddorp: TNO Kwaliteit van Leven.

Beck, A. T., Steer, R. A. & Brown, G. K. (1996). Manual for the Beck Depression Inventory-II. San Antonio TX: Psychological Corporation.

Beck, A. T., Steer, R. A. & Brown, G. K. (2002). Beck Depression Inventory-II. Dutch version: Van der Does A.J.W. Lisse: Swets Test Publishers.

Bekker, M. H. J., Croon, M. A. & Bressers, B. (2005). Childcare involvement, job characteristics, gender and work attitudes as predictors of emotional exhaustion and sickness absence. *Work & Stress.*, *19*, 221-237

Blonk, R. W., Brennikmeijer, S., Lagerveld, S. & Houtman, I. L. D. (2006). Return to work: a comparison of two cognitive behavioural interventions in cases of work-related psychological complaints among the self-employed. *Work & Stress.*, *20*, 129-144

Blustein, D. L. (2008). The role of work in psychological health and well-being. *American Psychologist.*, *63*, 228-240.

Cohen, J. (1988). Statistical power analysis for the behavioural sciences. Hillsdale, New Jersey: *Lawrence Erlbaum.*

Derogatis, L. R. (1977). SCL-90: administration, scoring and procedures manual-I for the R(evised) version. Baltimore: *John Hopkins University Scool of Medicine, Clinical Psychometrics Research Unit.*

De Vente, W., Kamphuis, J. H., Emmelkamp, P. M. G. & Blonk, R. W. B. (2008). Individual and group cognitive-behavioral treatment for work-related stress complaints and sickness absence: a randomized controlled trial. *Journal of Occupational Health Psychology.*, *13*, 214-231.

Glass, D. C. & McKnight, J. D. (1996). Perceived control, depressive symptomatology, and professional burnout: a review of the evidence. *Psychology and Health.*, *11*, 23-48.

Golden, R. N., Gaynes, B. N., Ekstrom, R. D., Hamer, R. M., Jacobsen, F. M., Suppes, T., Wisner, K. L. & Nemeroff, C. B. (2005). The efficacy of light therapy in the treatment of mood disorders: a review and meta-analysis of the evidence. *American Journal of Psychiatry.*, *162*, 656-662.

Gordijn, M. C. M., 't Mannetje, D. & Meesters, Y. (2006). The effects of blue enriched light treatment compared to standard light treatment in SAD. *SLTBR abstracts.*, *18*, 6.

Houtman, I., Van Hooff, M. & Hooftman, W. (2007). Arboblans 2006. Arbeidsrisico's, effecten en maatregeln in Nederland. Hoofddorp: TNO.

Leone, S. S., Huibers, M. J. H., Knottnerus, J. A. & Kant, I. J. (2007). Similarities, overlap and differences between burnout and prolonged fatigue in the working population. *Q J Med.*, *100*, 617-627.

Liu, L., Marker, M. R., Parker, B. A., Jones, V., Johnson, S., Cohen-Zion, M., Fiorentino, L., Sadler, G. R. & Ancoli-Israel, S. (2005).The relationship between fatigue and light exposure during chemotherapy. *Support Care Cancer.*, *13*, 1010-1017.

Maslach, C. & Jackson, S. E. (1981). The measurement of experienced burnout. *Journal of Occupational Behaviour.*, *2*, 99-113.

Maslach, C. & Schaufeli, W. B. (1993). Historical and conceptual development of burnout. In: W. B., Schaufeli, C., Maslach, T. Marek (Eds.), Professional burnout: recent developments in theory and research. 1-16 Washington DC: Taylor & Francis.

Maslach, C., Schaufeli, W. B. & Leiter, M. P. (2001). Job Burnout. *Annual Review of Psychology.*, *52*, 397-422.

Meesters, Y. & Lambers, P. A. (1990). Light therapy in patient with seasonal fatigue. *The Lancet.*, *336*, 745.

Meesters, Y., Jansen, J. H. C., Lambers, P. A., Bouhuys, A. L., Beersma, D. G. M., Van den Hoofdakker, R. H. (1993). Morning and evening light treatment of seasonal affective disorder: response, relapse, and prediction. *Journal of Affective Disorders.*, *28*, 165-177.

Meesters, Y. & Waslander, M. (2009). Burnout and light treatment. Stress & Health. Epub.

Meesters, Y., Horwitz, E. H. & Van Velzen, C. J. M. (2009, submitted): Day treatment of patients with severe work-related complaints.

Rosenthal, N. E., Sack, D. A., Gillin, C., Lewy, A. J., Goodwin, F. K., Davenport, Y., Mueller, P. S., Newsome, D. A., Wehr, T. A. (1984). Seasonal Affective Disorder: a description of the syndrome and preliminary findings with light therapy. *Archives of General Psychiatry.*, *41*, 72-80.

Rüger, M., Gordijn, M. C. M., Beersma, D. G. M., De Vries, B. & Daan, S. (2006). Time -of-day-dependent effects of bright light exposure on human psychophysiology: comparison of daytime and nighttime exposure.

Am-J-Physiol-Regul-Integr-Comp-Physiol. (2006). May; 290(5). R1413-20.

Schaap, C. P. D. R., Keijsers, G. P. J., Vossen, C. J. C., Boelaars, V. A. J. M. & Hoogduin C. A. L. (2001). Behandeling van burnout. In: C. A. L., Hoogduin, W. B., Schaufeli, C. P. D. R., Schaap, A. B., Bakker (Eds.), Behandelstrategieën bij burnout. Houten/Diegem: Bohn Stafleu Van Loghum.

Schaufeli, W. & Enzmann, D. (1998). The burnout companion to study & practice. A critical analysis. London: Taylor and Francis Ltd.

Schaufeli, W. B. & Van Dierendonck, D. (2000). UBOS: Utrechtse BurnOut Schaal. Manual. Lisse: Swets & Zeitlinger B. V.

Schaufeli, W. B., Bakker, A. B., Hoogduin, K., Schaap, C. & Kladler, A. (2001). On the clinical validity of the Maslach Burnout Inventory and the burnout measure. *Psychology and Health.*, *16*, 565-582.

Sheehan, D. V., Lecrubier, Y., Sheehan, K. H., Amorim, P., Janavs, J., Weiller, E., Hergueta, T., Baker, R. & Dunbar, G. C. (1998). The Mini-International Neuropsychiatric Interview (M.I.N.I.): The development and validation of a structured diagnostic psychiatric interview for DSM-IV and ICD-10. *Journal of Clinical Psychiatry.*, *59*, suppl, *20*, 22-33.

Schreurs, P. J. G., Van de Willige, G., Brosschot, J. F., Tellegen, B., Graus, G. M. H. (1993). De Utrechtse CopingLijst: UCL. Manual. Lisse: Swets & Zeitlinger B.V.

Sonnenschein, M., Sorbi, M. J., Van Doornen, L. J. P., Schaufeli, W. B.,Maas, C. J. M. (2007a). Evidence that impaired sleep recovery may complicate burnout improvement independently of depressive mood. *Journal of Psychosomatic Research.*, *62*, 487-494.

Sonnenschein, M., Sorbi, M. J., Van Doornen, L. J. P., Schaufeli, W. B. & Maas, C. J. M. (2007b). Electronic diary evidence on energy erosion in clinical burnout. *Journal of Occupational Health Psychology.*, *12*, 402-413.

Taris, T. W. (2006). Is there a relationship between burnout and objective performance? A critical review of 16 studies. *Work & Stress.*, *20*, 316-334.

Van Dam-Baggen, C. M. J. & Kraaimaat, F. W. (1987). Inventarisatielijst Omgaan met Anderen IOA. Manual. Lisse: Swets & Zeitlinger, B. V.

Van Rhenen, W., Schaufeli, W. B., Van Dijk, F. J. H. & Blonk, R. W. B. (2008). Coping and sickness absence. *Int Arch Occup Environ Health.*, *81*, 461-472.

Wileman, S. M., Eagles, J. M., Andrew, J. E., Howie, F. L., Cameron, I. M., McCormack, K. & Naji, S. A. (2001). Light therapy for seasonal affective disorder in primary care. *British Journalof Psychiatry.*, *178*, 311-316.

Willert, M. V., Thulstrup, A. M.,Hertz, J. & Bonde, J. P. (2009). Changes in stress and coping from a randomized controlled trial of a three-month stress management intervention. *Scand J Work Environ Health.*, *35*, 145-152.

World Health Organisation (WHO) (1994). De ICD-10. Classificatie van Psychische Stoornissen en Gedragsstoornissen. Klinische beschrijvingen en diagnostische richtlijnen. Nederlandse Vereniging voor Psychiatrie, M.W. Hengeveld. Lisse:Swets en Zeitlinger.

In: Nursing Issues: Psychiatric Nursing, Geriatric Nursing...   ISBN: 978-1-60741-598-5
Editors: C. D. McLaughlin et al., pp. 213-228   © 2010 Nova Science Publishers, Inc.

Chapter VII

Poverty and Mental Health: The Role of Community Development in Addressing Mental Health Variables through the Lifespan

David M. M. Sharp[*]

Louisiana College, 1140 College Drive,
Pineville, Louisiana 71360, U.S.A.

Abstract

The mental health of an individual throughout the lifespan is influenced by a range of factors that can either protect the individual from mental health problems or make them more vulnerable to those problems. The interdependency between health issues and social/economic issues is most acutely experienced by people who are in poverty. In the USA this often involves communities of the non-white population .

An approach highlighted by the WHO to tackling the complex range of social, environmental and health issues is Community Development. The basic components of community development are outlined with reference to two community development projects; one in a third word country; the other in a western society. The projects are used to examine the inter-relationships between community involvement, empowerment and subsequent changes in living conditions and health status.

Promotion of, and barriers to, effective community development in the U.S. are explored in relation to the needs of the vulnerable members of society who live in poverty and who are at increased risk of developing mental health problems.

Keywords: Mental Health; poverty; vulnerability factors; community development.

[*] Corresponding author: Phone, 318-487-7127, Email: dsharp@lacollege.edu

Introduction

The World Health Organization (WHO) notes that worldwide mental, behavioral and neurological disorders are major contributors to disability and death. These disorders are common in all countries and if left untreated cause immense suffering, producing significant economic and social hardships that affect one in four families at any point in time (WHO 2008). There is an ethnic/cultural dimension to the poverty variable that influences the mental health dimension (Davis 1995).

In the most recent source of official poverty estimates in the USA, the Current Population Survey (CPS) , 2005 Annual Social and Economic Supplement, the official poverty rate for 2004 was 12.7%, up from 12.5% from 2003 (U.S. Census Bureau, 2005). This equated to 37 million people in poverty, of these 24.7% were Blacks, 21.9% Hispanics, 9.8% Asians, and 8.6 % were Whites. The vast majority of the population affected by poverty is therefore nonwhites, and it is worth bearing this in mind when the impact of poverty on mental health issues in the U.S.A. is discussed. In addition, there is an ethnic/cultural dimension to the poverty variable that is bound to influence the mental health dimension (Davis 1995).

Although poverty rates show a downward trend, down 9.7 percentage points from 1959 (U.S. Census Bureau, 2005), there are still large amounts of people in our communities who suffer the adverse affects of poverty. The link between health and poverty is well known and well-documented (for example Townsend et al 1992; Waitzman and Smith 1998), and can be summarized in Gomm's (1996:110) statement :

> For nearly every kind of illness, disease or disability, 'physical' and 'mental', poorer people are afflicted more than rich people: more often, more seriously and for longer – unless, of course, they die from the condition, which they do at an earlier age.

Brugha et al (1988) pointed out that people who have mental health problems are also often physically unwell, while Broome (1989) noted that those who are physically unwell or handicapped are more likely to be mentally distressed. Therefore the influence of poverty on health will be multi-dimensional, it is to be anticipated that if poverty influences the physical health of a person there will be a good chance that their mental health will also be impacted. The WHO notes that care delivery must be holistic to ensure that the mental health needs of people with physical disorders is met as well as the physical needs of people with mental disorders (WHO 2008). The relationship between variables such as poverty with physical mental health is brought sharply into focus when we consider the plight of poorer sections of the elderly population. For this group there is a strong association between physical ailments, loss of ambulation, incontinence, hearing loss and depression (Arie, 1988); and Holland and Rabbitt (1991) have linked dietary deficiencies in the elderly and poorly controlled diabetes with depression.

When the social demographics are examined they routinely demonstrate a link between social group, or neighborhood, with high rates of premature death, coronary heart disease, long-term illness, childhood accidents and poverty. The social group, or neighborhood will also show high rates of depression, suicide , anxiety states and schizophrenia (Gomm 1996).

Community integration within neighborhoods was found by Yanos et al (2007) to be diagnosed with mental illness.

Although the links between physical ailments and mental health conditions appear to be many and complex, Gomm (1996:112) suggests that they can be represented in a simple triangular relationship linking social and economic conditions with physical illness and psychological stress:

This triangular representation realizes the definition of health contained within the first principle of the WHO Alma Ata Declaration in that health is a state of complete physical, mental and social well-being and not merely the absence of disease or infirmity (WHO 1978). Wong and Solomon (2002) describe community integration for people with severe mental illness as multidimensional involving these physical, social and psychological dimensions. They state that the physical dimension is "the extent to which an individual ... participates in activities, and uses goods and services in the community outside his/her home in a self initiated manner"; the social dimension related to the "extent to which the individual engages in community interactions"; and the psychological dimension is "the extent to which an individual perceives membership of his/her community", (2002, 14).

Gomm points out that researchers working within this triangle often fail to explore the dynamic of the relationship created, missing an opportunity to explore a holistic approach to health issues:

> Thus studies which investigate only the social correlates of coronary heart disease fail to note the way in which the same circumstances predict high levels of mental distress. Studies which focus on the epidemiology of mental illness may miss the fact that populations vulnerable to 'depression' or 'anxiety states' are also vulnerable to 'physical' diseases and handicaps. (Gomm 1996:117).

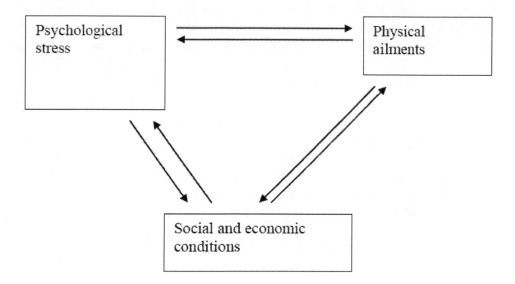

Figure 1. Three interconnected causes of mental health. (Based on Gomm 1996).

Casualty therefore can run in all directions within this triangular relationship. The ANA (1997) has pointed out that high degrees of poverty and stress result in an increased incidence of physical and mental illness. Those in poverty are more likely to develop physical illnesses; being physically ill, or disabled, a person is more likely to experience anxiety and depression; these mental health conditions make a person more prone to a lowered immunity level; which in turn makes the person more susceptible to physical illness; and so the cycle continues and the health problems increase. (Lewis et al 1994). Added to this cycle is a lifestyle dimension whereby poorer people are more likely to indulge in health damaging behaviors such as excessive smoking and drinking (Jones-Webb et al 1997; Flint and Novotny 1997), which can create or exacerbate physical conditions which in turn impinge on mental health conditions creating a greater possibility of susceptibility to physical illness and so on.

However, the link between poverty and mental health problems is not automatic and depends on a range of social variables, for example in the USA it is estimated that there are approximately 110,000 chronically homeless individuals with serious mental health problems (Culhane, Metraux and Hadley 2002). Although the non-white population forms the majority of people in the U.S. suffering from poverty, the highest suicide rate is amongst whites (CDC 2004). Therefore, although there is no automatic link between material conditions and physical and mental ill-health, "poor people are vulnerable in multiple ways by comparison with the better off" (Gomm, 1996:114). Adults who are considered to be poor, under U.S. federal guidelines, have a greater probability for the development of new psychiatric disorders than the non-poor population (Bruce et al. 1991).

Unemployment is a vulnerability factor related to poverty that has a well documented relationship to mental health problems. For example, unemployment rates are positively related to suicide rates, with the probability of suicide increasing as people's expectations of future income decreases (Yang 1992). Measures of relative wealth, such as unemployment rates, have been found to be a good predictor of the mental health status within a neighborhood (Kammerling and O'Connor, 1993) and poorer paid jobs have been linked to physical problems such as coronary illness, which in turn is correlated with mental health problems (Karasek and Theorell, 1990). Wilkinson (1992) pointed out the relationship between life expectancy and income distribution, showing a strong link between rising and falling death rates with similar rises and fall and income levels. Low weight gain in infants is often used as a simple indicator of poverty, Barker et al (1995) used this to point out triangular nature of the relationship between poverty and physical and mental health by establishing a link between childhood poverty and the likelihood of men committing suicide fifty years later. Gulcur et al (2007) note that the integration of adults with psychiatric disabilities into communities has psychological, physical and social dimensions that underpin the challenges in investigating the variables that impinge on health status. The link between social circumstances and mental health would appear to be a factor that is therefore present throughout the lifespan.

	Protective factors	**Vulnerability factors**
Children	Good Parenting skills and parents with good coping skills	Poor parenting skills Parents unable to cope with problems
	Family cohesion and good sibling relationships	Martial disharmony Domestic violence, sexual abuse
	Good parental mental health (especially of mother)	A mentally ill parent or a parent with a drug or an alcohol problem
	Good parent-child relationships	Fraught or distant parent-child relationships
	Positive peer relationships	Isolation and/or bullying
	Positive recognition for a skill or an activity	Lack of achievement or of recognition for achievement
Adolescents	Childhood as above and:	Childhood as above and:
	Successful move from one school to another or into new social situations	Poor adaptation to a new school (especially for girls)
	Ability to cope with day-to-day problems	Lack of coping skills
	Support with bereavement or life-threatening illness of a parent, or no parental bereavement or illness	Parental bereavement or illness without support Sexual abuse
	Family harmony	Marital discord or other family disharmony
	No depression or alcoholism in parents	Depression or alcoholism in a parent
	Higher socio-economic status, or personal ability to cope with poverty	Lower socio-economic status, or inability to cope with poverty
	Good Physical health	Poor physical health
Adults	Childhood and adolescence as above and:	Childhood and adolescence as above and:
	Social support and good social networks	Isolation or oppressive social networks
	Good coping skills and high self-esteem	Low self-esteem, poor coping skills
	Employment and low occupational stress	Unemployment or employment with high stress
	Fewer stressful life events or high resilience	More stressful life events or low resilience
	Marital harmony	Marital discord
	Good physical health	Poor physical health
	Coping successfully with death of a parent, spouse or child, or no such death	Failure to cope with death of a parent, spouse or child
	No severe financial problems	Severe financial problems
	Fulfilling social role responsibilities	Playing no or few valued social roles

Figure 2. Protective and Vulnerability Factors by stage of life. Source: based on Hodgson, R. And Abbasi, T. (1995).

Vulnerability Factors and Lifespan Development

Mental health issues can impact on an individual during any phase of their life long development. As noted above, poverty can influence the mental health of that individual, not just in respect to the immediate stress placed upon an individual at that particular moment in their life, but also in relation to factors that influence mental health issues throughout the life of the individual.

Hodgson and Abbasi (1995) summarize the factors that influence the mental health throughout the lifespan, pointing out that there are some factors that protect or preserve the individual's mental health status whilst other factors create vulnerability to mental health problems in the individual. As protective factors decrease, and vulnerability factors increase, then the individual is more at risk of developing severe mental health problems.

These protective and vulnerability factors can be outlined in relation to the stage of life of the individual:

Mental health problems may impact on a person throughout their lifespan and the impact of protective and vulnerability factors at one stage of a person's life might be felt at a later stage. Mental health problems in one stage may carry over, or influence the development of problems, at later stages (Rutter, 1985).

Many of the vulnerability factors have a compounding influence on mental health. For example, childhood factors such as marital disharmony, bullying and lack of achievement are compounded in adolescence if there is a lack of coping skills, sexual abuse or parental illness. This built up of factors through childhood and adolescence may, in adulthood, lead to isolation, low self-esteem and failure to cope with bereavement or loss. Therefore the protective and vulnerability factors throughout the lifespan form a matrix of possible mental health outcomes for the individual depending on the impact of social circumstances, such as poverty. Thus childhood poverty might not, in itself, have a long term, lifelong impact on an individual if they have family cohesion, good parental relationships and positive peer relationships. The person does not have to move out of poverty in later life to avoid developing mental health problems. It may be that the protective factors dominate and exclude the vulnerability factors; therefore it is of interest to investigate strategies whereby this can be encouraged.

The challenge in addressing mental health problems throughout the lifespan is therefore to reduce vulnerability factors whilst increasing protective factors. This often has to take place in health care systems where the development of mental health services is inadequate, especially in low-income and middle-income countries (Saraceno et al 2007). How best can a society, through various health care agencies achieve such a complex and multi-faceted task of social engineering? How can the resources and expertise to deal with the dynamic in the triangular relationship between mental health, physical health and social/economic conditions be provided? Given that health care professionals can not remove poverty, how can they concentrate on strategies to promote protective factors and ameliorate vulnerability factors in mental health? One strategy to do so is to identify those areas in the life cycle where they can make the most impact on individuals whose physical and mental health is impacted by poor social/economic conditions. Health professionals are not in a position to change society, but there are areas in society where a meaningful impact on the health status of individuals can be made. One approach worth pursuing is in the implementation of community development projects where real attempts to address the impact of social/economic conditions, such as poverty, on physical and mental health, have successfully been made in a variety of different social realities.

Community Development

The World Health Organization (2004) describes community development as a peoplecentered approach to promoting the well being of individuals within a society.

It aims to develop social, economic, environmental, and cultural well-being of communities with a particular focus on marginalized members. (WHO, 2004: 52).

In applying this approach the social/economic variables that impact on the physical and mental health status of the individual can be addressed, thus impacting on the triangular relationship described by Gomm (1996) previously. It is anticipated that through community development the protective factors that can promote mental well being throughout the life span can be promoted. The WHO (2004) points to work carried out in rural areas of India an example of how community development projects can impact on mental health issues, even when they were not intended to. Poverty, inequality, gender discrimination, and domestic violence were identified as some of the major vulnerability factors contributing mental illness within village settings in rural India. Mumford (1997) identified vulnerability factors, such as low self-esteem, learned helplessness, low security, social isolation, economic deprivation and low social status which might also be said to have an impact on mental health in these communities.

The WHO (2004) demonstrates how when Indian villages have targeted poverty, inequality and gender discrimination this has led indirectly to significant gains in mental wellbeing. As the interventions put into place were seen to be working, and people felt empowered to solve their own problems, people in the village often became more open approaching broader issues such as health needs. This is summarized by Arole et al. (2004) Figure 3 .

In this example the impact on mental health status through community development mediated via a range of economic interventions such as improved water resources, housing, health care and education. Social interventions such as improved social capital and social safety nets have been tied into cultural changes. Such interventions targeted increased empowerment and economic independence for women and equality for marginalized groups to produce empowerment across the community that led to improvements in health status. These improvements in health status accompanied, or led to, decreases in alcohol abuse and violence; corruption and crime; fear of dying from pregnancy or illness; and inequalities such as caste discrimination.

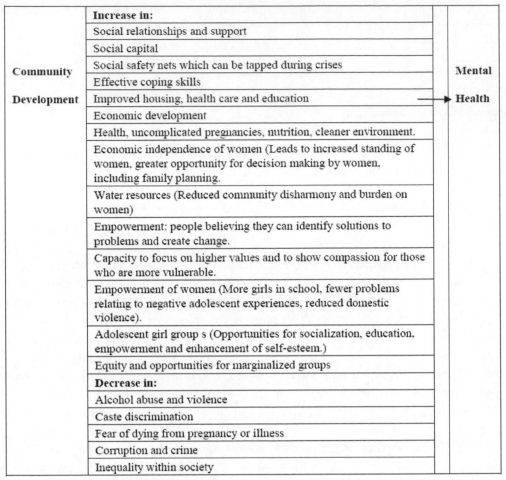

Community Development	**Increase in:**	Mental Health
	Social relationships and support	
	Social capital	
	Social safety nets which can be tapped during crises	
	Effective coping skills	
	Improved housing, health care and education	
	Economic development	
	Health, uncomplicated pregnancies, nutrition, cleaner environment.	
	Economic independence of women (Leads to increased standing of women, greater opportunity for decision making by women, including family planning.	
	Water resources (Reduced community disharmony and burden on women)	
	Empowerment: people believing they can identify solutions to problems and create change.	
	Capacity to focus on higher values and to show compassion for those who are more vulnerable.	
	Empowerment of women (More girls in school, fewer problems relating to negative adolescent experiences, reduced domestic violence).	
	Adolescent girl group s (Opportunities for socialization, education, empowerment and enhancement of self-esteem.)	
	Equity and opportunities for marginalized groups	
	Decrease in:	
	Alcohol abuse and violence	
	Caste discrimination	
	Fear of dying from pregnancy or illness	
	Corruption and crime	
	Inequality within society	

Source: Arole, Fuller and Deutschman. (2004).

Figure 3. The relationship between community development and mental health in rural villages in India.

This provides an example of the complexity of factors associated with mental health issues in community development models. The range of issues to be addressed included a raft of economic, social, and cultural variables making the outcomes related to mental health in the community difficult to define and measure. Hodgson and Abbasi (1995) point out that most of the mental health promotion projects that can be claimed to have been successful are those where the people being helped to develop coping skills would not be said to have pre-existing mental health problems. Whilst it is easy to identify and address vulnerability factors within a developmental model, such as bereavement through counseling, it is more difficult and contentious to tackle the vulnerability factors created by unemployment, homelessness or poverty. Interventions related to these social based vulnerability factors require intervention at a higher level than is possible solely through the delivery of health promotion initiatives.

The social interventions required in community development projects are compelling when they can be identified and implemented to provide obvious solutions in third world environments. However, there are similar community development projects that have been initiated in Western society that mirror in many ways those of the villages in India described above. Although the identification of vulnerability factors within a third world environment might be easier to identify , and the possible solutions may be easier to promote and measure, the application of similar approaches within Western society is no less compelling in its potential for dealing with mental health issues within the community.

For example in the early 1980's in the Granton neighborhood in Edinburgh, UK, a project was established to tackle topics that were of concern to residents in this deprived area. Staffed by a community development worker, a health visitor and a research worker, several community groups, such as a women's health group, were established. Although this women's health group started by examining topics such as stress, childbirth and communication with doctors, the agenda quickly moved on to focus on damp housing conditions, the major concern for the group. Pressure from the group via information sessions presented at the local university led to research studies of damp housing and health status in this, as well as two other cities. These studies established a link between damp housing conditions and emotional distress in women and respiratory and gastrointestinal problems in children (Martin et al. 1987, Platt et al. 1989).

The women in this community development project also addressed the issue of tranquillizer dependence. They formed a mutual support group the members of which eventually all gave up their addiction to drugs. They also recruited new members as a means of preventing the development of mental health problems in the community (Whitehead 1995). The group also established a community drop-in stress centre and set up an elderly forum to improve service delivery to elderly residents.

As with the previous example cited in India, women were again used as the key players in identifying the areas that required to be changed within the community. In both situations the improvement in physical conditions, such as housing and water, demanded social and economic changes that brought about improved physical and mental health.

Models and Policies

The Granton Project emphasizes the fact that the communities with the highest prevalence of mental illness are often areas of multiple deprivation where people have a poor general level of health and the fewest physical resources for caring. Thomas (1995) points out that it is not uncommon to find whole communities suffering from stress, perhaps as the result of the closure of a local factory; a run down in housing conditions; or fear of escalating crime. In Granton tackling damp-related illness and depression was successful because the local expertise in the community was utilized to identify the causes of problems and tackle them at source. It was noted that although the project was not set up to specifically target mental health problems, by identifying, and tackling, the problems that were causing stress in the community mental health issues were also addressed. Therefore, when the environmental/social variables were addressed so the health status of the population increased. As with the case in India, much more was happening than just the tackling of the initial problem. In both locations there were developments in new and worthwhile social relationships, new skills were learnt, self-esteem was improved and people began to feel in control of their own lives. All of these improvements can be viewed as the promotion of protective factors which will lower the vulnerability to mental health problems throughout the life span.

As noted previously, most of the poor in our American society are non-white. In 2006 Thomas et al pointed out the effectiveness of community development projects in overcoming the inequalities in mental health care experienced by members of local black and minority ethnic communities. Projects such as the Urban Justice Center in New York have a focus in community development in urbanized western society that provided "legal, technical and policy assistance to grassroots community groups engaged in a range of community development efforts throughout the city" (Urban Justice Center 2008). In working through the complexities of poverty it is necessary to use a range of local resources "to build the capacities of individuals, groups and organizations to include people with mental disorders in the developmental process" (BasicNeeds 2008).

Gilchrist (2004) drawing on research within community development, highlights two models of community development: the 'consensus' and 'radical' models. A consensus model might be employed where an improvement in service provision is desired for marginalized groups but there are no fundamental changes made to the way in which the services operate. The radical model suggests that simply improving the services for black and minority groups will be insufficient and it may be appropriate to instigate alternative, culturally sensitive, approaches to complement the usual therapies and counseling.

Funk, Drew and Faydi (2008), use the Optimal Mix of Services for Mental Health pyramid (see Figure 4) , developed by the WHO, to point out that:

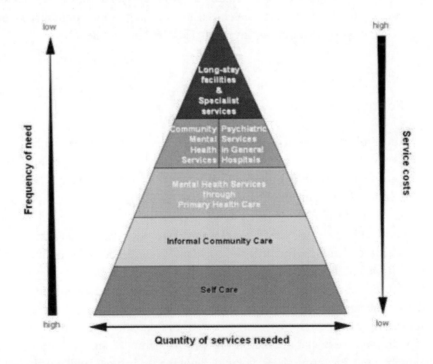

Figure 4. The Optimal Mix for Services for Menatl Health: WHO Pyramid Framework (Source Funk, Drew and Faydi (2008).

the majority of mental health care can be self managed or managed by informal community mental health services (… community groups, religious organizations, and schools). Where additional expertise and support is needed a more formalized network of services is required. In ascending order these include primary care services, followed by specialist community mental health services and psychiatric services based in general hospitals and lastly by specialist and long stay mental health services. Funk, Drew and Faydi (2008, p1).

For people with a mental health problem, the informal and self-care services at the bottom of the pyramid address the highest frequency of need for lowest cost. The WHO (2008) reports that for adequate development of mental health services "collaboration with other government non-health sectors, nongovernmental organizations, village and community health workers, and volunteers is required." (WHO 2008, p9).

Community Development, as defined by its own professional bodies, (Community Development Exchange, 2001), involves local people identifying the problems to be addressed and helping to shape the solutions. This is an empowering process that involves (as in India and Granton), a redistribution of power and resources and helps to build social capital in socially excluded communities (Thomas et al 2006). Although the actual impact on consumer driven interactions is on psychological outcomes for mentally ill individuals is difficult to measure, Greenwood et al note that there is a "strong and inverse relationship between perceived choice and psychiatric symptoms," (2005, p223).

In an editorial in the August 2003 edition of 'Health and Social Work', Galambos argues that in the challenging times we are currently facing, an examination of policy development and community intervention need to be emphasized. Policy development this decade would seem to suggest that this is slowly coming to fruition. There are many projects in the USA that improve health through participation and involvement of the health care consumer, promoting empowerment through consumer advocacy and client organizational change (Talbott and Hales 2001). Increasing empowerment through initiatives such as consumer choice enhances mastery thereby decreasing psychiatric symptoms (Greenwood et al 2005).

The Healthy People 2010 campaign was launched by The U.S. Department of Health and Human Services in January 2000 (U.S. Department of Health and Human Services 2000). The second goal identified in this health promotion initiative is "to eliminate health disparities among different segments of the population," with mental health, mental disorders and substance abuse being identified as amongst the 28 focus areas that should receive priority. Within the Department of Human Health and Services is located the Center for Faith-Based and Community Initiatives (CFBCI), a potential platform for developing Community development projects (Centers for Disease Control and Prevention 2003). Although this Center leads the Department's efforts to better utilize faith-based and community-based organizations in providing effective human services, the emphasis appears to be on accessing administrative resources, such as funding opportunities, scheduling conferences and obtaining technical assistance from the Centers for Disease Control and Prevention (CDC) and the Agency for Toxic Substances and Disease Registry (ATSDR) rather than influencing policy change or empowering communities.

A comprehensive community development initiative was initiated by Tommy G. Thompson, the U.S Secretary for Health and Human Services, in April 2003 when he convened a national summit of community leaders, policymakers and health officials (Galambos 2003). This summit led to the development of a five-year cooperative agreement that focused on community development programs to improve the health of those U.S. citizens with the greatest need. It is anticipated that the proposed changes in social and economic factors will have a positive impact on the physical and mental health of some of our poorest communities, as per the triangle of influence previously outlined. In so doing the protective factors relating to mental health will be potentiated whilst vulnerability factors through the lifespan will be ameliorated.

Care however must be exercised however when the desire is to involve communities in participation. In the early '70s Arnstein (1971) pointed out that there is a 'ladder of participation' made up of six rungs.

A. Citizen control
B. Delegated power
C. Partnerships (sharing of planning and decision making powers)
D. Placation or tokenism (given minor influence over some less important decisions)
E. Consultation (one-sided)
F. Information.

The lower levels on the ladder, D, E and F have little exchange of power or influence and are termed 'Community Engagement'. This is a reactive process that might include user involvement, consultation and some service improvement, but the agenda is set by the statutory authorities. In comparison, A, B and C, the three top levels on the ladder are part of 'Community Development' where the people themselves identify problems and shape the solutions. This is an empowering process bringing about the redistribution of power and resources, requiring statutory authorities to give priority to legal concerns and help build social capital in excluded communities. (Thomas et al 2006). This is the process of community involvement highlighted in the examples from India and Granton which provide models of the effectiveness in increasing the physical and mental health status of the communities involved when 'Community Development' is applied appropriately.

Hopefully recent initiatives identified under the Health People 2010 umbrella will focus on Community Development rather than the tokenism implied in Community Engagement. Developing partnerships, delegating power and giving citizens control over the health issues that matter to them will (as in India and Granton) change the social environment. This change in social and economic factors will have a profound positive impact on the physical and mental health of some of our poorest communities.

Conclusions

In examining the link between poverty and mental health there is a connection between social and economic conditions and physical and mental health (Gomm 1996). If mental health is dependent on physical health, which in turn is dependent on social and economic conditions, then the protective and vulnerability factors associated with mental health that exist throughout the lifespan are an integral part of this triangular relationship. Therefore, to holistically tackle issued relating to mental health and poverty, strategies employed must be developed that address a raft of factors that impinge on the individual. The WHO suggests that one way to do so is through Community Development projects, such as those discussed above. Using this approach enables statutory authorities to reach out and support the expertise of local groups in order that they can work with these statutory authorities to not only achieve better services but also to create viable alternatives that meet the specific cultural and spiritual needs of the community. (Seebohm et al 2006). This approach is therefore particularly appropriate for addressing the mental health needs of non-white populations, groups that experience some of the lowest levels of poverty in our society. As initiatives that move toward community development are put in place care must be taken that the nature of the projects that are initiated are truly 'Community Development' rather than the easier to apply, but tokenistic approach suggested by Community Engagement" (Arnstein 1971).

Examples from various parts of the world demonstrate that through involving and empowering communities to address their own health needs the mental health status of some of the poorest and most vulnerable members of society can be improved throughout the lifespan.

References

[1] ANA (1997). American Nurses Association: Improving minority health outcomes through culturally specific care. *Nurs Trends Issues.*, *2(3)*, *1*, 1997.

[2] Arie, T. (1988). Questions in the psychiatry of old age. In D. Evered and J. Whelan (eds.) (1988) *Research and the aging population*, Ciba Foundation Symposium., *134*, Chichester, Wiley.

[3] Arnstein, S. (1971). A ladder of citizen participation. *Journal of the American Institute of Planners*, *69*, 216-24.

[4] Arole, Fuller and Deutschman (sic) (2004). In World Health Organization (2004) *Promoting Mental Health: Concepts, Emerging Evidence, Practice.* France, WHO.

[5] Barker, J., Osmond, C., Rodin, I., Fall, C. & Winter, P. (1995). Low weight gain in infancy and suicide in later life. *British Medical Journal.*, *vol. 331*, 1203-1204.

[6] BasicNeeds (2008).. Menal Health and Development. Avialable at http://www.mentalhealthanddevelopment.org/about%20us.html (Accessed on 12/2/2008).

[7] Broome, A. (ed.) (1989). *Health Psychology: process and applications.* London, Chapman Hall.

[8] Bruce, M., Takeuchi, E. & Leaf, P. (1991). Poverty and psychiatric status: Longitudinal evidence from the New Haven Epidemiologic Catchment Area Study, *Arch Gen Psychiatry.*, *48*, *470*, 1991.

[9] Burgha, T., Wing, J. & Smith, B. (1988). Physical health of long-term mentally ill in in the community. *British Journal of Psychiatry*, *vol. 155*, 777-781.

[10] Centers for Disease Control and Prevention, (2003). Faith Based and Community Initiatives. Available at http://www.phppo.cdc.gov/dphsdr/FaithBase/ (Accessed 4/19/2007).

[11] CDC (2004). Centers for Disease Control and Prevention, National Center for Injury Prevention and Control (producer). Web-based Injury Statistics Query and Reporting System (WISQARS) [Online]. (2004). Available online from: URL: http://www.cdc.gov/ncipc/wisqars/default.htm. (Accessed 10/12/2008).

[12] Community Development Exchange, (2001). *The startaegic framework for community development.* Available from www.cdx.org.uk (Accessed 11/28/2008).

[13] Culhane, D., Metraux, S. & Hadley, T. (2002). Public service reductions associated with placement of homeless persons with serious mental illness in supportive housing. *Housing Policy Debate., 13(1)*, 107-163.

[14] Davis, K. (1995). Mental health training and black colleges: Identifying the need. Keynote speaker at the September *African-American Behavioral Health Conference*, Atlanta,.

[15] Flint, A. J. & Novotny, T. E. (1997). Poverty status and cigarette smoking prevalence and cessation in the United States, 1983-1993: the independent risk of being poor. *Tobacco Control., Vol. 6, 14-18*, 1997.

[16] Funk, M., Drew, N. & Faydi, E. (2008). The Optimal Mix of Services for Mental Health. Geneva, World Health Organization. Available at https://www.who.int/mental_health/policy/services/2_Optimal%20Mix%20of%20Services_Infosheet.pdf(Accessed 12/07/08).

[17] Galambos, C. M. (2003) Building Healthy Environments: Community-and Consumer-Based Initiatives, *Health and Social Work*, August., *28(3)*, 171-173.

[18] Gilchrist, A. (2004) *The well-connected community: a networking approach to community development.* Bristol: The Polity Press.

[19] Gomm, R. (1996) Mental health and inequality. In T. Heller, J. Reynolds, R. Muston and S. Pattison (eds.) (1996). *Mental Health Matters: A Reader.* Basingstoke, MacMillan Press Ltd.

[20] Greenwood, R. M., Schaefer-McDaniel, N. J., Winkel, G. & Tsemberis, S. J. (2005). Decreasing psychiatric symptoms by increasing choice in services for adults with histories of homelessness. *American Journal of Community Psychology, Vol. 26, Nos 3-4*, December, 223-238.

[21] Gulcur, L., Tsemberis, S., Stefancic, A. & Greenwood, R. M. (2007). Community integration of adults with psychiatric disabilities and histories of homelessness. *Community Mental Health Journal., Vol 43, No. 3*, June. 211-228.

[22] Hodgson, R. & Abbasi, T. (1995) *Effective Mental Health Promotion*, Technical report 13, Cardiff, Health Promotion Wales/Hybu Iecyd Cymru.

[23] Holland, C. & Rabbitt, P. (1991). The course and causes of cognitive change with advanced age. *Reviews in Clinical Gerontology, vol I*, 79-94.

[24] Jones-Webb, R., Snowden, L., Herd, D., Short, B. & Hannan, P. (1997). Alcohol-Related Problems among Black, Hispanic and White Men: The Contribution of Neighborhood Poverty. *Journal of Studies on Alcohol., Vol. 58*, 1997.

[25]Kammerling, R. & O'Connor, S.(1993) Unemployment rate as a predictor of psychiatric admission. *British Medical Journal*, *vol. 307*, 1538-1539.

[26]Karasek, J. & Theorell, T. (1990) *Healthy Work: stress, productivity and the reconstruction of working life*, New York, Basic Books.

[27]Lewis, C., Sullivan, C. & Barraclough, J. (1994) *The Pschoimmunology of Cancer*, Oxford, Oxford University Press

[28]Martin, C., Platt, S. and Hunt, S. (1987) Housing conditions and ill-health. *British Medical Journal.*, 294, 1125-1127.

[29]Mumford, D. B. (1997) Stress and psychiatric disorder in rural Punjab: a community survey. *British Journal of Psychiatry.*, *170*, 473-478.

[30]Platt, S., Martin, C., Hunt, S. & Lewis, C. (1989) Damp housing, mould growth and symptomatic health state. *British Medical Journal.*, *298*, 1673-1678.

[31]Rutter, M. (1985) Resilience in the face of adversity: protective factors and resistance to psychiatric disorder. *British Journal of Psychiatrl.*, *vol. 147*, 598-611.

[32]Saraceno, B., van Ommeren, M., Batniji, R., Cohen, A., Gureje, O., Mahoney, J., Sridhar, D., & Underhill, C. (2007). Barriers to improvement of mental health services in low-income and middle-income countries. *The Lancet , Volume, 370 , Issue 9593*, 1164-1174.

[33]Seebohm, P., Henderson, P., Munn-Giddings, C., Thomas, P. & Yasmeen, S. (2006) Power to the community. *Mental Health Today*, Feb 31-34.

[34]Talbott, J. A. & Hales, R. E. (Eds.) (2001). *Textbook of administrative psychiatry: New concepts for a changing behavioral health system (2nd ed.)*, Washington, DC: American Psychiatric Association.

[35]Thomas, D. (1995) *Helping Communities to Better Health: the Community Development Approach*, Cardiff, Health Promotion Wales/Hybu Iechyd Cymru.

[36]Thomas, P., Seebolm, P., Henderson, H., Munn-Giddings, C. & Yasmeen, S. (2006) Tackling race inequalities: Community development, mental health and diversity. *Journal of Public Mental Health*, June *5(2)*, 13-19.

[37]Townsend, P., Whitehead, M. & Davidson, N. (eds) (1992). *Inequalities in Health: the Black Report and the health divide*, Harmondsworth, Penguin.

[38]U.S. Census Bureau, Housing and Household Economic Statistics Division, last revised August 30, 2005. Available at http://www.ceb=nsus.gov/hhes/www/poverty/ poverty04/ pov04 hi.html. (Accessed 2/12/2007).

[39]Urban Justice Center (2008). Projects- Community Development. Available at http://www. urbanjustice.org/ujc/projects/community.html (Accessed 11/30/2008).

[40]U.S. Department of Health and Human Services (2000) Healthy People 2010. Available at http://www.healthypeople.gov/ (Accessed 4/19/2007).

[41]Waitzman, N. J & Smith, K. R. (1998). Phantom of the area: poverty-area residence and mortality in the United States. *American Journal of Public Health.*, *Vol. 88, Issue 6*, 973-976

[42]Whitehead, M. (1995) Tackling inequalities: a review of policy initiatives. In M., Benzeval, K. Judge & M. Whitehead (Eds.), *Tackling Inequalities in Health: an Agenda for Action.* London, King's Fund.

[43]Wilkinson, R. (1992) Income Distribution and Life Expectancy. *British Medical Journal*, *vol. 304*, 165-168.

[44]Wong, Y. I. & Solomon, P. L. (2002) Community integration of persons with psychiatric disabilities in supportive independent housing: A conceptual model and methodological considerations. *Mental Health Services Research.*, *4(2)*, 13-28.

[45]World Health Organization (1978) Declaration of Alma-Ata. International Conference on Primary Health Care, Alma-Ata, USSR, 6–12 September 1978. Available at http://www.who.int/hpr/archive/docs/almaata.html (Accessed 11/29 2008).

[46]World Health Organization (2004) *Promoting Mental Health: Concepts*, *Emerging evidence*, *Practice.* France, WHO.

[47]World Health Organization (2008). *Integrating mental heath into primary care: A global perspective.* World Health Organization and World Organization of Family Doctors (Wonca), Singapore, Wonca Press.

[48]Yang, B. (1992) Sociological and economic theories of suicide: a comparison of the USA and Taiwan. *Soc Sci Med.*, *34*, *333*, 1992.

[49]Yanos, P. T., Felton, B. J., Tsemberis, S. & Frye, V. A. (2007). Exploring the role of housing type, neighborhood characteristics, and lifestyle factors in the community integration of formerly homeless persons diagnosed with mental illness. *Journal of Mental Health*, December., *16(6)*, 703-717.

In: Nursing Issues: Psychiatric Nursing, Geriatric Nursing...   ISBN: 978-1-60741-598-5
Editors: C. D. McLaughlin et al., pp. 229-242   © 2010 Nova Science Publishers, Inc.

Chapter VIII

Nursing Burnout in the Era of Evidence Based Practice

[1]Stefanos Mantzoukas and [2]Mary Gouva
Highest Technological Educational Institute of Epirus, GREECE.

Abstract

Superimposed organizational demands, work overload and limited decision-making capacities are often associated with the development of occupational stress by nurses that eventually create a sensation of professional burnout. In the current era of evidence-based practice, health organizations and regulatory bodies impose further demands on practicing nurses as to implement research evidence in practice setting. Also, evidence-based practice requires that nurses search the electronic literature as to find the best available evidence for practice. Lastly, in accordance to the traditional view of evidence-based practice, decisions relating to patient care are not the product of the practitioners' intellect, but the result of research findings deriving from randomized control trials that the practicing nurses merely implement. This traditional view of evidence based practice appears to create further organizational demands, work overload and limited decision-making potentials for practicing nurses that is bound to intensify the burnout feelings. Therefore, the current chapter will conclude that the traditional view on evidence-based practice needs to be abandoned as to avoid the perpetuation of burnout sensations in nurses. A more radical view will be proposed that conceptualizes evidence-based practice as an ideology of individual emancipation, where daily practice is based on the individual nurse's critical and reflexive analysis of singular situations and contexts taking into consideration the feasibility, appropriateness, meaningfulness and effectiveness of all types of evidence and developing a line of thought that has logical validity and argumentative coherence. This radical view will empower individual practitioners and enable them to undertake rational decisions based on the various types of knowledge that they possess leading to a notion of ownership of nursing praxis and a sense of professional fulfillment. Finally, this radical conceptualization of evidence-based practice not only fits in with the current trend in nursing, but also facilitates nurses to overcome the burnout feelings.

Introduction

The concept of burnout amongst practicing nurses is a well documented phenomenon in the nursing literature. Furthermore, a series of literature reviews and research studies have identified a variety of underlying etiological factors that contribute to burnout sensations in nurses. However, what appears to be missing from the relevant literature is the analysis that links burnout and the current era of evidence based practice and how this current era of evidence based practice can affect burnout feelings amongst nurses. The aim of the current chapter is to provide an overview on burnout and on the underlying factors that lead to burnout. Consequently, we will go on to develop the links between burnout and evidence based practice as to identify potential factors of perpetuating burnout by the use of evidence based practice and mechanisms for overcoming burnout if evidence based practice is re-conceptualized as to become more relevant and appropriate for nursing practice.

The Concept of Burnout in Nursing

The notion of burnout has been regarded by the literature as an occupational hazard that exhibits multidimensional, complex and commingled characteristics with a dynamic and developmental nature that has, when present, deleterious effects on both the individual and the organization (Kanste et al. 2007, Jennings 2008b). The initial coiner of the term "burnout" is considered to be Freudenberger (1974) and his study on frontline human service workers and the various manifestations of chronic stress that these workers displayed due to the numerous and direct interactions they had with large numbers of people. Consequently, Maslach & Jackson (1981, 1982) conceptualized burnout as a syndrome typified by negative feelings, such as emotional exhaustion, depersonalization and reduced personal accomplishment, and went on to develop a burnout inventory as to measure the emerged and self-reported psychological, physical and behavioral strain indicators, which amongst others included tension, irritability, fatigue, headache, backache, extreme tiredness, sleep disorders, indifference, cynicism and negative self-image (Duquette et al. 1994, Kilfedder, 2001).

Duquette et al. (1994) in a comprehensive review on burnout in the nursing profession identified the work of Jenkins and Ostchega (1986), and Topf and Dillon (1988) as the first two studies that have documented workplace stressors as contributing factors to nursing burnout. Duquette et al. (1994) concluded that the stressful environment along with the constant state of alertness required create conditions of physical and mental exhaustion for the nurses that lead to burnout sensations. Since the work of Deuquette et al. a series of other studies have similarly identified that nursing practice can significantly increase the levels of occupational stress impacting negatively on nurses' physical and psychological well-being (Sutherland & Cooper 1992, Caplan 1994, Morita & Shima 2004, Gouva et al. 2009). The nursing literature defines burnout as the index of the dislocation between what people are and what they have to do. Such a dislocation consequently is anticipated to create an erosion of values, dignity, spirit and a haemorrhaging of oneself leading to depletion of both energy and personal resources, leaving individuals helpless and with negative feelings (Gillespie & Melby 2003, Laschinger & Leiter 2006).

Three different sources have been identified that potentially can create stress for nurses and could lead to the development of burnout sensation. Firstly, the context in which nursing occurs is usually intense and emotionally charged (McVicar, 2003;Yam & Shiu, 2003;Winwood & Lushington, 2006) typified by superimposed organizational demands, by nurses' lack of authority with limited decision-making capacities, and by aggressive and violent behavior including both verbal and physical assaults (Sawatzky, 1996; Corley *et al.*, 2001; Bakker *et al.*, 2005, Isaksson et al. 2009). Secondly, the nature of the nursing profession that includes intimate involvement with individual situations, human suffering and patient mortality, along with the development of interpersonal relationships and the use of empathy as a caring and therapeutic technique, coupled with extended working hours and physical work demands, such as lifting, carrying or moving weighty objects, or having to walk extensive distances for extended periods with little rest (Freshwater 2002, Mann & Cowburn 2005, Winwood & Lushington 2006, Jennings 2008b). Thirdly, the personality of individual nurses, the reasons for entering the nursing profession and the educational provision have been identified as potential factors for developing burnout sensation. Nurses that suffer burnout usually display inadequate personal and social coping mechanisms, dissonance between their personal ambitions and daily reality, along with a dissonance between their education and their inability to implement the acquired knowledge in practice (Kilfedder et al. 2001, Gillespie & Melby 2003, Gouva et al. 2009).

What is equally interesting and possibly of greater significance is that burnout sensation not only creates a series of negative consequences for the individual nurse, but has as well a negative effect on the professional and caring activities that the nurse conducts for the patients. It is extensively reported in the literature that overexposure to stressful experiences can induce maladaptive, dysfunctional and exhaustive behaviors diminishing nurses' confidence to practice nursing and reducing the sense of personal accomplishment, hence inciting tempered and irritable reactions (Tavares, 1994, Gillespie & Melby 2003, Mrayyan 2006, Winwood & Lushington 2006). This can result to irrational thinking patterns leading to cynical attitudes, destructive behaviors and detachment from work, which eventually breeds feelings of ineffectiveness, routinization, depersonalization and lack of professional autonomy and authority (Bonell 1999, Balvere 2001, Laschinger & Leiter 2006).

These attitudes can seriously compromise patient outcomes, patient safety, and quality care (Jennings 2008). For instance, Laschinger and Leiter (2006) identified that burnout played a major role in the relationship between nursing and patient outcomes. Jennings (2008) expanded on this, by explicitly linking nurses' high state-anxiety and burnout feelings with an increase of medical errors by nurses. Moreover, a set of other authors correlated burnout with inflexible practice, with difficulty of admitting error, with denial of failing to solve problems, with detachment from patients, with increased falls and nosocomial infections, and with proliferation of adverse events and patient mortality (Schmitz et al., 2000, Gillespie & Melby 2003, Laschinger & Leiter 2006). Also, feelings of burnout are associated with malpractice and unethical practice, with disempowerment sensation and with lack of control over the practice setting (Laschinger & Leiter 2006, Jennings 2008, Gouva et al. 2009)

Such practice provision, renders nursing not merely problematic but questionable and unacceptable. Unreasonable lack of skills by the nurse, omission to perform expected duties and caring activities or perform them below the required standard, and improper conduct in the performance of caring activities due to carelessness or ignorance are all considered cases of nurse malpractice (Graves-Ferrell, 2007, Brooke 2008, Keian-Weld & Garmon-Bibb 2009). Malpractice is conceptualized as a type of practice that is below the standards of care as defined by law, regulatory nursing bodies, policies and position statements by specialty societies, health care institutions and organizations, current nursing literature, and job descriptions. Such practice is unacceptable and entails serious consequences such as patient physical and/or psychological injury, financial harm to both patient and nurse, defamation of the nurse, the hospital and the profession, and even legal persecution of the nurse (Keian-Weld & Garmon-Bibb 2009).

The Era of Evidence-Based Practice Nursing

Perhaps the most basic framework currently underlying and shaping nursing practice is the concept of evidence based practice. Evidence based practice has acquired a prominent position in the strategic planning of nursing regulatory and accreditation bodies and this eminence is echoed in the educational, practice, policy and competence frameworks developed by these governing bodies (Jutel, 2008; Hudson et al., 2008). Evidence-based practice requires that nurses implement rational, moral and superior decision-making processes that prevent clinical errors or the provision of suboptimal care (Djulbegovic 2006, Borry et al. 2006, De Simone 2006). The current health literature asserts that clinical practice should be based on evidence as to promote standardization, certainty and consistency in practice that would eventually lead to high quality of care and avoidance of clinical errors (Mantzoukas 2007, Nolan and Bradley 2008, Rolfe et al. 2008). Moreover, the literature seems to inextricably align EBP with best practice (Walker 2003, Tolson et al. 2005), with doing the right thing (Muir-Gray 1997), with avoiding harmful interventions (Brocklehurst & McGuire 2005) and with transparent, accountable and legally defensible decisions (Page & Meerabeau 2004, Parahoo 2006).

The very inception of the evidence based practice movement in the early 1990s was based on the attempt to avoid hearsay, ritual, route and intuitive practice and base practice on more scientific, legitimate and rational approaches, hence increasing effectiveness and minimizing the possibility of error. One of the most quoted definition of evidence-based medicine, which is the forerunner of the evidence based practice movement, suggests the de-emphasis of "intuition, unsystematic clinical experience and pathologic rationale" for clinical decision making and instead places emphasis on "the examination of evidence from clinical research" (EBMWG 1992). This initial view of evidence based practice considered as most eminent and valid evidence those emerging from randomized control trials, which were termed as the golden standard for practice (Walker 2003, Franks 2004, Mistiaen et al. 2004, Berwick 2005, Rycroft-Malone 2006).

Furthermore, the eminence attributed to evidence emerging from randomized control trials is mirrored in the hierarchy of evidence as developed by the proponents of this initial view of evidence based practice. At the top of the hierarchy are the findings from systematic reviews of randomized control trials and the next level down the hierarchy are evidence from at least one well conducted randomized control trial. The next three levels down the pyramid are evidence from controlled research that lack randomization, research without a control group and opinions of respected authorities. Interestingly, the last three levels are not recommended to inform practice, thus assuming that they are not sufficient evidence to base practice (Sackett 1993, McKenna et al. 2000, Morse 2006). The positioning of evidence emerging from randomized control trials at the top of the hierarchical structure of evidence and the very language used to characterize these types of evidence are indicative of both the validity and significance attributed to evidence emerging from randomized control trials. Moreover, the significance attributed to evidence emerging from randomized control trials is portrayed in the guidelines and clinical protocols that are developed and which are based on the most updated randomized control trials. Furthermore, the proponents of this type of evidence based practice have developed RCT databases (such as Cochrane's database), created a series of evidence based journals that contain primarily RCT abstracts and currently are experimenting with computerized decision supporting systems that are based on RCT reviews (Mistiaen et al. 2004, Brocklehurst & McGuire 2005, Haynes 2005, Walker- Dilks 2005).

In a sense, it is not at all surprising that the nursing profession has rushed to adapt the evidence based practice discourse as it resonates with nurses long-standing calls for the development of a research based profession and actual research-based clinical information taking precedence over traditional modes of care (Bonell 1999, Hudson et al. 2008). More importantly, evidence based practice evangelizes increased effectiveness in practice provision, minimization of error and standardization of practice (Rashotte & Carnevale 2004, Parahoo 2006). Such a promise clearly counteracts the negative outcomes that relate to nurses' burnout sensations that include adverse effects on patient safety, clinical errors, substandard nursing care and high rates of patient mortality.

Moreover, it appears that there is no reason for burnout sensation to be present if the evidence based practice discourse is implemented. Part of the literature anticipates evidence based practice as a prescriptive process for making decisions, which is typified by the use of a series of predefined steps or processes that the practitioner merely follows (Mantzoukas 2008). Such an explicit decision-making mechanism can eradicate role ambiguity and role conflict that are primary contributing factors for nurses' burnout. Also, this view of evidence suggests that clinical decision-making and problem solving derive from objective and generalizable sources such as research findings from randomized control trials, which purport to provide definitive, accurate, and truthful evidences enabling nurses to practice in a predictable, objective, and standardized manner (Mantzoukas 2007). Hence, seriously limiting clinical unpredictability, practice complexity and context specific intricacies that are again primary sources of stress and burnout for nurses. Also, the traditional view of evidence based practice does not require intimate patient involvement, but merely requires that nurses can adequately search databases as to find existing evidence on treating specific patient problems and implement these evidences, therefore removing another element that contributes to the creation of burnout sentiments (Kessenich 1997, Thompson et al. 2005). In summation, the traditional view of evidence based practice via objectification and standardization of practice not only secures efficient, effective and safe practice, but also eradicates clinical complexity, practice ambiguity, role conflict and nurses intimate involvement with singular patient situations, thus removing all those contributing factors that have been identified as responsible for developing nursing burnout.

Critique of Traditional Evidence-Based Practice and its Role in Perpetuating Burnout

Whilst the above traditional view on evidence based practice seem to be able to deal with nursing burnout, nonetheless the nursing literature is replete with a continuum of authors that on one end of the spectrum raise cautionary voices with regards the usefulness of the traditional view of evidence based practice (Bonell, 1999) and on the other end of the spectrum a set of authors that are waging a polemic against the fascist attitude of evidence based practice (Walker 2003, Holmes et al. 2006). This criticism leveled against evidence based practice and its relevance and usefulness in nursing has direct implications with the development of burnout sensation for nurses. If evidence based practice is unable to achieve the goals in nursing as explicated above, than it is appropriate to assume that it would be very unlikely that it would be able to extricate the burnout sensation for nurse professionals.

The critique that evidence based practice has attracted from nurse authors relate to its basic premises and aims that are considered to be incongruent with nurses and nursing practice. The notion of objective, detached and generalisable evidence as propounded by the traditional view of evidence based practice via the use of research findings emerging from randomized control trials is considered a simplistic, questionable and superficial approach unable to achieve efficiency and optimum care (Geanellos 2004, Mantzoukas 2008, 2009). In fact, evidence based practice is accused of discounting the importance and complexity of human encounters in the provision of services (Geanellos 2004).

Moreover, it is argued that evidence-based practice does not increase objectivity but rather obscures the subjective elements that inescapably enter all forms of human inquiry (Goldenberg 2006). Thus, the problem with evidence based practice is that, at best, it downplays, and at worst, it utterly disavows the subjective elements operating at the heart of nursing (Holmes et al. 2007). In other words, nursing is the practice of the unique that requires personal knowing of the individual, with contextual knowledge and the ability to carry out specific and unique activities as to care and cater for specific patient needs (Carper 1978, Edwards 2001, Rolfe 2006, Mantzoukas & Jasper 2008). The fact that the traditional view of evidence based practice does not consider these essential types of nursing knowledge as valid forms of knowledge creates for nurse practitioners conflicting messages where the practice requirements of evidence based practice become incompatible with professional values and demands.

Furthermore, the use of evidence emerging from randomized control trials has as well practical limitations. Practitioners are busy professionals dealing with complex and unique clinical problems that require on the spot decisions to be made. It is, therefore, virtually impossible for practitioners to stop before every decision is to be made and retreat back to the library to retrieve all relevant evidence emerging from randomized control trials (Rolfe 2005,

Mantzoukas 2008). Also, the limited number of experimental studies conducted by nurses and the ''antitrial'' cultural permeating the nursing discipline further limits the numbers of evidence deriving from randomized control trials available to clinical nurses (Cullum, 1997; Droogan and Cullum, 1998, Mantzoukas 2009). Additionally, the notion of singular and absolute evidence that randomized control trials evangelize cannot solve daily clinical problems because answers and solutions for daily practice need to be constructed or fabricated as to fit individual cases (Forbes et al. 1999, Edwards 2001, Weaver & Olson 2006). Hence, if nurses base their practice only on evidence from randomized control trials they will be running the serious risk of being unable to deal and solve daily patient problems.

Finally, basing practice on evidence emerging from randomized control trials can make practice appear as a cookbook activity with the restrictive effect that this has on practitioners' initiative and autonomy (McKenna et al. 2000, Lorenz et al. 2005). In fact, it is argued by parts of the literature that the value attributed to evidence emerging from randomized control trials is an intentional distortion by highly established researchers, nurse academics, nurses' with authoritative positions in governmental posts, economical imperatives, other professional groups, and the epistemology of positivism (Forbes *et al.*, 1999; Walker, 2003; Freshwater & Rolfe, 2004; Mantzoukas, 2007). The fundamental explanation for such a distortion appears to be the need of these powerful groups to maintain and increase their powerful and hegemonic positions and they can achieve this by basing their status on their ability to develop, conduct, and disseminate randomized control trials (Rolfe, 2000; Murray *et al.*, 2007, Mantzoukas 2007). Moreover, evidence developed by groups far removed from the clinical environment pre-packaged in the form of evidence-based practice guidelines has a silencing effect on practitioners' intellectual and critical voices on methodology, philosophy, theory and practice issues transforming practitioners into mute, docile, unaccountable and without autonomy professionals (Freshwater and Rolfe, 2004; Holmes et al., 2008; Rolfe et al., 2008).

In summation, the critique of the traditional view of evidence based practice is founded on the dissonance that exists between the professional ideals of the nursing profession that advocates for unique and singular patient care, and the practice requirements of evidence based practice that strive for objective and generalisable evidence and practice. Consequently, this dissonance is furthered by the impracticality of acquiring evidence deriving from randomized control trials and the inappropriateness of this evidence in solving daily clinical problems. The result of implementing evidence in practice that is both impractical and inappropriate often leads to patient dissatisfaction and reduces patients' confidence in nursing care. Finally, the critique of the traditional view of evidence based practice concludes that the preponderance of standardized practice as developed by individuals removed from the ward context can lead to routinization of practice and seriously curtail nurse autonomy.

The dissonance between the ideal and the real, the depersonalization of practice, the inability to implement learned practices in the clinical context, patient dissatisfaction and anger for not solving their problems, routinazation of practice and lack of autonomy in the clinical environment make up not only a critique towards the traditional view of evidence based practice, but also constitute the foundational blocks for developing burnout sensation. While the rhetoric of the traditional view of evidence based practice as already demonstrated appear to be removing all those contributing factors that have been identified as responsible for developing nursing burnout, nevertheless its actual implementation perpetuates and further cultivates nursing burnout.

Radical Conceptualization of Evidence-Based Practice as Means of Overcoming Burnout

From the heretofore analysis the answer begging question is if there is hope in the current era of evidence based practice for nurses to avoid or overcome burnout feelings. Whilst the traditional view of evidence based practice seems to perpetuate burnout feelings in nurses, nonetheless this is not to suggest that there is no hope. Indeed, if evidence based practice is re-conceptualized or re-described in a radical, but more useful manner, then burnout would not be an issue for nursing. This re-conceptualization entails what the Kant termed as "sapere aude", which freely translates as *dare to think for yourself* (Critchley 2001, Mantzoukas & Watkinson 2008). In other words, nurses cannot expect of others to think for them and provide them with ready made answers for their own practice, but each nurse practitioner needs to think for their own self.

This radical view of evidence based practice does not imply that the nurse will know a lot of evidence or indeed even be proficient in finding evidence, but that s/he would be able to think about the value of evidence, critique the evidence and reason on the conditions of the possibility of implementing specific evidence in specific cases in specific contexts (Murray et al 2007, Mantzoukas 2007). Hence, the radical re-conceptualization of evidence based practice entails the identification of the potentials and limitations through reflexive and critical analysis of singular situations and contexts taking into consideration the feasibility, appropriateness, meaningfulness and effectiveness of all types of evidence and developing a line of thought that has logical validity and argumentative coherence (Avis & Freshwater, 2006; Pearson et al., 2007; Mantzoukas, 2007).

Furthermore, such critical and reflexive approach does not only identify the limits and usefulness of the available evidence, but also critiques the potentials and limits of the individual and the context within which s/he operates. Murray et al. (2007) suggest that practical application of knowledge will always be inadequate or in bad faith if "the practitioner does not avow the political and ethical dimensions of his or her own power/knowledge" (p. 515). Eventually, evidence based practice is not a product that can be passed from knower to would be knower, but a process involving well-reasoned and justified sets of action that relate logically and coherently to previous actions and signify in a contingent manner the actions that would follow. The greater the sophistication of the justified actions and the more critical the reasoning of the implemented practice, the greater their value and validity becomes. Finally, evidence that emerge from the reflexive, critical and reasoned faculties of individual practitioners will be more applicable and relevant to specific patient cases and practice contexts. Even in the cases that the practice context may not be conducive to the suggested evidence, the practitioner using reflexive, critical and reasoned approaches is appropriately positioned as to change the context of her or his practice.

Of course this requires a different kind of practitioner and a different kind of educational provision. In this radical conception of evidence based practice the educational system needs to prepare nurses not with ready made knowledge prepackaged in the form of theories and definitive evidence, but instead needs to have a developmental nature where the practitioner is enabled to ask questions, to critically scrutinize theories and evidence for their logical coherence, to look at practice with a questioning mode as to identify how things are, why they are as such and imagine how they can be different. Such a questioning, critical and reflective mode of practice allows and requires a culture of freedom. A thinking-culture where there is no right answer or correct practice. In other words, everything is possible and anything goes as long as it is rationally argued, logically justified and critical reflected upon.

This radical view of evidence based practice can become the means for overcoming the burnout sensation. The practitioners that base their practice on this radical view of evidence will not be entrapped in the dissonance between ideal and real because there is no ideal or even real for that matter. Both the ideal and real will be a creation each time of the individual practitioner that will be based and developed on critical reflexivity. Furthermore, such a practitioner has a sense of ownership of his/her practice as each time the practitioner creates a new micro-theory as to fit the specific needs of a specific patient. Even if the organizational environment is not conducive to such practices this new type of practitioner that implements a radical version of evidence based practice will be able to use his/her skills as to change the conditions of the context and function as a change agent. Finally, this radical view of evidence based practice has an emancipatory role for the nurse as it provides a sense of freedom and autonomy in the decision making of patient care. Furthermore, such practice allows for the constant development of practitioner as it is required that s/he constantly has to logically justify all choices made.

Conclusion

In conclusion this chapter has summarized the detrimental effects that burnout has for both the practitioner and the patient. Moreover, it has identified as primary contributors to burnout sensation the dissonance between the ideal notion of nursing and the reality of daily practice, practitioners' lack of authority and limited decision-making capacity, and the limitations of nurses' professional autonomy. Furthermore, the current era of evidence based practice further perpetuates nurses' burnout sensation, since the traditional view of evidence based practice contributes to the disillusionment of practitioners and to the delimitation of nurse autonomy in the practice setting. The objective and generalisable evidence produced by researchers far removed from the reality of the clinical setting, along with the alleged catholicity of this evidence and its projection as the most effective and optimal knowledge for patient treatment creates a greater sense of dissonance to practitioners that are educated and cultured in caring for individuals as unique and singular beings in unique and specific contexts requiring personal knowledge and understanding of their caring needs. Also, superimposing evidence in practice that are the result of electronic searches in various evidence based practice databases transforms practitioners from decision makers to mere technicians capable only of finding ready made solutions to practice situations. However, if evidence based practice is re-described as a critical, reflexive and reasoned approach to practice and re-conceptualized as a process that the practitioner undertakes as to shape practice, rather than a product that is imposed on practice, than the notion of dissonance, the lack of ownership of practice and the limitation of autonomy would cease to be an issue and therefore evidence based practice will become a mechanism for overcoming burnout in nursing.

References

Avis, M. & Freshwater, D. (2006). Evidence for practice, epistemology, and critical reflection. *Nursing Philosophy.*, *7*, 216-224.

Balvere, P. (2001). Professional nursing burnout and irrational thinking. *Journal for Nurses in Staff Development.*, *17*, 264-271.

Berwick, D. M. (2005). Broadening the view of evidence-based medicine. *Quality and Safe Health Care.*, *14*, 315-316.

Bonell, C. (1999). Evidence-based nursing: a stereotyped view of quantitative and experimental research could work against professional autonomy and authority. *Journal of Advanced Nursing.*, *30*, 18-23.

Borry, P., Schotsmans, P. & Dierickx, K. (2006). Evidence-based medicine and its role in ethical decision-making. *Journal of Evaluation in Clinical Practice.*, *12*, 306-311.

Brocklehurst, P. & McGuire, W. (2005). Evidence based care. *British Medical Journal.*, *330*, 36-38.

Brooke, P. (2008). Malpractice maladies. *Nursing Management*, *39*, 20-26.

Caplan, R. P. (1994). Stress, anxiety and depression in hospital consultants, general practitioners and senior health service managers. *British Medical Journal.*, *309*, 1261-1263.

Carper, A. B. (1978). Fundamental patterns of knowing in nursing. *Advances in Nursing Science.*, *1*, 13-23.

Critchley, S. (2001). *Continental Philosophy: A Very Short Introduction*. Oxford: Oxford University Press.

Cullum, N. (1997). Identification and analysis of randomised controlled trials in nursing: a preliminary study. *Quality in Health Care.*, *6*, 2-6.

De Simone, J. (2006). Reductionist inference-based medicine, i.e. EBM. *Journal of Evaluation in Clinical Practice.*, *12*, 445-449.

Djulbegovic, B. (2006). Evidence and decision making. *Journal of Evaluation in Clinical Practice.*, *12*, 257-259.

Droogan, J. & Cullum, N. (1998). Systematic reviews in nursing. *International Journal of Nursing Studies.*, *35*, 13-22.

Duquette, A., Kerouac, S., Sandhu, B. & Beaudet, L. (1994). Factors related to nursing burnout: a review of empirical knowledge. *Issues in Mental Health Nursing.*, *15*, 337-358.

Edwards, D. S. (2001). *Philosophy of Nursing: An Introduction*. Basingstoke: Palgrave.

Evidence-Based Medicine Working Group (EBMWG) (1992). Evidence-based medicine: a new approach to teaching the practice of medicine. *JAMA.*, *268*, 2420- 2425.

Forbes, D., King, K., Kushner, K. E., Letourneau, N., Myrick, A. F. & Profetto-McGrath, J. (1999). Warrantable evidence in nursing science. *Journal of Advanced Nursing.*, *29*, 373-379.

Franks, V. (2004). Evidence-based uncertainty in mental health nursing. *Journal of Psychiatric and Mental Health Nursing.*, *11*, 99-105.

Freshwater, D. & Rolfe, G. (2004). *Deconstructing Evidence Based Practice.* Basingstoke: Palgrave.

Freudenberger, H. J. (1974). Staff burn-out. *Journal of Social Issues.*, *30(1)*, 159-185.

Geanellos, R. (2004). Nursing based evidence: moving beyond evidence-based practice in mental health nursing. *Journal of Evaluation in Clinical Practice.*, *10*, 177- 186.

Gillespie, M. & Melby, V. (2003). Burnout among nursing staff in accident and emergency and acute medicine: a comparative study. *Journal of Clinical Nursing.*, *12*, 842-851.

Goldenberg, M. J. (2006). On evidence and evidence-based medicine: lessons from the philosophy of science. *Social Science and Medicine.*, *62*, 2621-2632.

Gouva, M., Mantzoukas, S., Mitona, E. & Damigos, D. (2009). Understanding nurses' psychosomatic complications that relate to the practice of nursing. *Nursing and Health Sciences.*, *11*, 154-159.

Graves-Ferrell, K. (2007). Documentation, part 2: the best evidence of care: complete and accurate charting can be crucial to exonerating nurses in civil lawsuits. *The American Journal of Nursing.*, *107*, 61-64.

Haynes, B. R. (2005). Of studies, summaries, synopses and systems: The 4S evolution of services for finding current best evidence. *Evidence Based Nursing.*, *8*, 4-6.

Holmes, D., Murray, S. J., Perron, A. & Rail, G. (2006). Deconstructing the evidence-based discourse in health sciences: truth, power, and fascism. *International Journal of Evidence-Based Healthcare.*, *4*, 180-186.

Holmes, D., Murray, S., Perron, A. & McCabe, J. (2008). Nursing best practice guidelines: reflecting on the obscene rise of the void. *Journal of Nursing Management.*, *16*, 394-403.

Hudson, K., Duke, G., Haas, B. & Varnell, G. (2008). Navigating the evidence-based practice maze. *Journal of Nursing Management.*, *16*, 409-416.

Isaksson, U., Graneheim_Hallgren, U., Richter, J., Eisemann, M. & Astrom, S. (2008). Exposure to violence in relation to personality traits, coping abilities, and burnout among caregivers in nursing homes: a case-control study. *Scandinavian Journal of Caring Sciences.*, *22*, 551-559.

Jenkins, I. F. & Ostchega, Y. (1986). Evaluation of burnout in oncology nurses. *Cancer Nursing.*, *9*, 108-116.

Jennings, B. (2008). Work Stress and Burnout Among Nurses: Role of the Work Environment and Working Conditions. In R. G. Hughes (Eds.), *Patient Safety and Quality: An Evidence-Based Handbook for Nurses* (1-22). Rockville, MD: Agency for Healthcare Research and Quality. http://www.ahrq.gov/qual/nurseshdbk/

Jutel, A. (2008). Beyond evidence-based nursing: tools for practice. *Journal of Nursing Management.*, *16*, 417-421.

Kanste, O., Kyngas, H. & Nikkila, J. (2007). The relationship between multidimensional leadership and burnout among nursing staff. *Journal of Nursing Management.*, *15*, 731-739.

Keian-Weld, K. & Garmon-Bibb, S. (2009). Concept analysis: malpractice and modern-day nursing practice. *Nursing Forum.*, *1*, 2-10.

Kessenich, C. R., Guyatt, G. H. & DiCenso, A. (1997). Teaching nursing students evidence-based nursing. *Nurse Educator.*, *22*, 25-29.

Kilfedder, C., Power, K. & Wells T. (2001). Burnout in psychiatric nursing. *Journal of Advanced Nursing.*, *34*, 383-396.

Laschinger, H. & Leiter, M. (2006). The impact of nursing work environment on patient safety outcome: the mediating role of burnout/engagement. *Journal of Nursing Administration.*, *36*, 259-267.

Lorenz, A. K., Ryan, W. G., Morton, C. S., Chan, S. K., Wang, S. & Shekelle, G. P. (2005). A qualitative examination of primary care providers' and physician managers' uses and views of research evidence. *International Journal for Quality in Health Care.*, *17*, 409-414.

Mantzoukas, S. (2007). The evidence-based practice ideologies. *Nursing Philosophy.*, *8*, 244-255.

Mantzoukas, S. (2008). A review of evidence-based practice, nursing research and reflection: leveling the hierarchy. *Journal of Clinical Nursing.*, *17*, 214-223.

Mantzoukas, S. & Jasper, M. (2008). Types of nursing knowledge used to guide care of hospitalized patients. *Journal of Advanced Nursing.*, *62*, 318-326.

Mantzoukas, S. & Watkinson, S. (2008). Redescribing reflective practice and evidence-based practice discourses. *International Journal of Nursing Practice.*, *14*, 129-134.

Mantzoukas, S. (2009). The research evidence published in high impact nursing journals between 2000 and 2006: a quantitative content analysis. *International Journal of Nursing Studies.*, *46*, 479-489.

Maslach, C. & Jackson, S. E. (1981) The measurement of experienced burnout. *Journal of Occupational Behaviour.*, *2*, 99-113.

Maslach, C. & Jackson, S. (1982). Burnout in Health Professions: A Social Psychological Analysis. In G. Sanders, & J. Suls (Eds.), *Social Psychology of Health and Illness* (79-103). Hillsdale, NJ: Lawrence Erlbaum.

McKenna, H., Cutcliffe, J. & McKenna, P. (2000). Evidence-based practice: demolishing some myths. *Nursing Standards.*, *14*, 39-42.

McVicar, A. (2003). Workplace stress in nursing: a literature review. *Journal of Advanced Nursing.*, *44*, 633-642.

Mistiaen, P., Poot, E., Hickox, S. & Wagner, C. (2004). The evidence for nursing interventions in the Cochrane database of systematic reviews. *Nurse Researcher.*, *12*, 71-80.

Morita, T. & Shima, Y. (2004). Emotional burden of nurses in palliative sedation therapy. *Palliative Medicine.*, *18*, 550-557.

Morse, M. J. (2006). The politics of evidence. *Qualitative Health Research*, *16*, 395-404.

Murray, S., Holmes, D., Perron, A. & Rail. G. (2007). No Exit?: Intellectual Integrity Under the Regime of 'Evidence' and 'Best-Practices'. *Journal of Evaluation in Clinical Practice.*, *13*, 512-516.

Nolan, P. & Bradley, E. (2008). Evidence-based practice: implications and concerns. *Journal of Nursing Management.*, *16*, 388-393.

Parahoo, K. (2006). *Nursing Research: Principles, Process and Issues* (2nd edition). Basingstoke: Palgrave Macmillan.

Pearson, A., Wiechula, R., Court, A. & Lockwood, C. (2007). A reconsideration of what constitutes evidence in the healthcare professions. *Nursing Science Quarterly.*, *20*, 85-88.

Rashotte, J. & Carnevale, F. A. (2004). Medical and nursing clinical decision making: a comparative epistemological analysis. *Nursing Philosophy.*, *5*, 160-174.

Rolfe, G. (2006). *Nursing* Praxis and the *Science of the Uni*que. *Nursing Science Quarterly*, *19*, 39-43.

Rolfe, G. (2005). The deconstructing angel: nursing, reflection and evidence-based practice. *Nursing Inquiry*, *12*, 78-86.

Rolfe, G., Segrott, J. & Jordan, S. (2008). Tensions and contradictions in nurses' perspectives of evidence-based practice. *Journal of Nursing Management*, *16*, 440-451.

Rycroft-Malone, J. (2006). The politics of the evidence-based practice movements. *Journal of Research in Nursing*, *11*, 95-108.

Sackett, D. L. (1993). Rules of evidence and clinical recommendations. *Canadian Journal of Cardiology*, *9*, 487-489.

Schmitz, N., Neuman, W. & Opperman, R. (2000). Stress, burnout and loss of control in German nurses. *International Journal of Nursing Studies*, *37*, 95-99.

Sutherland, V. J. & Cooper, C. L. (1992). Job stress, satisfaction and mental health among general practitioners before and after introduction of new contract. *British Medical Journal*, *304*, 1545-1548.

Tavares, M. (1994). Burnout in AIDS care. *Professional Nurse*, *12*, 24-27.

Thompson, C., McCaughan, D., Cullum, N., Sheldon, T. & Raynor, P. (2005). Barriers to evidence-based practice in primary care nursing - why viewing decision-making as context is helpful? *Journal of Advanced Nursing*, *52*, 432-444.

Topf, M. & Dillon, E. (1988). Noise-induced stress as a predictor of burnout in critical care nurses. *Heart & Lung*, *17*, 567-574.

Walker, K. (2003). Why evidence-based practice now? A polemic. *Nursing Inquiry*, *10*, 145-155.

Walker-Dilks, C. (2005). Contribution of the Cochrane library to the evidence-based journals. *Evidence Based Nursing*, *8*, 7.

Weaver, K. & Olson, K. J. (2006). Understanding paradigms used for nursing research. *Journal of Advanced Nursing*, *53*, 459-469.

Winwood, P. C. & Lushington, K. (2006). Disentangling the effects of psychological and physical work demands on sleep, recovery and maladaptive chronic stress outcomes within a large sample of Australian nurses. *Journal of Advanced Nursing*, *56*, 679-689.

Yam, B. M. & Shiu, A. N. Y. (2003). Perceived stress and sense of coherence among critical care nurses in Hong Kong: a pilot study. *Journal of Clinical Nursing*, *12*, 144-146.

In: Nursing Issues: Psychiatric Nursing, Geriatric Nursing…   ISBN: 978-1-60741-598-5
Editors: C. D. McLaughlin et al., pp. 243-255   © 2010 Nova Science Publishers, Inc.

Chapter IX

Exploring the Use of Emerging Technologies to Enhance Interdisciplinary Collaborative Practice in Palliative Care

[1]Emma J. Stodel[*] and [2]Colla J. MacDonald[**]
[1]Learning 4 Excellence, Canada.
[2]University of Ottawa, Canada.

Abstract

Organisational and financial policies in the long-term care sector make it hard for caregivers to justify time away from caring for residents to participate in continuing education programs (Romanow, 2002). ELearning offers appropriate and useful methods to deliver convenient and flexible education that fits within the constraints of the healthcare workplace. The growing popularity of emerging technologies presents new opportunities for delivering engaging and effective learning. However, if these technologies are going to be used in education they need to be examined in that regard. Consequently, the purpose of this project was to explore the use of emerging technologies to develop an online learning resource for caregivers that require palliative care and collaborative practice expertise to care for terminally ill residents in long-term care homes.

Introduction

Residents in long-term care settings have co-morbid chronic conditions and are a frail and vulnerable population. These individuals become terminally ill and wish to die in their long-term care home without having to move to a hospital or other care facility. In order to provide effective palliative care, teams of caregivers must come together to care for the resident holistically. The importance of collaborative practice in healthcare has been emphasised in numerous reports and policy documents (Health Canada, 2004; Health Council of Canada, 2006). Many have suggested that improving collaborative practice among healthcare professionals will require them to learn together in order to work together (Areskog, 1994). However, organisational and financial policies in the long-term care sector make it hard for caregivers to justify time away from caring for residents to participate in continuing education programs (Romanow, 2002). ELearning and evolving technologies (e.g., digital storytelling, 3D software, artificial intelligence, interactive voice response systems) may provide the solution by offering appropriate and useful methods to deliver convenient and flexible education that fits within the constraints of the healthcare workplace. However, the effectiveness and viability of these new tools as a means of creating engaging and effective learning remains unclear and requires further research. Consequently, the purpose of this project was to explore the use of emerging technologies to develop an online learning resource for caregivers that require palliative care and collaborative practice expertise to care for terminally ill residents in long-term care homes. The use of emerging technologies was explored and the impact on learners' experiences and learning outcomes examined.

Methodology

Participants

The learning resource was piloted in two long-term care homes in a mid-sized city in Ontario, Canada with 55 (48 females, 7 males; 17 from Home A, 38 from Home B) caregivers from 19 disciplines. Most (31%) were in the 45-54 year old age group. Ninety-six percent ($n = 52$) of the participants indicated they had a computer at home and/or had access to a computer at work. On the computer the learners used most frequently, 51 (94%) had high-speed Internet, 2 (4%) had dial-up, and 1 (2%) did not have an Internet connection at all. In general, the learners rated their computer abilities quite highly. Thirty-one learners (57%) reported that they use a computer every day for email, word processing, games, and/or searching the web and eight (15%) indicated they were very experienced with computers. However, five learners (9%) had never used a computer before and ten (19%) rated their abilities as novice and indicated they only use a computer occasionally. However, no participants indicated they had a negative attitude towards computers. Only three learners indicated they had concerns regarding learning online.

The Learning Resource

The resource was designed to facilitate the development of palliative care and collaborative practice skills and knowledge to improve the quality of care and life of terminally ill individuals. The resource uses case-based learning activities to permit the integration of clinical theory and practice, which situates learning in the workplace and fosters the development and application of work-related skills. The resource presents discipline-specific knowledge essential to resident care so learners can identify with their own field, while also learning about other disciplines and perspectives.

The possibilities afforded through the availability of broadband technologies were used to create a rich multimedia resource employing technologies designed to immerse learners in the learning environment through interaction with the content and an engaging design. The decision was made to develop a Flash-based product to allow the development of a highly tailored multimedia learning resource that meets the needs of the learners and can support interactive learner-centred activities. The resource employs digital storytelling; interactive online activities and tools learners can share and print; animations to show learners how to use the resource and highlight concepts; 3D objects that can be manipulated by the learners to obtain the information they need and want; videos to illustrate practice points and encourage reflection; audio clips from experts in the field; an artificial intelligence "expert" who responds to learners' questions about grief and mourning; an interactive voice response system; and interactive game-based activities to help learners test their knowledge and monitor their learning.

Evaluation

Research design

The Staged Innovation Design (Campbell, 1969; Wagner, 1984) was adopted as the research design to assess the learning outcomes (Fig. 1). The Staged Innovation Design involves the use of an experimental group and a control-replication group. The program is first introduced to the experimental group and the other group serves as a control. Then, the program is introduced to the control-replication group. The results from the control-replication group can be compared to those of the experimental group, as well as serve as a replication. This research design allows research to be conducted in a natural setting, thereby strengthening external validity, while also maximising internal validity (Feldon & Yates, 2007).

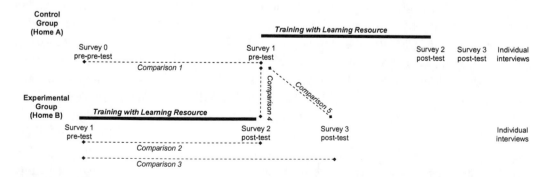

Figure 1. Research design.

Table 1. Summary of evaluation surveys.

Survey	Content
Survey 0 (pre-pre-test)	Section A: Identifying information Section B: Tool to assess skills and knowledge of collaborative practice that aligned with the learning objectives Section C: 14-item Quality of Care/Process subscale from the Attitudes Toward Health Care Teams Scale (Heinemann et al., 1999). Tool to assess attitudes towards collaborative practice. Section D: Jones and Way's Collaborative Practice Survey (Way et al., 2001). Tool to assess collaborative practice behaviour.
Survey 1 (pre-test)	Section A: Demographic information Section B: Tool to assess skills and knowledge of collaborative practice that aligned with the learning objectives Section C: 14-item Quality of Care/Process subscale from the Attitudes Toward Health Care Teams Scale (Heinemann et al., 1999). Tool to assess attitudes towards collaborative practice. Section D: Jones and Way's Collaborative Practice Survey (Way et al., 2001). Tool to assess collaborative practice behaviour.
Survey 2 (post-test)	Section A: DDLM evaluation tool (adapted from MacDonald et al., 2002). Tool to assess eLearning resource in terms of content, delivery, service, and outcomes. Section B: Tool to assess skills and knowledge of collaborative practice that aligned with the learning objectives Section C: 14-item Quality of Care/Process subscale from the Attitudes Toward Health Care Teams Scale (Heinemann et al., 1999). Tool to assess attitudes towards collaborative practice.
Survey 3 (post-test)	Section A: Jones and Way's Collaborative Practice Survey (Way et al., 2001). Tool to assess collaborative practice behaviour. Section B: DDLM evaluation tool (adapted from MacDonald et al., 2002). Tool to assess eLearning resource in terms of content, delivery, service, and outcomes.

Data collection and analysis

Various tools were used to collect data that allowed the participants' experiences and learning outcomes to be determined. Data were collected from four surveys, as well as individual interviews with 15 participants. The four surveys were compiled from existing survey tools and included demographic questions, an adaptation of the Demand-Driven Learning Model (DDLM) evaluation tool (MacDonald, Breithaupt, Stodel, Farres, & Gabriel, 2002), the Quality of Care/Process subscale from the Attitudes Toward Health Care Teams Scale (Heinemann, Schmitt, Farrell, & Brallier, 1999), and Jones and Way's Collaborative Practice Survey (Way, Jones, & Baskerville, 2001). Table 1 outlines the composition and purpose of each survey. T-tests and 2 HOME x 2 TESTTIME mixed factorial ANOVAs were used to compare participants' scores from the surveys as described in the research design.

The interviews were designed to determine the participants' experiences with the technologies used, as well identify the learning outcomes. The interviews took 20-45 minutes and were audio-taped and transcribed verbatim. Qualitative data analysis involved searching the transcripts for relevant information. A preliminary list of relevant emergent categories was developed. Once the categories were created satisfactorily, the data were assigned to the categories and the findings compiled. Direct quotations were used to preserve the voice of the participants.

Findings

Learners' Experiences with the Technology

Overall, learners expressed excitement over the variety of activities and effectiveness of the learning resource. The praise not only came at the level of the learners, but also from the organisation. One Director of Care expressed her delight in being involved with the project: "I thought [the leaning resource] was great and it was lucky that [our long-term care home] was chosen and [we] had the opportunity to take the learning resource. The home is very proud of what we have done as well".

The learning resource employed a number of different media to present the content and deliver the different learning activities in an online format. The learners' reactions to learning online, the different activities and resources, and the usability of the resource will be highlighted in the ensuing sections.

Learning Online

Learners enjoyed learning online. One learner indicated, "It was new and interesting. I like this way of learning" (Personal Support Worker). Another learner noted, "I love cutting edge stuff. I love new stuff. I think you have to find other ways to go after thing[s]. I was so enthusiastic and very proud of the fact that we want to be innovative and ... try something else, anything that could reach out to more people and turn more people on [to continued professional development]" (Executive Director). The learners appreciated the flexibility, convenience, and self-paced nature of learning online. However, one emphasised the need to chunk the learning into even smaller segments than it already was: "You want things that people could do in 10-15 minutes. This is really [all] the time they have" (Physician). There is no doubt that many of the learners struggled to find time to complete the learning resource. One learner noted: "It was hard to find the time to do it here at work. I know some staff had to do it at home, during their lunch hour and after hours. The organisation gave a lot of time to do it, but ... everyone is very, very busy here" (Administrator). In addition, the team activity they were asked to complete with co-workers face-to-face in order to apply what they had learned in the workplace proved to be a stumbling block due to time and scheduling constraints.

Activities and Resources

Learners continually commented on how impressed they were with the variety of resources presented to them through the program. However, one learner still indicated she would like more activities and less reading and another stated she would have liked more videos as she found them helpful. The use of different technologies led one learner to comment: "I found it energising. It really made you think. ... You start hearing how the families are thinking.... It gives you a notion of the dynamics of each family ... and how they [interpret] things because this was based on the whole family history" (Executive Director). Learners' experiences with the technologies are described below.

A digital story, presented in the form of a photo album, is used to introduce "Rose", the fictional patient in the case study. The story highlights who Rose is as a person, the things she accomplished in her life, and the main events in her life. One learner attested how this approach was effective in getting caregivers to think of those they are caring for as whole people: "Sometimes you get desensitised in long-term care. By seeing [Rose's] regression, the pictures from when she was younger to the end, it really reaffirmed her as a person. It happens when you read someone's obituary. You feel, 'Wow this person was really a person, not just somebody you cared for'" (Life Enrichment Coordinator).

As learners view the story they are asked to think about Rose's needs at the end of her life. One learner noted, "That helped me to take a lot from the pictures. The change from where she entered the nursing home. You could see how she declined. That was sad. That is why we need to give them the best life possible in their last days of life" (Chaplin). It was clear that learners connected with Rose. One noted, "I was curious to see what was going to happen with Rose". Similarly, a Registered Nurse related: "It was enjoyable meeting Rose. It brought a personal touch to the palliative care training". A few learners talked about Rose as if she was a real person and not a case-study: "Rose was fascinating. What she has experienced we would have had no idea. Her story is a lesson to all of us. She was a fighter and a winner. She was brave and strong" (Personal Support Worker). The Director of Care from one of the homes commented on how the authenticity of the content affected the learners: "It was so real and it touched our lives. A lot of people here who went through the program dropped some tears. It was sad. People believed that Rose was real!" (Director of Care).

Another way content was provided was through video. Six learners indicated the videos were what they liked best about the learning resource. The learners felt the videos were beneficial, relevant, and interesting: "I wish I could take the videos out and show them to the [other] staff…. They were a very good demonstration of the attitude you have to have—the presence, the respect, and the dignity" (Registered Nurse). Similarly an Executive Director reported, "I really liked the video portion…. When you started to see things, you started to feel things. That was the closest you could get to experiencing something without actually experiencing something". Although the learners reported the videos were interesting, interactive, and authentic, four of the learners interviewed noted that the care providers portrayed in the videos were insensitive to Rose. One of the Directors of Care indicated she used this video as a teachable moment with her staff: "I … asked my staff, 'How would you feel if you were a family member and the palliative care staff were being so impersonal?' I believe people live up to their last breath. They can hear and feel. We can't judge that they are not there". This comment amplifies the importance of paying attention to every detail when creating educational videos as the learners may pick up on omissions and subtle actions. Others noted the importance of making the videos more culturally sensitive.

Flash was used to create a resource library in the form of an interactive bookshelf. As learners move their mouse over the books a description of the resource appears. The resource can then be accessed through a simple mouse click. This was the favourite element of the resource for many of the participants. Learners indicated it had "great reading material", "great information and guidelines", "great links to additional resources", "the information to be able to help me within my own practice", and "opportunities to learn more about palliative care". In an interview, one learner elaborated: "The value of the bookshelf overshadowed other sections of the learning resource [for me]" (Life Enrichment Coordinator).

A number of interactive learning activities were also developed using Flash. For example, a "hangman" game is used to review elements of collaborative practice. Initially, learners had to complete this activity in order to move on but it became apparent that this impacted the learners' experiences and so this feature was disabled so users could move more freely through the resource. Another example of a Flash-based activity is an interactive pie chart that is used to help learners think about patients' needs at the end of life from a holistic perspective. A Personal Support Worker indicated how helpful this learning activity was: "I liked the pie. I had to choose which [quadrant of the pie] is more important. I had to think [about the end of my life] and put myself into that position to decide what was important to me when the time comes, whether it is physical, emotional, or spiritual. It really made me think".

As a means of exploring the use of other technologies, voice recognition, 3D imaging, and artificial intelligence (AI) were integrated into the resource. Dragon Naturally Speaking was installed on the computers at the long-term care homes. This enabled learners to navigate through the resource using voice recognition without having to use a mouse or keyboard. The technology was new and complicated and very few learners took the time to experiment with it. None of the learners commented on this feature during the evaluation. Another approach for presenting content that was explored was the use of 3D images that learners could manipulate. However, rather than facilitating learning, the inclusion of these 3D objects detracted from it as specific software was required to view them. Although the long-term care homes had been asked to load this software on the computers learners would use they still had trouble accessing content in this form. Lastly, the use of artificial intelligence was used to create an expert who responds to learners' questions about grief and mourning. The technology was easy to use; learners simply had to type their questions into a text box and click 'submit'. Again, none of the learners commented on this feature, suggesting it was not of interest to them. Data gathered on the use of this feature revealed that fewer than 30 questions were submitted during the first six months of implementation.

Usability

When asked what they liked most about the learning resource, eight learners mentioned that it was easy to use. With the support of the site coordinators, even learners with little or no computer experience successfully completed the learning. One of the site coordinators discussed these learners' successes: "I had a couple of people who had absolutely no computer skills [and] giggled all the way saying 'How silly I am'.... After they did it, they felt very proud of themselves" (Director of Care). One Registered Nurse noted, "Although my computer skills are not very advanced, I found it easy". Another learner said, "I think the technology was very cool; cool and usable" (Executive Director). There were, however, a couple of technical glitches that were a source of frustration for some learners. These included problems completing surveys; seeing and/or hearing the videos; accessing resources on the bookshelf; losing responses and having to start an activity again; and downloading software.

Learning Outcomes

Did the learners acquire new knowledge and skills regarding palliative care and collaborative practice?

In order to determine whether the learning resource met its objectives of improving palliative care and collaborative practice knowledge and skills, a questionnaire was developed that asks learners to rate how confident they are in various aspects of palliative care and collaborative practice that relate to the learning objectives of the resource. A paired sample t-test was conducted with the Home B (the experimental group) participants' scores from the learning objectives questionnaire in Survey 1 and Survey 2 (Comparison 2, Fig. 1) to determine whether the palliative care and collaborative practice knowledge and skills of participants in the experimental group changed as a result of completing the learning resource. Participants' scores were significantly higher after the training ($t = -4.059$, $df = 34$, $p < .05$). These findings provide preliminary evidence that the learning resource was effective in meeting the learning objectives.

Next, an independent sample t-test was conducted with Home B (the experimental group) participants' post-test scores and Home A (the control-replication group) participants' pre-test scores from the learning objectives questionnaire (Comparison 4, Fig. 1). The purpose of this was to determine whether Home B's post-test scores were significantly higher than Home A's pre-test scores, thereby providing further evidence for the effectiveness of the learning resource. Home B participants' scores following the completion of the learning resource were significantly higher than Home A participants' scores prior to the training ($t = -4.944$, $df = 49$, $p < .05$). These findings provide further confirmation regarding the effectiveness of the learning resource in meeting the learning objectives.

A 2 HOME x 2 TESTTIME mixed factorial ANOVA with repeated measures on the second factor was conducted on the participants' scores from the pre- and post-test of the learning objectives questionnaire to compare the pre- and post-test scores of both groups. There was no TESTTIME by HOME interaction ($F(1, 49) = 2.417$, $p = .126$, MSError = 65.50) nor a significant main effect for the home ($F(1, 49) = .957$, $p = .333$, MSError = 137.26). This latter finding indicates that there were no differences in participants' scores between the two homes. However, there was a significant main effect for the test time ($F(1, 49) = 37.87$, $p = .000$, MSError = 65.50) indicating that learners' knowledge and skills with regards to palliative care and collaborative practice improved after completion of the learning resource.

In the post-test, learners were asked whether they felt it was the learning resource that contributed to their improved palliative care and collaborative practice skills and knowledge in terms of each of the learning objectives. For each learning objective, 73-92% of the learners indicated that they felt it was the learning resource that helped them improve in these areas. Lastly, in order to provide further evidence that it was the learning resource that was the cause of the change in participants' scores, paired sample t-tests were conducted on the participants' scores from Home A (the control group) for the learning objectives questionnaires in Survey 0 and Survey 1 (Comparison 1, Fig. 1). There were no significant differences between the learners' scores on the learning objective questionnaire ($t = 0.912$, $df = 15$, $p > .05$) during this control period. In short, the knowledge and skills of participants not exposed to the learning resource did not change over time without training. The interview data supported these findings. In the interviews, learners reported they acquired new information related to both palliative care and collaborative practice.

Was there a change in the learners' attitudes towards the value and use of collaborative practice?

The Attitudes Toward Health Care Teams Scale (Heinemann et al., 1999) was used to determine whether there was a change in the learners' attitudes towards the value and use of collaborative practice as a result of using the learning resource. A paired sample t-test was conducted with the Home B (the experimental group) participants' scores from the Attitudes Toward Health Care Teams Scale in Survey 1 and Survey 2 (Comparison 2, Fig. 1) to determine whether the participants in the experimental group changed their attitudes as a result of completing the learning resource. There was no significant difference in participants' scores after the training ($t = -0.670$, $df = 34$, $p > .05$). These preliminary findings suggest that the learning resource was not effective in changing the participants' attitudes.

A 2 HOME x 2 TESTTIME mixed factorial ANOVA with repeated measures on the second factor was conducted on the participants' scores from the pre- and post-test of the Attitudes Toward Health Care Teams Scale (Heinemann et al., 1999) to compare the pre- and post-test scores of both groups. There was no TESTTIME by HOME interaction ($F(1, 49) = 0.197$, $p = .659$, MSError = 101.73) nor significant main effects for neither the home ($F(1, 49) = 1.112$, $p = .297$, MSError = 179.77) nor the test time ($F(1, 49) = 0.089$, $p = .766$, MSError = 101.73). These findings indicate that there were no differences in participants' scores depending on which home they worked in and that there were no changes in the participants' scores on the Attitudes Toward Health Care Teams Scale following completion of the learning resource. When asked during the interviews if their attitude towards collaborative practice changed, most learners indicated that they felt they already had a positive attitude towards working as a team prior to their learning.

Was learning transferred to the workplace? If so, did this result in an increase in interprofessional collaboration?

In the DDLM evaluation tool learners completed after they had finished the learning resource, learners were asked whether they had applied new knowledge and skills in the workplace. Eighty-five percent of the learners agreed or strongly agreed they had applied new knowledge and 79% agreed or strongly agreed they had applied new skills. However, there was little evidence to support the transfer of learning to the point of patient care in the data collected from the interviews. When asked if they had transferred learning to the workplace learners often responded "not yet", "it is too soon to tell", or "no, but I think I will in the future". There were, however, indications that what learners learned will impact how they deliver care in the future. One learner noted, "The [pie] is something I can take with me [and use] for any resident" (Chaplin). Another indicated that she is going to use what she learned in this module to educate other staff.

Way et al.'s (2001) Collaborative Practice Survey was used to assess whether there were any changes in the learners' collaborative practice behaviours as a result of using this learning resource. A paired sample t-test was conducted with the Home B (the experimental group) participants' scores (Comparison 3, Fig. 1) to determine whether the participants in the experimental group changed their collaborative practice behaviours as a result of completing the learning resource. There was no significant difference in participants' scores (t = -0.045, df = 33, p >.05). These preliminary findings suggest that the learning resource was not effective in changing the participants' collaborative practice behaviours. However, when asked in the DDLM evaluation survey, 79% of the learners indicated they worked more effectively as a team as a result of their participation in the learning resource.

A 2 HOME x 2 TESTTIME mixed factorial ANOVA with repeated measures on the second factor was conducted on the participants' scores from the pre- and post-test of Way et al.'s Collaborative Practice Survey to compare the pre- and post-test scores of both groups. There was no TESTTIME by HOME interaction ($F(1, 45)$ = 0.962, p = .332, MSError = 89.15) nor significant main effects for neither the home ($F(1, 45)$ = 0.506, p = .481, MSError = 115.57) nor the test time ($F(1, 45)$ = 0.859, p = .359, MSError = 89.15). These findings indicate that there were no differences in participants' scores depending on which home they worked in and that there were no changes in the participants' scores following completion of the learning resource.

The interview data supported the findings from the survey. Most learners interviewed reported that they felt they already worked well as a team and therefore the learning resource did not have a big impact on their practice in this regard. However, a few learners did suggest they were working better as a team as a result of participating in the resource. This was because they felt they better understood the importance of teamwork. A few administrators discussed how after completing the learning resource they made more of an effort to include all team members and make them feel valued: "I think it made me make a more conscious effort to include them more. Just to make them more aware of collaboration: 'maybe you could do this, she could do that'… making them feel more valuable" (Director of Care).

Discussion

Overall, learners had a positive reaction to the learning resource and it was effective in meeting the learning outcomes of improved collaborative practice and palliative care skills and knowledge. We were also able to gain some insight into the use of emerging technologies in education. Partnerships with individuals and organisations afforded us access to software (e.g., 3D software) and specific skills (e.g., filming and editing, 3D imaging) that allowed us to experiment with presenting content in various ways. Throughout the development of the resource we struggled with the competing needs of research and education. While it was extremely important to us to create a pedagogically sound learning resource that would meet the learning objectives outlined by the content experts, we were also being funded by a research grant to explore the use of emerging technologies in education. Therefore, not all our technology decisions were driven by pedagogy as advocated in the literature (Ascough, 2002; Roblyer, 2006).

Our findings were varied. Some technologies, such as the digital storytelling and videos, facilitated an emotional connection with the learning for many of the learners. The use of sound and image allowed the learners to "live" the experience with Rose and her family.

Other technologies, however, detracted from the learners' experiences. In order to view and interact with the 3D images specific software needed to be installed. This proved to be a roadblock for many of the learners despite the fact the long-term care homes had been asked to load the software onto the computers for the learners. Since the completion of the pilot we have created step-by-step instructions on how to download the software using screenshots. Nonetheless, having to download software takes time away from learning and time is a premium for this population. Alternative means of presenting this content need to be explored. Technologies that were not integral to the functioning and completion of the resource, such as using voice recognition to navigate through the resource or the artificial intelligence "expert" that was used as an additional resource, saw little to no use.

The integration of multiple different technologies into the resource required the skills of multiple programmers who could create the elements using these technologies. In addition to the Flash developer who programmed the majority of the resource, we also needed someone who could create 3D images and program the interactive features on them, as well as someone who could program the artificial intelligence component of the resource. Increasing the number of programmers and finding people with the necessary skills added to the budget and time required for development and compounded complications related to logistics and the management of the project. Given the minimal use of these elements the cost-benefit ratio was low. That is not to say that these elements may not be effective learning tools, just that how they were used in this resource did not add to the learning experience. These findings emphasise the importance of it being the pedagogy that drives the technological decisions and not vice versa. They also attest to Berge's (1998) belief in technological minimalism, which he defined as "the unapologetic use of minimum levels of technology, carefully chosen with precise attention to their advantages and limitations" (p. 74).

Despite our sometimes unsuccessful attempts to integrate emerging technologies into this resource, overall, the functionality and effectiveness of the resource was apparent. The demographics of learners in the pilot group revealed that most (72%) use a computer on a daily basis. However, nine percent of the learners had never used a computer before. The need to create a resource with a simple, non-threatening design and easy navigation was apparent. Indeed, we appeared successful in achieving this as learners found the resource was well laid out and easy to navigate. Navigation comprised 'Next' and 'Back' buttons and an animated inukshuk that allowed learners to navigate to the different sections. Learners were provided with animated (video capture) instructions that provide an overview of the resource and how to navigate through it.

Not only were learners' reactions to the usability of the learning resource generally positive, but learners acquired new palliative care and collaborative practice skills and knowledge. The use of the Staged Innovation Design (Campbell, 1969; Wagner, 1984) controlled for some threats to internal validity and provided strong evidence for the effectiveness of the learning resource in achieving the learning objectives in terms of skills and knowledge developed. Learners specifically commented that they had developed an appreciation and respect for those working in other disciplines, as well as learned about the importance of working as a team, new perspectives about resident care, and the signs and symptoms of dying.

In terms of whether the learners' attitudes towards collaborative practice changed and learning was transferred to the point of care, the data do not provide a conclusive picture. Quantitative analyses revealed that learners' attitudes did not change as a result of completing the learning resource. Indeed, the learners who were interviewed indicated they already had positive attitudes towards collaborative practice. Perhaps there was no change due to a ceiling effect. Indeed, further analyses conducted to explore this revealed this might be a possible explanation. A paired sample t-test was conducted on pre- and post-test scores on the Attitudes Toward Health Care Teams Scale (Heinemann et al., 1999) for the learners who had scores in the bottom 50% on the pre-test ($n = 27$ including ties). Although there was still no significant difference between pre- and post-test scores the differences between responses was much larger for this group. Furthermore, data from the interviews did provide examples of how learners' attitudes towards collaborative practice and providing palliative care had changed.

In terms of whether the new knowledge and skills acquired by the learners had been applied in the workplace the results are again inconclusive. Data from the quantitative survey tools indicated that learners believed they had applied new knowledge and skills in the workplace. However, there was little evidence to support the transfer of learning to the point of resident care in the data collected from the interviews, though many indicated they intended to in the future. Preliminary findings regarding whether collaborative practice had improved as a result of the training were not positive. However, given the short time frame from completion of the learning resource to the evaluation, this is perhaps not surprising. It is reasonable to expect changes in behaviour will require time to take effect. Follow-ups at a later date are suggested.

To conclude, this project filled an important need in healthcare and eLearning and benefited all the organisations involved in this project. Many of the project partner organisations will continue to benefit from having a learning resource they can integrate into their academic programs or clinical practices to enhance palliative care and collaborative practice. Others have benefited from gaining a deeper understanding of the complexities of using emerging technologies in the healthcare field.

Acknowledgments

This project was funded in part by Inukshuk Wireless and developed in conjunction with Faculty of Education, University of Ottawa; Palliative Care, Bruyère Continuing Care; Élisabeth Bruyère Research Institute; School of Rehabilitation Sciences, Faculty of Health Sciences, University of Ottawa; Primary Health Care Nurse Practitioner Program, University of Ottawa; NGRAIN; Learning 4 Excellence; The Bess and Moe Greenberg Family Hillel Lodge; Palliative Care Multidiscipline Post Graduate Certificate Programs, Algonquin College.

References

Areskog, N. H. (1994). Multiprofessional education at the undergraduate level-the Linköping model. *Journal of Interprofessional Care, 8*(3), 279-282.

Ascough, R. S. (2002). Designing for online distance education: Putting pedagogy before technology. *Teaching Theology and Religion, 5*(1), 17-29.

Berge, Z. L. (1998). Guiding principles in web-based instructional design. *Educational Media International, 35*(2), 72-76.

Campbell, D. T. (1969). Reforms as experiments. *American Psychologist, 24,* 409-429.

Feldon, D. F. & Yates, K. A. (2007). Increasing validity in the evaluation of new distance learning technologies. *Computers in Human Behaviour, 23,* 2355-2366.

Health Canada, (2004). *Interprofessional education for collaborative, patient-centred practice.* Retrieved March 11, 2004 from http://www.hc-sc.gc.ca/english/hhr/inter professional/index.html

Health Council of Canada. (2006). *Health care renewal in Canada: Clearing the road to quality.* Retrieved May 11, 2006 from http://www.healthcouncilcanada. ca/en/index.php?option =com_content&task=view&id=70&Itemid=72.

Heinemann, G., Schmitt, M., Farrell, M. & Brallier, S. (1999). Development of an attitudes toward health care teams scale. *Education and the Health Profession, 22(1),* 123-142.

MacDonald, C. J., Breithaupt, K., Stodel, E. J., Farres, L. G. & Gabriel, M. A. (2002). Evaluation of web-based educational programs via the Demand-Driven Learning Model: A measure of web-based learning. *International Journal of Testing, 2*(1), 35-61.

Roblyer, M. D. (2006). *Integrating educational technology into teaching.* Upper Saddle River, NJ: Pearson.

Romanow, R. (2002). Commission on the future of health in Canada. Building on values: The future of healthcare in Canada (Cat. CP 32-85/2002E-IN). Government of Canada.

Wagner, N. (1984). Instructional product evaluation using the Staged Innovation Design. *Journal of Instructional Development, 7*(2), 24-27.

Way, D., Jones, L. & Baskerville, N. B. (2001). *Improving the effectiveness of primary health care delivery through nurse practitioner/family physician structured collaborative practice.* Final Report to the Health Transitions Fund, Ottawa, Ontario.

In: Nursing Issues: Psychiatric Nursing, Geriatric Nursing…   ISBN: 978-1-60741-598-5
Editors: C. D. McLaughlin et al., pp. 257-270   © 2010 Nova Science Publishers, Inc.

Chapter X

The Impact of Emotional Intelligence on Nursing Burnout

José María Augusto Landa and Esther López-Zafra
Department of Social Psychology, University of Jaén (Spain).

Abstract

Several studies analyze the importance that stress has on nursing professionals. However, several emotional variables, such as Emotional Intelligence, play a role in its impact. In this book chapter for *Nursing Burnout* we focus on the role that Emotional Intelligence has in Burnout. Specifically, we summarize a series of studies that analyze the modulator impact of emotional intelligence on nursing burnout, occupational stressors and their impact on the health of nursing professionals. Our studies show that those nursing professionals that have clear feelings about their emotions and situations that occur, and are capable of dealing with those emotions, have lower levels of stress in their work. Also, those nurses who show a high ability to curtail their negative emotional states and prolong positive emotional states show higher levels of overall health than those individuals who have trouble regulating their emotions.

Our results imply that the emotional and cognitive dimensions related to emotional breakdown and burnout have to be taken into account in future training programs for nursing professionals.

Keywords: Emotional Intelligence, Burnout, Occupational stressors, Health, Nursing.

Introduction

Research into stress at work has found that individuals who have direct contact with patients, clients, users or students, develop over a longer or shorter period of time the so-called *Burnout Syndrome*. This syndrome refers to the fact that a professional may be overwhelmed by the situation they are suffering (in family, social or working context) and that their capacity for adaptation has been exceeded.

The concept of Burnout was firstly mentioned by Herbert Freudenberger (1974) to describe the physical and mental state that he observed among young volunteers working in a detox clinic. A year later many of them felt exhausted, were easily irritated, had developed a cynical attitude towards their patients and tended to avoid them. Afterwards, Maslach (1976) used the term in psychological science in 1977 at a convention of the APA. Since then the term has been used to describe the burnout experienced by workers in human services (education, health, and public administration). At the present time it is possibly one of the most used concepts in hospitals, schools and businesses.

Maslach and Jackson (1986) conceptualize burnout as a tridimensional syndrome that is developed in professionals whose work targets are people. They add three characteristic dimensions: 1) Emotional Exhaustion; 2) Depersonalization and c) Personal Accomplishment. *Emotional Exhaustion* (EE) is characterized by the progressive tiredness, fatigue or loss of energy that may be evident in physical, mental or combined aspects. It implies an exhaustion of energy, the experience of being emotionally exhausted due to daily and continued contact with individuals whose work deal with (patients, students…). *Depersonalization* refers to the development of feelings, attitudes, and negative responses (both distant and cold) to other people, especially to the beneficiaries of their work. This depersonalization is followed by an increase in irritability and a decline in motivation. Workers view the patients in a dehumanized way, due to affective hardening, blaming them for their problems (e.g.: the patient deserves the illness, the student the failure, the prisoner his conviction…). *Lack of Personal Accomplishment* (PA) is manifested by negative answers to him/her-self and to work. There is a tendency for professionals to be negatively assessed and this negativity affects especially their performance at work and the relationship with the people they serve.

While the burnout syndrome arises as a response to chronic stress at work, it is noteworthy that it is a result of an ongoing process in which coping strategies, often used by the subject, fail. Coping strategies serve as mediating variables between the perceived stress and its consequences, and when they fail, the problem continues. This syndrome can have very negative results for both the individual who suffers it and for the organization in which they perform a professional role. For the individual it may affect their physical and/or mental health, resulting in psychosomatic disorders (e.g., cardio disorders, headaches, gastritis, ulcers, insomnia, dizziness or even states of anxiety, depression, and alcoholism). However, although all these stressors are general for all nurses, some people are affected more than others, showing major consequences of this stress. An individual skill that would help to better understand why certain subjects are more susceptible to the negative consequences of stress than others is Emotional Intelligence.

Job Stressors that Cause the Occurrence of Burnout Syndrome in the Field of Nursing

Work-related stress leads to a situation of dissatisfaction that could be one of the causes of demotivation experienced by health professionals, especially nurses. Nursing is, by nature, a profession subject to high degrees of stress, partly due to the specific nature of tasks and those under their care. If we add the lack of autonomy of these professionals in their work, the lack of clarity of some tasks, the high pressure that they face and the lack of support from superiors, these professionals are a "perfect target" for the burnout syndrome in their work. Authors such as Cherniss (1980) or Stevens and O'Neil (1983) suggest that nursing professionals have no realistic expectations about the service they work for and the incongruity between their expectations and reality influences the stress they experience. Also, Maslach and Jackson (1986) indicate that healthcare professionals are asked to engage intensively with people who usually are in a problematic situation in which they show feelings such as frustration, fear and despair. In these cases, the resulting tension can have an effect of emotional exhaustion and the emotional response is not itself a variable of burnout, but the definition of the phenomenon.

Several studies (Cottrell, 2001; Demeuroti, Bakker, Nachreiner & Schauferi, 2000; Humpel, Caputi & Martin, 2008) found that nursing professionals are the group most prone to stress in their work, with the negative consequences that this entails for their health. Among the main causes of stress among nurses are: contact with suffering and death, conflicts with peers, lack of preparedness to deal with the emotional needs of patients and their families, uncertainty about the effectiveness of treatment, tiredness and fatigue, fear of incurring negligence or inability, and night work.

In Florida, Stechmiller and Yarandi (1993) carried out research at nine hospitals on stress, job satisfaction and burnout among nurses in charge of more critical care. They found that the responsibility of the profession, dealing with other people at work, problems of health, satisfaction with the amount of work, job security, psychological resistance and job satisfaction had a significant effect on emotional exhaustion, which is a component of burnout. The study by Parker and Kulik (1995) found that the levels of employment support and job stress were significant factors in predicting burnout. The highest levels of exhaustion were in close relationship with a poor appraisal of the work done by the same person or the supervisor, with a greater number of working days lost due to sick leave and with a greater number of absences for mental health reasons. Along the same lines, the study by Collins (1996) examined the relationship between job stress, resistant personality and burnout in nurses at hospital. The results they found were that to promote resistance through training programs for nurses could be useful in dealing with stress and might reduce the burnout that occurs in the environment of health services. A study carried out by Avalos Gimenez and Molina (2005) using the Maslach Burnout Inventory found that between 27% and 39% of the nurses had scores indicative of burnout in one of the three subscales. Likewise, their results indicated a greater deterioration among the nurses who worked in in-patient and general services, and lower in surgical nurses. The study by Albaladejo, Villanueva Ortega, Anastasio, Calle and Dominguez (2004) with 622 nurses found that the majority of participants had symptoms of burnout, and that the most affected were young people with only a few years of service, working in emergency departments or in oncology. A recent study conducted by Augusto-Landa, López-Zafra, Berrios-Martos and Aguilar-Luzón (2008) using *The Nursing Stress Scale* with a sample of nurses showed that the largest occupational stressors among nurses were workload, death and suffering, followed by insufficient training, uncertainty regarding treatment, problems with hierarchy and lack of support. Other incidents that in other professions can be more stressful but that in nursing were minor stressors, were problems between the nursing staff, the concern to move temporarily to other services owing to lack of staff and not knowing well how to operate and manage specialized machine.

The effects of stress in nursing practice lead to absenteeism (Wheeler & Riding, 1994), somatic diseases (Lindop, 1999), coronary artery disease, and alcoholism (Cavlheiro, Moura Junior & Lopez, 2008). With regard to the working timetable, it is important to note that the constant changes of schedule in this work have an influence on biological rhythms, disrupting the sleep-wake cycle and pace, and affecting the social relationships of the subject (Piotrokowsky, 1987). We also must take into account the importance of socio-demographic and labor variables. Some studies (Hamaideh, Mryyan, Mudallal, Faouri & Kahsawneh, 2008) have stressed the relationship between demographic variables and work with the appearance of responses to different stressors.

Among the demographic variables, some studies (Duran, Fernandez & Rodriguez, 2006; Maslach & Jackson, 1985; Schwartzmann, 2004) found that single people or people without family responsibilities were more prone to the appearance of burnout syndrome than people who were married or in a stable relationship. In terms of labor variables, the assignment of unit or service, and the possibility of the worker to choose and to be comfortable in that unit has been considered one of the most important indicators of job satisfaction (Chen, Chen, Tsai & Lo, 2007).

Emotional Intelligence

Salovey and Mayer are considered the pioneers in coining the construct Emotional Intelligence (EI), after publishing an article in 1990 in which the term first appeared. It was defined as *"the ability to monitor one's own and others' feelings and emotions, to discriminate among them and use this information to guide one's thinking and actions"* (Salovey & Mayer, 1990, p. 189). However, this construct became enormously popular after the publication of Daniel Goleman's book entitled "Emotional Intelligence" (1995). Following this work, scientists became increasingly interested in the concept, giving rise to numerous studies in various areas of psychology (education, work, health, laboratory contexts, etc.). All contributions made by researchers have led to two lines of research and definitions of the Emotional Intelligence construct: a) First, the *ability model*, known as emotional intelligence conceived as genuine intelligence in the use of our adaptive emotions so that the subject can solve problems and adapt effectively to the environment (Mayer & Salovey, 1997); b) Second, *mixed models or personality models* that focus on stable traits or behavioral variables, such as welfare, motivation or the ability to engage in relationships (Bar-On, 2000; Goleman, 1995).

Figure 1. Percentage of occupational stressors in a nursing sample.

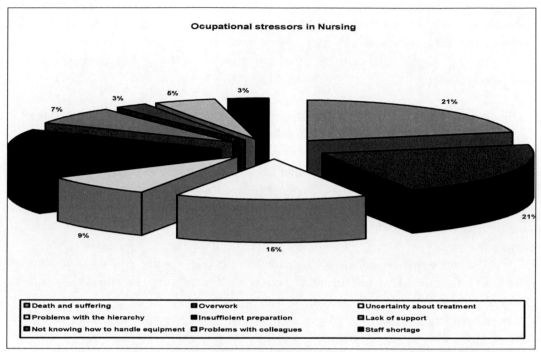

Source: Adapted from Augusto-Landa, López-Zafra, Berrios-Martos & Aguilar-Luzón (2008)

We focus on the model postulated by Mayer and Salovey (1997), whereby Emotional Intelligence refers to four aspects or elements that are ordered hierarchically: 1) the ability to perceive, glean and express emotions accurately (emotional perception) 2) the ability to access and / or generate feelings that facilitate thought (emotional integration), 3) the ability to understand emotions and emotional knowledge and reasoning to emotions (emotional comprehension) and 4) the ability to regulate emotions to promote one's own and others' emotional and intellectual growth (emotional regulation). These skills continue a sequence, from the most basic psychological processes (the first) to the more complex or integrated (the last).

Emotional Perception comprises three kinds of skills: 1) the ability to respond, identify and record one's own and others' emotional messages in different contexts, based on physical condition, behavior, objects, architecture, art, expressions and / or use of language; 2) the ability to express one's own and others' emotions and feelings in an appropriate manner, and the needs associated with them, through verbal and nonverbal language and 3) the ability to recognize true emotions in others and to distinguish between honest and dishonest emotional expressions.

Emotional Integration refers to the ability to generate emotions to facilitate cognitive processes such as memory, reasoning, decision making, problem solving or creative thinking.

In fact, different emotional states may promote approaches to specific problems (e.g. happiness facilitates inductive reasoning and creativity), make us consistent with our mood states (e.g. to see things one way when you're optimistic and happy and in a pessimistic way when you are sad and in a threatening way when experiencing anger or rage), facilitate the formation of judgments and memories and/or encourage the consideration of multiple viewpoints (e.g. people with changing moods show more creativity than those who have a stable mood state).

Emotional Understanding includes four types of skills: 1) the ability to understand the nature and implications of emotions, such as how some lead to others, how they change over time, how they affect relationships and what are the short and long term consequences, 2) the ability to label emotions and understand the relationships between words (e.g. the relationship between love and like), 3) the ability to understand complex emotions and ambivalent feelings (e.g. love - hate or fear - surprise) and, 4) the ability to recognize the transitions between emotions (e.g. the transition from anger to satisfaction or from anger to shame).

Finally, emotional regulation is the ability to receive equally positive and negative emotions, reflect on them and monitor their way of expression in oneself and others, moderating the negative feelings and enhancing the positive ones.

In subsequent publications, Mayer and Salovey (2007) supplement and enrich the concept of IE, diminishing the importance of the perception and regulation of emotions, and placing a greater emphasis on the influence of emotions on thought and intelligence.

This model has led to many publications and has produced great interest in the scientific community. Among its main advantages we can highlight its solid theoretical basis and good empirical support in basic and applied areas.

The Role of Emotional Intelligence over Stress and Health in the Nursing Context

We now have a large body of research related to work environments that have analyzed the role of emotional intelligence related to welfare, health and stress management. Ciarrochi, Deane and Anderson (2002) found that emotional intelligence had a moderating role in the relationship stress-psychological health, such that subjects with high Emotional Intelligence are better predisposed to cope with environmental demands than subjects with a low score in this variable.

One of the self-reports most commonly used in the measurement of EI from the perspective on which we focus is the Trait Meta-Mood Scale (TMMS) developed by Salovey, Mayer, Goldman, Turvery and Palfai (1995) and adapted to Spanish by Fernández -Berrocal, Extrermera and Ramos (2004). This self-report fits into the term known to researchers as Perceived Emotional Intelligence (PEI), which refers to the knowledge that individuals have about their own emotional abilities, and which does not always coincide with their actual ability (Salovey, Woolery, Stroud & Epel, 2002). The TMMS provides an estimate of the reflective aspects of our emotional experience. It is made up of three key dimensions (subscales) of Intrapersonal Emotional Intelligence: 1) *Attention to feelings*, which refers to the tendency of individuals to observe and think about their emotions, feelings, assess and review their affective states, focusing and maximizing their emotional experience (Gohm & Clore, 2000). Its extreme levels (high vs. low attention) are related to emotional imbalance. 2) *Emotional Clarity* refers to the ability of individuals to control their emotions as opposed to knowing only that one feels good or bad. 3) *Repair of one's own emotions* deals with the person's ability to stop their negative emotional states and extend their positive emotional states.

From the above, it follows that emotions play a decisive role and that the ability to reason about them, and to perceive and understand them may allow us to develop emotional regulation processes that would help to moderate the negative effects of stress and lead to better health (Extremera, Fernández-Berrocal y Durán, 2003). Moreover, as the syndrome of burnout stems from social interaction between those who offer their services and those who receive them, the proper management of the emotions arising from such interactions is a key factor in explaining why some individuals are more resistant to appearance of the syndrome than others. This approach has led to the fact that the prevention and treatment of burnout acquires special relevance the concept of emotional intelligence as predictor of quality that can predict success and cope with setbacks that may arise in such professions. From this, we can deduce that a nurse is an emotionally intelligent person who can work in harmony with their thoughts and feelings (Freshwater & Stickley, 2004). The importance of the development of empathy (as an aspect of emotional competence) appears as a central factor in many nursing theories (Peplau, 1992; Newman, 1994; Parker, 2002). A recent study performed by Aguilar-Luzón and Augusto Landa (2009) investigated the relationship of the PEI measured by the TMMS and the personality traits measured by the NEO-FFI as predictors of empathy (measured by the Interpersonal Reactivity Index (IRI scale)) in nursing students, and found that emotional attention and repair were predictors of involvement empathy (one dimension of the IRI). Specifically, high scores in emotional repair predict the tendency of individuals to experience feelings of compassion and concern for others, that is, the meta-cognition of their emotions would act as a basis in the understanding of the emotions of others. Thus, it is possible for people with a good understanding of their emotions to extrapolate this ability to the interpersonal field. In this sense, people who give excessive attention to their emotions would perform the same process when it comes to addressing the feelings of others. This would explain the positive relationships between their own and others' emotional attention.

Other studies have shown that emotional intelligence allows nurses to develop therapeutic relationships to deal with patients and their families and to better manage stress (Cadman & Brewer, 2001; Simpson & Keegan, 2002). The results of the studies presented lead us to believe that emotional intelligence is positively associated with health and negatively with stress. Thus, Limonero, Tomás-Sábato, Fernández-Castro and Gómez-Benito (2004) analyzed the relationship between the stress suffered by nursing professionals and the TMMS. Their results showed that stress correlated negatively with Clarity and Emotional repair. That is, nursing professionals that are clear about what emotions they are feeling and the situations that provoke them are able to regulate these emotions and have lower levels of stress in their work. Along the same lines, the study carried out by Augusto-Landa, Berrios-

Martos, López-Zafra and Aguilar-Luzón (2006) analyzed the predictive ability of PEI and positive and negative affects to explain levels of burnout and mental health in nurses. Thus, attention to emotions accounted for part of the variance of the components of burnout (emotional exhaustion and depersonalization), while low attention and high clarity and emotional regulation of emotions accounted for part of the variance of a component of the burnout called personal fulfillment. In fact, the subjects with low attention and high emotional clarity and emotional regulation reported greater personal fulfillment. With regard to mental health, the scales of positive and negative affect (Bradburn`s scale of positive and negative affect) accounted for part of the variance in mental health. This can be explained by the positive association of positive affect with social contacts and extraversion, whereas negative affect is associated with interpersonal problems, anxiety and neuroticism. Regarding the components of PEI, we found that an adequate attention to feelings, high clarity and emotional regulation are predictors of good mental health. A more thorough examination of the hierarchical regression analysis conducted on the criterion variable revealed that PEI influenced burnout in different ways. Firstly, a direct influence was found in the percentage of variance accounted for by each dimension (emotional exhaustion: 9%; depersonalization: 10%; personal fulfillment: 41%), but there was also an indirect influence through the scale of affect, as the analysis showed that PEI factors influence the tendency to suppress negative affect and enhance positive affect, and in turn this trend accounts for part of the variance of the dimensions of burnout. We also note that the probability of burnout is lower in subjects who score high in emotional clarity or comprehension and emotional repair.

Along the same lines, but with nursing students, the study performed by Montes-Berges and Augusto-Landa (2007) analyzed the role of PEI in relation to social support, coping strategies and mental health. The results showed that Clarity and emotional regulation were outlined as predictors of social support of the subjects, and emotional regulation also appeared as the only predictor of mental health. These studies are consistent with the findings of Tsaousis and Nikolaou (2005) who found that high levels of emotional intelligence were good predictors of physical and psychological health.

Graphic 1

Differences in Health dimensions by High or Low Emotional Regulation

Health Dimensions	PF	RP	BP	GH	VT	SF	MH
Low Regulation	28.68	7.49	9.05	18.05	15.15	8.21	20.68
High Regulation	29.41	7.82	9.82	20.07	17.97	8.76	23.84

Note: PF: Physical Function; RP: Physical role; BP: Body Pain; GH: General Health; VT: Vitality; SF: Social Function; MH: Mental Health.
Adapted from Augusto-Landa, López-Zafra, Berrios-Martos and Aguilar-Luzón, 2008.

Graphic 2. Differences in quality of life and psychological well-being dimensions by high vs. Low emotional regulation.

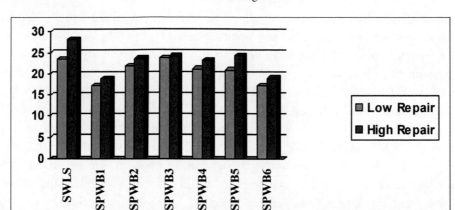

Note: SWLS: Life quality; SPWB1: Self-acceptance: SPWB2: Positive relationships with others: SPWB3: Autonomy; SPWB4: Environment domination; SPWB5: Life Project; SPWB6: Personal Growth.

Source: Adapted from Augusto-Landa & Montes-Berges (2009)

Similarly, the study carried out by Augusto-Landa et al. (2008) analyzed the role that PEI has on occupational stress (measured by the Nursing Stress Scale) and health (measured by the SF.36 questionnaire) in nursing professionals. Their results showed that those nursing professionals with high clarity and emotional regulation reported lower levels of stress, but those with high emotional attention reported higher levels of stress. Emotional regulation is shown as an important variable in the dimensions of health measures through the health questionnaire SF-36. As may be seen in the following graphic, individuals with high emotional regulation showed better levels of health in its various dimensions than those subjects with low emotional regulation.

Similar results have been found in nursing students by Augusto-Landa and Montes-Berges (2009), showing that emotional regulation appeared as the main predictor of the variance in different dimensions of the health questionnaire SF-36 (Vitality, Mental Health, Social Functioning and General Health) and somatic symptoms. Data from the above-mentioned studies suggest that emotional intelligence could be a personal ability of nursing staff that leads to a better perception of subjective well-being, self-efficacy and self-evaluation at work and helps to maintain high levels of dedication to work. Thus, a recent study by Augusto-Landa & Montes-Berges (submitted) analyzed the role of PEI on the quality of life and dimensions of psychological well-being in a sample of 85 nurses. Analysis of variance results showed that emotional regulation (high vs. low) had an effect on life satisfaction and psychological well-being, confirming the importance of this factor in quality of life and the dimensions of psychological well-being. These data allow us to extend and corroborate those found in this type of samples.

Conclusions of the Studies and Future Research

In our studies, presented above, we show the role that emotional intelligence has as a modulator variable of stress and as an important variable in nurses' health. We have analyzed the differential role played by the three components (Attention, Clarity and Regulation) of PEI. In general, the characteristic pattern is that people with higher levels of psychological adaptation and lower levels of stress and burnout are those characterized by moderate to low scores in emotional attention and high scores in the other two dimensions of TMMS (emotional Clarity and Repair). It is important to summarize the importance of the dimensions of TMMS and their role in individual well-being as well as its influence on the different criteria that we have discussed throughout the chapter. Emotional attention is a dimension whose ends are usually characterized by emotional imbalance. Individuals who usually pay attention to emotions are characterized by their monitoring at all times the progress of their moods in an effort to try to understand, which is not always productive to the subject, especially when this high level of attention is not accompanied by the discrimination of the causes, reasons and consequences. The real danger for these people is that they could develop an emotional spiral that leads to a ruminative process outside their control, rather than alleviating their mood, and this would perpetuate a negative state of mood.

This hypothesis endorses the findings that show that high emotional attention is associated with high levels of stress, lower job satisfaction and low self – concept (Augusto-Landa, et al. 2006; Augusto-Landa, et al. 2008; Augusto-Landa, López-Zafra, Aguilar-Luzón & Salguero de Ugarte, 2009) in nursing professionals. In terms of the clarity factor, the evidence shows that individuals who easily identify their specific emotions during stressful situations spend less time dealing with their emotional reactions. In addition, they invest fewer cognitive resources, which allows them to evaluate alternatives for action, to keep their thoughts on other tasks or to perform more adaptive coping strategies. In fact, high scores in emotional clarity were associated with different dimensions of overall health and greater adaptation to stressful situations at work (August-Landa et al. 2006, 2008), greater life satisfaction (Augusto-Landa & Montes-Berges, submitted) and positive coping strategies (Montes-Berges & Augusto-Landa, 2007).

Finally, emotional regulation emerges as the main predictor of health in nursing professionals, so that those who are able to regulate their emotional states (interrupt negative emotional states and prolong positive ones) show higher levels of health. Catanzaro and Mearns (1990) demonstrated the importance of expectations in capacity to regulate emotional and protective factors in our mental health and wellbeing.

The findings provided by research involve a range of evidence about cognitive and emotional factors related to the occurrence of burnout and emotional imbalance that must be taken into account in future training programs aimed at the prevention and monitoring of work stress both in students and nurses.

For all these reasons, we think that the training of emotional intelligence in professionals, not only in nursing professionals but also in nursing students, is necessary to prevent occupational stress and its impact on health. In current Higher education, which emphasizes a high profile development of interpersonal skills, training in the dimension of emotional intelligence is essential.

Increasingly, our students of nursing and physiotherapy reach higher education with a serious deficiency in the skills required during the academic year, the uptake and implementation of clinical practice, and their incorporation into the world of work. Moreover, the adaptation of degree programs to make them suitable for the framework of the European Higher Education Area means rethinking these degrees from a dual perspective. On the one hand, the EHEA will soon require our students to develop a set of core competencies in order to be competitive in the labor market. In addition, teachers are inevitably required to adapt their programs and contents to the introduction of these skills both in the curriculum of the students and in the proposal and performance of training programs that promote the development of such skills. In some universities, as for example the University of Málaga (Spain), students are being trained in competencies such as Emotional intelligence. Previous studies have performed training programs of social skills with nursing students (Marín & León, 2001), but there are no studies about training other competencies with these students. Thus, it is essential to create materials totally adapted to the needs of these students, especially in their clinical training. Our research team is deeply involved in creating these materials dealing with the skills of emotional intelligence in order to enhance attention to emotions, clarity and emotional repair, to promote social and emotional support of male and female future nurses, and to provide training in communication with non-experts in the field and interpersonal skills in general.

References

Aguilar-Luzón, M. C. & Augusto-Landa, J. M. (2009). Relación entre inteligencia emocional percibida, personalidad y capacidad empática en estudiantes de enfermería. *Psicología Conductual, 17(2)*, 351-364.

Albaladejo, R., Villanueva, R., Ortega, P., Astasio, P., Cale, M. E. & Domínguez, V. (2004). Burnout sindrome among nursing staff at a hospital in Madrid. *Revista Española de Salud Pública, 78*, 505-516.

Augusto-Landa, J. M., Berrios-Martos, M. P., López-Zafra, E. & Aguilar-Luzón, M. C. (2006). Relación entre burnout e inteligencia emocional y su impacto en salud mental, bienestar y satisfacción laboral en profesionales de enfermería. *Ansiedad y Estrés, 12*, 479-493.

Augusto-Landa, J. M., López-Zafra, E., Aguilar-Luzón, M. C. & Salguero de Ugarte, M. F. (2009). Predictive validity of perceived emotional intelligence on nursing students' self-concept. *Nurse Education Today, 29*, 801-808.

Augusto-Landa, J. M., López-Zafra, E., Berrios-Martos, M. P. & Aguilar-Luzón, M. C. (2008). The relationship between emotional intelligence, occupational stress and health in nurses: A questionnaire survey. *International Journal of Nursing Studies, 45*, 888-901.

Augusto-Landa, J. M. & Montes-Berges, B. (submitted). Inteligencia Emocional Percibida e intensidad afectiva como predictores de la satisfacción vital y el bienestar psicológico. Un estudio con profesionales de enfermería.

Augusto-Landa, J. M. & Montes-Berges, B. (2009). Perceived emotional intelligence, health, and somatic symptomatology in nursing students. *Individual Differences Research, 7,* 197-211.

Avalos, F., Giménez, I. & Molina, J. M. (2005). Burnout en enfermería de atención hospitalaria. *Enfermería Clínica, 15(5),* 275-282.

Bar-On, R. (2000). Emotional and Social intelligence. Insights from the Emotional Quotient Inventory. In R. Bar-On, & J. D. A. Parker (Eds.), *The Handbook of Emotional Intelligence.* San Francisco: Jossey-Bass.

Cadman, C. & Brewer, J. (2001). Emotional intelligence: A vital prerequisite for recruitment in nursering. *Journal of Nursering Management, 9,* 321 324.

Calvalheiro, A. M., Moura Junior, D. F. & Lopes, A. C. (2008). Stress in nurses working in intensive care units. *Revista latino-americana de enfermagem, 16(1),* 29-35.

Catanzaro, S. J. & Mearns, J. (1990). Measuring general expectancies for negative mood regulation: Initial scale development and implications. *Journal of Personality Assessment, 54,* 546-563.

Chen, Y. M., Chen, S. H., Tsai, C. Y. & Lo, L. Y. (2007). Role stress and job satisfaction for nurse specialists. *Journal of Advanced Nursing, 59(5),* 497-509.

Cherniss, C. (1980). *Profesional burnout in human service organizations.* New York: Praeger Publishers.

Ciarrochi, J., Deane, F. & Anderson, S. (2002). Emotional intelligence moderates the relationship between stress and mental health. *Personality and Individual Differences, 28,* 539-561.

Collins, M. A. (1996). The relations of work stress, hardiness, and burnout among full-time hospital staff nurses. *Journal Nurses Staff Dev., 12(2),* 71-75.

Cottrell, S. (2001). Occupational stress and job satisfaction in mental health nursering: Focused interventions through evidence based assessment. *Journal of Psychiatric and Mental Health Nursering, 8,* 157 164.

Demeuroti, E., Brakker, A. D. & Schauferi, W. B. (2000). A model of burnout and life satisfaction amongst nurses. *Journal Advanced Nursing, 32(2),* 24-38.

Durán, M. M., Rodríguez, A. & Fernández, L. (2006). Prevalencia del Síndrome del quemado y estudio de factores relacionados en las enfermeras del CHUVI (Complexo Hospitalario Universitario de Vigo). *Enfermeria Global, 8,* 1-18.

Extremera, N., Fernández-Berrocal, P. & Duran, A. (2003). Emotional intelligence and burnout in teachers. *Encuentros en Psicología Social, 1,* 260-265.

Fernández-Berrocal, P., Extremera, N. & Ramos, N. (2004). Validity and reliability of the Spanish modified version of the Trait Meta-Mood Scale. *Psychological Reports, 94,* 751-755.

Freshwater, D. & Stickley, T. (2004). The heart of the art: Emotional intelligence and nursering education. *Nursering Inquiry, 11(2),* 91 98.

Freudenberger, H. J. (1974). Staff burn-out. *Journal of Social Issues, 30(1),* 159-165.

Gohm, C. L. & Clore, G. L. (2000). Individual differences in the emotional experience: Mapping available scales to process. *Personality and Social Psychology Bulletin, 26,* 679-697.

Goleman, D. (1995). *Emotional Intelligence.* New York. Bantam.

Hamaideh, S. H., Mrayyan, M. T., Mudallal, R., Faouri, G. I. & Khasawneh, N. A. (2008). Jordanian nurses'job stressors and social support. *International Nursing Review*, *55(1)*, 40-7.

Humpel, N. & Caputi, P. (2001). Exploring the relationship between work stress, years of experience and emotional competency using a simple of Australian mental health nurses. *Journal of Psychiatric and Mental Health Nursing*, *8*, 399-403.

Limonero, J., Tomás-Sabato, J., Fernández-Castro, J. & Gómez-Benito, J. (2004). Influence of perceived emotional intelligence in nursing job stress. *Ansiedad y Estres*, *1*, 29-41.

Lindop, E. (1999). A comparative study of stress between pre and post project 2000 students. *Journal of Advanced Nursing*, *29*, 967-973.

Marín, M. & León, J. M. (2001). Entrenamiento en Habilidades Sociales: un método de enseñanza-aprendizaje para desarrollar las habilidades de comunicación interpersonal en el área de enfermería. *Psicothema*, *13*, 247-251.

Maslach, C. (1976). Burned-out. *Human Behavior*, *5(9)*, 16-22.

Maslach, C. & Jackson, S. E. (1981). The measurement of experienced Burnout. *Journal of Occupational Behavior*, *2*, 99-113.

Maslach, C. & Jackson, S. E. (1982). Burnout in health professions: A social psychological analysis. In G. Sancers, & J. Suls, (Eds,), *Social psychology of health and illness*. Hillsdale, NJ: Erlbaum.

Maslach, C. & Jackson, S. E. (1985). The role of sex and family variables in burnout. *Sex Roles*, *12*, 835-851.

Maslach, C. & Jackson, S. E. (1986). Burnout research in the social services: A critique. Special issues: Burnout among social workers. *Journal of Social Service Research*, *10*, 95-105.

Mayer, J. D. & Salovey, P. (1997). What is emotional intelligence? In P. Salovey y, & D. Sluyter (Eds.), *Emotional Development and Emotional Intelligence: Implications for Educators (3-31)*. New York: Basic Books.

Mayer, J. D. & Salovey, P. (2007). ¿Qué es la inteligencia emocional? In J. M. Mestre Navas, & P. Fernández-Berrocal, (Coords.), *Manual de inteligencia emocional*, (25-45). Madrid: Pirámide.

Montes-Berges, B. & Augusto-Landa, J. M. (2007). Exploring the relationship between perceived emotional intelligence, coping, social support and mental health in nursing students. *Journal of Psychiatric and Mental Health Nursing*, *14*, 163-171.

Newman, M. (1994). *Health as expanding consciousness*. Boston: Jones and Bartlett.

Parker, M. (2002). Aesthetic ways in day to day nursering. In D. Freshwater (Ed.), *Therapeutic nursering*, (100 120). London: Sage.

Parker, P. A. & Kulik, J. A. (1995). Burnout, self an supervisor-rated job performance, and absenteeism among nurses. *J. Behav. Med.*, *18(6)*, 581-599.

Peplau, H. (1992). *Interpersonal relations in nursering*. London: Macmillan.

Piotrokowsky, C. (1987). Families and work. In A. Susman, & C. Stenmetz (Eds.), *Handbook of marriage and the family*. New York. Plenium Press.

Salovey, P. y. & Mayer, J. D. (1990). Emotional intelligence. *Imagination, Cognition, And Personality*, *9*, 185-211.

Salovey, P., Mayer, J. D., Goldman, S., Turvey, C. & Palfai, T. (1995). Emotional attention, clarity, and repair: Exploring emotional intelligence using the Trait Meta Mood Scale. In J. W. Pennebaker (Ed.), *Emotion, disclosure and health*, *(125-154)*. Washington, D. C.: American Psychological Association.

Salovey, P., Woolery, A., Stroud, L. & Epel, E. (2002). Perceived emotional intelligence, stress reactivity and symptom reports: Furthers explorations using the Traid Meta-Mood Scale. *Psychology and Health*, *17*, 611-627.

Schwartzmann, L. (2004). Estrés laboral. Síndrome de Desgaste (quemado), Depresión: ¿Estamos hablando de lo mismo? *Ciencia y Trabajo*, *6(14)*, 174-182.

Simpson, R. L. & Keegan, A. J. (2002). How connected are you? Employing emotional intelligence in a high tech world. *Nursering Administration Quaterly*, *26(2)*, 80 86.

Stechmiller, J. K. & Yarandi, H. N. (1993). Predictors of burnout in critical care nurses. *Heart-Ling*, *22(6)*, 534-541.

Stevens, G. & O´Neill, P. (1983). Expectation and burnout in the developmental disabilities field. *American Journal of Community Psychology*, *11*, 615-627.

Tsaousis, I. & Nikolaou, I. (2005). Exploring the relationship of emotional intelligence with physical and psychological health functioning. *Stress and Health*, *21*, 77 86.

Wheeler, H. H. & Riding, R. (1994). Occupational stress in general nurses and midwives. *British Journal of Nursing*, *3*, 52.

In: Nursing Issues: Psychiatric Nursing, Geriatric Nursing...   ISBN: 978-1-60741-598-5
Editors: C. D. McLaughlin et al., pp. 271-283   © 2010 Nova Science Publishers, Inc.

Chapter XI

Is Caring for the Elderly a Health Risk? A Qualitative Study on Work Experience, Coping and Health Behaviours of Nurses

Brigitte Jenul[1], Ingrid Salem[2] and Eva Brunner[3]
[1]Department of Psychology, Alps-Adria-University Klagenfurt,
Universitaetsstrasse 65-67, 9020 Klagenfurt, Austria.
[2]Department of Psychology, Alps-Adria-University Klagenfurt,
Universitaetsstrasse 65-67, 9020 Klagenfurt, Austria.
[3]Carinthia University of Applied Sciences, Hauptplatz 12, 9560 Feldkirchen, Austria.

Abstract

Caring for elderly and disabled people poses a challenge not only for society but for each person working in this domain. This study addresses individual work experiences, coping strategies and health behaviour of nurses in the elderly care.

Interviews (N = 52) were conducted and analyzed using qualitative content analysis (Elo & Kyngäs, 2008; Patton, 2002). The reliability of the developed category system was evaluated by providing interrater agreement which led to a very good result.

The interviews showed that daily routine in nursing homes was often made difficult by institutional standards and hampered by negative experiences with the residents. In addition to perceiving the hostile, egoistic and uncooperative behaviour of the residents as a burden, more than half emphasised time pressure and staff shortage as stressful. Positive working experiences were related to contacts with residents and their relatives who expressed gratefulness and appreciation but those experiences were outnumbered by unpleasant incidents. The most commonly mentioned coping strategies were taking exercises and seeking for social support. These strategies seemed to help reduce stress during leisure time. Coping with hassle during the working hours is mainly realized by communication with colleagues. On the other hand, delimitation which is defined as distancing oneself from the residents and work in general, plays an important role. About one third of the interview partners could only handle wearisome demands by taking (physical) revenge on the residents or sneering at them.

Health-risk behaviours such as smoking, unbalanced diet and high levels of drug use were frequently reported and multiple risk behaviour was observed. Eighty percent of the interviewed nurses were smokers and more than half of them reported the use of drugs in order to overcome working hours. Body mass index was between 19 and 41, most respondents were at least slightly overweight.

Work conditions in nursing homes seemed to lead to self-neglect and health-risk behaviour on the part of nurses and had negative impact on the interaction with the residents. Due to demographical changes in our society and the prospective increasing demand for nursing and health professionals, nursing homes should become a healthy workplace by focusing on workplace health promotion.

Keywords: Burnout, coping, social support, health behaviour.

Introduction

The need for care of the elderly is rapidly expanding due to higher life expectancy and aging of the oldest old population reaching 85 years and over (Lutz et al., 2008). Currently 80 % of elder care is provided by family members (Attias-Donfut, 2001; Schneekloth, 2006). Institutional care seems daunting to most of us. Media often covers appalling stories in nursing homes including abuse, neglect and the misuse of physical and chemical restraints. Studies show that shortage of staff, absenteeism and a high turnover are some of the main problems in nursing homes (Hasselhorn et al., 2005; Hsu et al., 2007; McGillis Hall & Kiesners, 2005). Best possible care would require patience, keeping in mind the individual needs of the elderly residents as well as interprofessional cooperation (Grond, 2003; Spichiger et al., 2006). These standards are difficult to achieve taking in consideration the pressure of daily work routine often manifested in physical and emotional stresses and strains. Attritions in the musculoskeletal system are frequently reported physical consequences (Jenull-Schiefer et al., 2007; Zimber, 2003), whereas psychological strains are emotionally burdening. The interpersonal contact with residents, their relatives and colleagues contributes to the mental vulnerability (Landau, 2004). In our study (Jenull-Schiefer et al., 2007) 23 % of the health care professionals within the long-term care for the elderly were emotionally exhausted, another 17 % had aversions to residents. The causes of these negative feelings were interactions with confused, aggressive or hostile persons who reacted in a non predictable and poorly adjusted way (Brodaty et al., 2003; Demir et al., 2003). Work strain is often explained by the construct of burnout by Maslach and Leiter (2001). This colloquialism substantially comprises three aspects: emotional exhaustion, depersonalisation or cynicism and a reduction of efficiency. Studies on burnout stated that exhaustion may result from loss of self-confidence in one's own profession and may lead to feelings of fatigue and weakness. Depersonalisation is defined as distancing behaviour and a reduction of efficiency can be seen as a lack of personal accomplishment (Bauer et al., 203; Maslach & Leiter, 2001). Effects of burnout are low job satisfaction and high staff turnover rates as well as individual psychosomatic symptoms (Burisch, 2006; Milisen et al., 2006).

The Effort-Reward Imbalance Model by Siegrist (1996) illustrates the correlation between work conditions and health. Individual health risks are boosted by the imbalance between demanding requirements exhausting the staff and an inadequately low appreciation for their work. This broad concept has to be supplemented by particular components related to the care for elderly, in the way Fillion et al. (2007) did for the field of palliative care.

Main stress factors were found to be time pressure, team conflicts and dealing with death and dying. Emotional support by the team was considered as the main resource. Psychological stress research links general fitness for work in a stressful job domain to coping strategies. Coping is defined as a cognitive and behavioural attempt to deal with internal and external difficult situations (Lazarus & Launier, 1981; Samaha et al., 2007). These difficulties are commonly handled by either problem-oriented or emotion-oriented coping strategies. To divide these strategies in adaptive and maladaptive strategies is regarded as futile due to the individuality of each case (Kaluza, 2003). It is widely agreed that the use of legal and illegal drugs is a health risk and can thus be considered as maladaptive. Based on these theoretical presumptions the present study focuses on job-related strains as well as individual coping strategies of staff in the elderly care.

Methods

The objective of the study was to generate information of individual work experiences, coping strategies and health related behaviour of staff members within the elderly health care. The investigating research strategy needed a qualitative approach for a better comprehension regarding the setting within the job, the perception and personal involvement of participants. Based on quantitative results (Jenull-Schiefer et al., 2007) and relevant studies (Badger, 2005; Brodaty et al., 2003; Demir et al., 2003; McGrath et al., 2003) we constructed an interview guide focussing on three domains: 1. work experiences within nursing homes, 2. individual coping strategies and 3. information on selected health related behaviour. In the first part of the interview participants were invited to report on positive and negative aspects of their daily working routine. The second part of the interview addressed the presentation of individual coping strategies within both, work and leisure time. A third part discussed health related behaviour such as smoking, nutrition, drug use.

Study Participants

We collected interview data in cooperation with nursing service supervision of six nursing homes in Carinthia (Austria). The design of this comprehensive research study addressed all fulltime nursing employees (registered nurses and aides). Based on the staff of the nursing homes the participation of nurses (N = 52) was about 38 %. The study participants were around 40 years old (range 22 - 57) and had on average 11 years of professional experience (range 0.5 to 38 years). Two-thirds of the study participants were female. The sample shared to the same extent in nurses and care attendants.

Ethical Directives

Participants were informed that participation was voluntary and the information provided would be treated confidentially. The first author gave full information about the aims, methods, and expected benefits of this study. This approach is consistent with the ethical principles and code of conduct of psychologists (APA, 2002).

Data Collection and data Evaluation

Two graduate students of psychology conducted the interviews. Interviewers were trained in a face-to-face setting by the research team. They were especially instructed to deal with different communication styles and interviews were practiced by role plays. During a pilot phase each of them conducted and transcribed three interviews, which were analyzed and discussed in cooperation with the research team. The interview guide proved to be applicable. Interviewers made appointments with the nurses to conduct the interviews at the workplace. They lasted for 37 to 90 minutes, with a mean duration of one hour. The interviews were taped, transcribed verbatim and analysed by using qualitative content analysis; structuring, deductive and inductive techniques were applied (Elo & Kyngäs, 2008; Patton, 2002). First the material was structured according to the three domains of the interview guide. Second we formulated theory driven main categories which is a mainly deductive procedure. Third we went through the interviews line by line defining inductive categories which were subsumed under the main categories. The process of developing the category systems was accompanied by research team meetings to discuss the progress and assure intersubjective comprehensibility (Steinke, 2004). To evaluate the quality of the category systems 22 interviews were randomly selected and another researcher independently coded them. We achieved a kappa between .79 and .83 which according to Fleiss and Cohen (1973) indicates a good interrater agreement.

Results

We present the results by defining the main categories within each domain giving some typical examples.

Work Experiences

Table 1 relates to negative work experiences.

Table 1. Negative work experiences in the long term care for the elderly.

Category	Definition	N (%)
Time pressure	Caring duties emphasising time pressure / under time pressure	28 (54 %)
Residents behaviour	Egoism, discontent, self-pity, aggression, ...	20 (38 %)
Patient-staff ratio	Staff shortage emphasising time factor	17 (33 %)
Behaviour of relatives	Discontent, effort, ...	14 (27 %)
Conflicts at the work place	Disputes with colleagues, bad atmosphere, ...	12 (23 %)

The main source of burden for 54 % of the participants is working under time pressure:

> "The permanent time pressure leaves our residents by the wayside." (21)
> "Care duties in the morning are very demanding and time consuming anywhere, some days we barely get to do more than change the swaddling pants." (27)

38 % denominated the work with difficult residents as exhausting. According to the statements those demanding residents are mostly old depressive persons which are little cooperative within the daily routine and behave in a maladadjusted way:

> "At the moment we have hard work days, the residents are very fidgety, some stream a lot and the place is very noisy. ... having ten arms would come in handy." (2)
> =..."well, then he doesn't want to get up, gets unruly, ... you try to motivate him but at some point you run out of energy ..." (26)

Furthermore the mostly chronic staff shortage lays a strain on 33 % of the interview partners:

> "Our department is dimensioned for 36 residents, sometimes they accommodate two or three residents more and we have to take care of them as well with nobody asking about how to manage." (19)
> "... by far too little staff, huge staff shortage, there is too little time for the individual resident, how can we manage if staff members leave and they are not replaced." (38)

Arguments and discussions with family members add to the already difficult work routine (mentioned by 27 %):

> "Family members are always burdening, because you can try as much as you can, you never seem to get it right." (8)
> "Relatives often have a bad conscience about shunting the parents off to the hospital or nursing home. This bad conscience is often taken out on us." (11)

A similar amount of the statements regarded conflicts at the workplace (23 %):

> "A lot of colleagues make your life miserable." (17)

"Some of the colleagues are hard to get along with; I think some of them really missed their vocation." (22)

Positive work experiences were mentioned infrequently as shown in table 2.
Only about a third of the nursing staff told about positive experiences with residents:

"You get a lot back. You realize it when you care for them or when you talk to them or spend time with them, it is great when they say, I missed you, that is when you feel that what you are doing is the right thing." (8)
"… when one of the residents give you a grateful look, that is always a wonderful experience." (10)

A small percentage brought up the recovery of residents

"We have a lot of patients who are brought in following a heart attack and a couple of days later you can meet them in the hallway and you can see that they are getting better." (18)
"It makes me happy if patients, who basically come to die, leave and go home." (19)

and the cooperation within the team:

"Some shifts are fun in spite of our high work load. I remember weekend shifts where everybody was in a good mood and everything flowed smoothly." (3)
"If I'm on duty with a colleague I get along with, this makes life easier." (12)

Table 2. Positive work experiences in the long term care for the elderly.

Category	Definition	N (%)
Grateful residents	Positive feedback by residents	15 (29 %)
Improvement of residents	Recovery of residents, regaining autonomy, …	6 (12 %)
Communication with colleagues	Positive cooperation and working climate	4 (8 %)

Table 3. Non-job-related coping strategies.

Category	Definition	N (%)
Physical activities	Sports, hiking, taking walks, swimming, …	29 (56 %)
Social support (Family, friends)	Recreational activities with friends and family members	28 (54 %)
Tranquillity	Relax and rest the mind	17 (33 %)
Leisure activities		9 (17 %)

Coping Strategies

Statements on individual coping strategies were divided into „job-related "and „non-job-related coping strategies".

Physical Acitivities (56 %)

"I do a lot of sports, anything outdoor really." (8)
"I do strength training; it helps me to get rid of all the stress, the negative energies and the frustration." (3)

and social support by family and friends (54 %) are the most commonly mentioned coping strategies used by the nurses to relax after closing time (s. table 3).

"I come home and play with my little daughter that helps me and relaxes." (7)
"Things put pressure on me - I need to talk about it when I come home." (10)

A third was able to reduce stress by chilling out and lazing around:

"… and then I need ten minutes of total peace and quiet in which nobody should talk to me." (24)
"Just sitting down and relaxing in my garden." (19)

The daily nursing routine is facilitated by intercommunication with colleagues (54 %) (s. table 4). The following interview sequences can confirm this aspect:

"To vent my anger by talking about it to a colleague."(8)
"Just to talk, to speak with a colleague, I need to talk about my problems."(21)

One third of the participants try to relax during the shift by taking some breaks:

"I look out for a quiet corner to get a bit of peace and quiet during the shift." (24)
"It's important to allow for breaks, I mostly go for a smoke." (14)

Table 4. Job-related coping strategies (cinst)

Category	Definition	N (%)
Communication with colleagues	To come to terms with stressful events by discussing the respective situations with your team	28 (54 %)
Breaks	Relax and rest the mind	18 (35 %)
Set boundaries, keep your distance	To distance oneself from others, …	17 (33 %)

The following category involves personal dissociation from residents:

"If the residents bother me, I slam the door and scoff at them, ..."(26)
"... then I turn on the radio really loud and then I try to take no notice of them ..."(29)

This shows that excessive demands and emotional dismay are met by sarcasm and revenge as well as not paying attention to the need of residents.

Health Behaviour

The major part of our interview partners considered their health to be good or at least adequate. A narrow third judged their health situation as scarcely sufficient or bad (s. table 5). The results regarding health behaviour showed multiple health risk behaviour.

Thirty-three nurses were smokers (63 %). They mostly smoked after intensive and highly demanding nursing chores and as a reaction to stress and high workload and frustration. Smoking also enabled them to take a break and get away from it all:

"When I'm stressed out I go and get a smoke. (6)
Smoking helps." (16)

58 % admitted to self-medication, mostly analgetica, in order to be able to overcome a stressful working day. Here are some examples from the interviews regarding the handling of self-medication:

"Yes, I often take analgetics or opioids, whatever comes along and helps me. I have to continue to work after all." (4)
"If I can't manage it any more, I do take some pills. Mostly not really the flimsy kind, I used to take them also in my previous job already. We all tend to be easy with self-medication, why should you bear up against pain?" (18)

In half of the cases medication was taken regularly.

Interview partners had BMI between 17.2 and 41.7, a few of them (13) in overweight range of 25 to 30 and seven of them were adipose. Nursing staff (38 %) were quite self-critically about their dietary habits, 62 % admitted to an extremely high consumption of sweets:

Table 5. Health behaviour.

Category	Definition	N (%)
Smoking	To distance oneself from others, ..., a cigarette allows a break, ...	33 (63 %)
Self-medication	To get along with stress and pain	30 (58 %)
Food	Eating as a coping strategy	20 (38 %)

"...I eat some chocolate, chocolate always helps." (10)
"I check myself some sweets, it boosts my blood sugar level and I feel better." (15)

Discussion

The findings from this study illustrate that daily working routine in the care of the elderly is characterized by a multiple amount of stressful experiences. Registered nurses and care attendants who participated in our study varied in age and profession but had very similar experiences. Positive moments seem to be the exception from the rule. This imbalance pointed to an elevated risk for burnout (Siegrist, 1996; McGillis & Kiesners, 2005). Institutional work conditions showed to be extremely burdening according also to comparable studies (Jenull-Schiefer et al., 2007; Mackintosch, 2006). Apart from time pressure and staff shortages the present study also broached the issue of residents' behaviours and attitudes. Confused elderly persons were depicted as egoistic, hostile, uncooperative and discontent. Most nurses have little training in understanding the cognitive and behavioural aspects of dementia, hardly anyone can handle the emotional expressions combined with this disease (Magai et al., 2002). Recent studies show, that recognition of happy faces is relatively unimpaired in patients suffering from dementia, but it is poor for negative emotions like sadness or anger (Lough et al., 2006; Rosen et al., 2006). One may assume that behavioural patterns and nonverbal emotional communication taking place in the process of dementia might be misinterpreted by nursing staff and thus perceived as personally offending (Inhester, 2005). A key aspect of social interaction is the ability to derive other people's mental state and emotional feelings. Nursing home residents with dementia cannot recognize negative emotions and adapt their behaviour accordingly, thus offending social norms. Frankly acknowledged punishments such as cutting out communication or sarcastic remarks can thus be seen as comprehensible coping strategies. Although such action is understandable and intelligible it clearly disagrees with our moral attitudes. Such incidents can be seen as one aspect of violence within care for the elderly (Schulz, 2005). Abuse and aggression within a caregiver-patient-relationship do mostly not happen intentionally (Bojak, 2001), but result from a chain of events and cannot be reduced to a simple victim-offender-interaction (Ostermann, 1999). Abuse of any kind is seen as one way of coping with stress (Meyer, 1998). The multifactorial model by Schwerdt (1994) describes such acts of violence and abuse by caregivers as malign decompensation and assigns such behaviour to the last of five stages in the process of burnout. Besides such critical and maladaptive strategies the participants also broached the issue of problem-oriented coping. Social support which comprises emotion- and problem-oriented aspects (Welbourne et al., 2007) plays an important role in job- and non-job-related areas of life. High level of social support correlates with a low level of stress (LeSergent & Haney, 2005). Mutual assistance between staff members in well functioning teams are assumed to be a good strategy to avoid stress and burnout in jobs related to the elderly care. Metz and Heimerl (2002) contradict this result by demonstrating that such well functioning teams are a rarity in the field of nursing and caregiving. In the present study 54 % reported about positive experiences, including active team communication as well as close collaboration with colleagues. Efforts towards teambuilding are of major importance. Most of our participants showed a risky health related behaviour. With a percentage rate of 63 the proportion of smokers was much higher as in former studies. In the study by Jenull-Schiefer et al. (2007) 50 % of the participants declared themselves as smokers which exceeds the Austrian population based rates of 23 % by far (BMGF, 2006). The functionality of smoking is perceived differently. Cigarettes serve as a reason to take a break and are used to relieve pressure; smoking also structures the work day and brings you back in contact with yourself after demanding time spans. Furthermore a majority of the participants referred to drug abuse. Half of the respondents regularly take pain medication. Storr et al. (1999) linked drug abuse by caregivers to the massive work load. Results, that corresponds with our study. Self-medication served as a way to cope with stress and strain. Our participants gave account of their eating habits in a self-critical way. Unbalanced diet, eating along the way and discontent with the staff cantina were regarded as reasons for weight problems. Many of the participants were bariatric. These results were also found in the study by Samaha et al. (2007). The investigated group rated their own state of health poorer than the corresponding group in the general population. Not only did general conditions in nursing homes lead to a neglectful und health risky behaviour by the caregivers but also had implications on the interaction with residents. Contrary to our expectations, nurses discussed abuse openly and in fact all types of abuse and neglect were confessed to in the course of the study. Occupational and residential characteristics such as under-staffing residents' behaviour contribute to a high stress level. The main problem is the under-staffing. The implementation of health promoting strategies is a pressing and necessary requirement within the setting of nursing care. Background checks on all staff members working in nursing homes are indispensable. Even the most minor abuse should be considered with alertness and nursing homes should be equipped with abuse prevention plans, including basic and advanced training for the staff as well as psychological training towards sensitivity to nonverbal communication.

References

APA, (2002). Ethical principles of psychologists and code of conduct 2002. Retrieved September, 23, 2008, from http://www.apa.org/ethics/code2002.pdf.

Attias-Donfut, C. (2001). The dynamics of elderly support. The transmission of solidarity patterns between generations. *Zeitschrift für Gerontologie und Geriatrie, 34*, 9-15.

Badger, J. (2005). A descriptive study of coping strategies used by medical intensive care unit nurses during transitions from cure- to comfort-oriented care. *Heart & Lung, 34*, 63-68.

Bauer, J., Häfner, S., Kächele, H., Wirsching, M. & Dahlbender, R. (2003). Burnout und Wiedergewinnung seelischer Gesundheit am Arbeitsplatz [Burnout and recovery of mental health at the workplace.] *Psychotherapie, Psychosomatik, Medizinische Psychologie, 53*, 213-222.

Bojak, B. (2001). *Gewaltprävention.* [Violence prevention.] München: Urban & Fischer.

Brodaty, H., Draper, B. & Low, L. F. (2003). Nursing home staff attitudes towards residents with dementia: strain and satisfaction with work. *Journal of Advanced Nursing, 44*, 583-590.

Bundesministerium für Gesundheit und Frauen (BMGF) (Hrsg.). (2006). Österreichischer Frauengesundheitsbericht. [Austrian women health report.] Wien: BMGF.

Burisch, M. (2006). *Das Burnoutsyndrom. Theorie der inneren Erschöpfung* (3rd ed.). [The burnout sydrom. Theory on the inner fatigue.] Berlin: Springer.

Demir, A., Ulusoy, M. & Ulusoy, M. (2003). Investigation of factors influencing burnout levels in the professional and private lives of nurses. *International Journal of Nursing Studies, 40*, 807-827.

Elo, S. & Kyngäs, S. (2008). The qualitative content analysis process. *Journal of Advanced Nursing, 62*, 107-115.

Fillion, L., Tremblay, I., Truchon, M. & Côté, D. (2007). Job satisfaction and emotional distress among nurses providing palliative care: Empirical evidence for an integrative occupational stress-model. *International Journal of Stress Management, 14*, 1-25.

Fleiss, J. & Cohen, J. (1973). The equivalence of weighted kappa and the intraclass correlation coefficient as measures of reliability. *Educational and Psychological Measurement, 33*, 613-619.

Grond, E. (2003). Die Pflege verwirrter alter Menschen. [The care of confused elderly persons.] Lambertus: Freiburg.

Hasselhorn, H. M., Tackenberg, P., Buescher, A., Simon, M. l., Kümmerling, A. & Müller, B. (2005). Work and health of nurses in Europe. Results from the NEXT-Study. University of Wuppertal and University of Witten, Deutschland. Retrieved September, 25, 2008, from http://www.next.uni-wuppertal.de

Hsu, H. C., Kung, Y. W., Huang, H. C., Ho, P. Y., Lin, Y. Y. & Chen, W. S. (2007). Work stress among nursing home care attendants in Taiwan: A questionnaire survey. *International Journal of Nursing Studies, 44*, 736-746.

Inhester, O. (2005). Gewalt gegen Senioren in pflegerischen Beziehungen – Vernachlässigung und Misshandlung. [Physical violence against elderly persons in caregiver-patient-relations. Neglect and abuse.] In D. Schröder, & R. Berthel (Eds.), *Gewalt im sozialen Nahraum*, (166-194). Frankfurt: Verlag für Polizeiwissenschaft.

Jenull-Schiefer, B., Brunner, E., Ofner, M. & Mayring, P. (2007). Stressbelastung von Wiener Altenpflegerinnen aus Österreich, Osteuropa und Asien. [Stress in registered nurses from Austria, Eastern Europe and Asia in Vienna] *Zeitschrift für Gesundheitspsychologie, 15*, 78-82.

Kaluza, G. (2003). Stress. [Stress.] In M. Jerusalem, & H. Weber (Eds.), *Psychologische Gesundheitsförderung*, (339-361). Göttingen: Hogrefe.

Landau, K. (2004). *Medizinisches Lexikon der beruflichen Belastungen und Gefährdungen. Definitionen, Vorkommen, Arbeitsschutz.* [Medical lexicon of job related pressure and hazards. Definition, sources, occupational safety.] Stuttgart: Genter.

Lazarus, R. & Launier, R. (1981). Streßbezogene Transaktion zwischen Person und Umwelt. [stress-related transaction between person and environment.] In J. Nitsch (Ed.), *Stress*, (213-259). Bern: Huber.

LeSergent, C. & Haney, C. (2005). Rural hospital nurses´ stressors and coping strategies: A survey. *International Journal of Nursing Studies, 42*, 315-324.

Lough, S., Kipps, C., Treise, C., Watson, P., Blair, J. & Hodges, J. (2006). Social reasoning, emotion and empathy in frontotemporal dementia. *Neuropsychologia, 44*, 950-958.

Lutz, W., Sanderson, W. & Scherbov, S. (2008). The coming acceleration of global population ageing. *Nature*, *451*, 716-719.

Mackintosh, C. (2006). Protecting the self: A descriptive qualitative exploration of how registered nurses cope with working in surgical areas. *International Journal of Nursing Studies*, *44*, 982-990.

Magai, C., Cohen, C. & Gomber, D. (2002). Impact of training dementia caregivers in sensitivity to nonverbal emotion signals. *International Psychogeriatrics*, *14(1)*, 25-38.

Maslach, C. & Leiter, M. (2001). *Die Wahrheit über Burnout. Stress am Arbeitsplatz und was Sie dagegen tun können.* [The truth about burnout. Stress on the job and what to do about it.] Wien: Springer.

McGillis Hall, L. & Kiesners, D. (2005). A narrative approach to understand the nursing work environment in Canada. *Social Science & Medicine*, *61*, 2482-2491.

McGrath, A., Reid, N. & Boore, J. (2003). Occupational stress in nursing. *International Journal of Nursing Studies*, *40*, 555-565.

Metz, C. & Heimerl, K. (2002) Was alle angeht, können nur alle angehen – Der Stellenwert von interdisziplinären Teams. [The concern of everybody has to do with everybody. The significance of interdisciplinary teams.] In S., Pleschberger, K. Heimerl, & M. Wild (Eds.), *Palliativpflege – Grundlagen für Praxis und Unterricht*, (301-314). Wien: Facultas.

Meyer, M. (1998). *Gewalt gegen alte Menschen in Pflegeeinrichtungen.* [Physical abuse against elderly persons in nursing homes.] Bern: Huber.

Milisen, K., Abraham, I., Siebens, K., Darras, E. & Dierckx de Casterlé, B. (2006). Work environment and workforce problems: A cross-sectional questionnaire survey of hospital nurses in Belgium. *International Journal of Nursing Studies*, *43*, 745-754.

Ostermann, B. (1999). *Arbeitsbelastungen in der Altenpflege bewältigen.* [To cope with stress on the job in nursing homes.] Weinheim: Beltz.

Patton, M. (2002). *Qualitative research and evaluation methods.* Thousand Oaks: Sage.

Rosen, H., Wilson, M., Schauer, G., Allison, S., Gorno-Tempini, M. L., Pace-Savitsky, C., Kramer, J., Levenson, R., Weiner, M. & Miller, B. (2006). Neuroanatomical correlates of impaired recognition of emotion in dementia. *Neuropsychologia*, *44*, 365-373.

Samaha, E., Lal, S., Samaha, N. & Wyndham, J. (2007). Psychological, lifestyle and coping contributors to chronic fatigue in shift-worker nurses. *Journal of Advanced Nursing*, *59*, 221-232.

Schneekloth, U. (2006). Entwicklungstrends und Perspektiven in der häuslichen Pflege. [Future trends and perspectives within family care settings.] *Zeitschrift für Gerontologie und Geriatrie*, *39*, 405-412.

Steinke, I. (2004). Quality criteria in qualitative research. In U. Flick, E v. Kardoff, & I. Steinke (Eds.), *A companion to qualitative research*, (184-190). London: Sage.

Schwerdt, R. (1994). Ausgebrannt. Enstehungsbedingungen für Burnout bei AltenpflegerInnen. [Burnout. Predictors for burnout in nursing home staff.] *Altenpflegeforum*, *1*, 110-119.

Schulz, P. (2005). *Gewalterfahrungen in der Pflege.* [Violence in nursing.] Frankfurt: Mabuse.

Siegrist, J. (1996). Adverse health effects of high effort-low reward conditions. *Journal of Occupational Health Psychology*, *1*, 27-41.

Spichiger, E., Kesselring, A., Spirig, R. & De Geest, S. (2006). Professionelle Pflege – Entwicklung und Inhalte einer Definition. [Professionell care – development and definition.] *Pflege*, *19*, 45-51.

Storr, C., Trinkoff, A. & Anthony, J. (1999). Job strain and non-medical drug use. *Drug and Alcohol Dependence*, *55*, 45-51.

Welbourne, J., Eggerth, D., Hartley, T., Andrew, M. & Sanchez, F. (2007). Coping strategies in the workplace: Relationships with attributional style and job satisfaction. *Journal of Vocational Behavior*, *70*, 312-325.

Zimber, A. (2003). Arbeit und Gesundheitsschutz. [Work and occupational safety.] *Pflege aktuell*, *7/8*, 380-384.

In: Nursing Issues: Psychiatric Nursing, Geriatric Nursing…   ISBN: 978-1-60741-598-5
Editors: C. D. McLaughlin et al., pp. 285-297   © 2010 Nova Science Publishers, Inc.

Chapter XII

Burnout of Public Health Nurses Involved in Mental Health Care

Hirohisa Imai[*]

Department of Epidemiology, National Institute of Public Health, 2-3-6 MINAMI,
WAKO, SAITAMA 351-0197, JAPAN.

Abstract

Aims

This study examined whether prevalence of burnout is higher among community psychiatric nurses working under recently introduced job-specific work systems than among public health nurses (PHNs) engaged in other public health services. Work environment factors potentially contributing to burnout were identified. In addition, correlations of burnout with emergency patient referral systems and the feelings of PHNs providing mental health services were examined.

Methods

Two groups were examined. The Psychiatric group comprised 525 PHNs primarily engaged in public mental health services at public health centers (PHCs) that had adopted the job-specific work system. The Control group comprised 525 PHNs primarily engaged in other health services. Pines' Burnout Scale was used to measure burnout. Respondents were classified by burnout score into three groups: A (mentally stable, no burnout); B (positive signs, risk of burnout); and C (burnout present, action required). Groups B and C were considered representative of "burn-out". A questionnaire was also prepared to investigate systems for supporting PHNs working at PHCs and to define emergency mental health service factors contributing to burnout.

[*] Corresponding author: Director and Chairman, Department of Epidemiology, National Institute of Public Health, 2-3-6 MINAMI, WAKO, SAITAMA 351-0197, JAPAN, Tel: +81-48-458-6167, Fax: +81-48-469-2677, E-mail: imaihiro@niph.go.jp

Results

Final respondents comprised 785 PHNs. Prevalence of burnout was significantly higher in the Psychiatric group (59.2%) than in the Control group (51.5%). Responses indicating lack of job control and increased annual frequency of emergency overtime services were significantly correlated with prevalence of burnout in the Psychiatric group, but not in the Control group. Also when analyzed in relation to several states of feeling of PHNs, prevalence of burnout among psychiatric PHNs was found to increase significantly as frequency of experiencing a feeling of restriction during overtime work.

Conclusions

Prevalence of burnout is significantly higher for community psychiatric nurses than for PHNs engaged in other services. Overwork in emergency services, lack of job control, and a feeling of restriction appear to represent work environment factors contributing to burnout. Inadequacy of emergency mental health service systems was identified as a cause of the high prevalence of burnout among these nurses.

Main Messages of this Chapter

- Prevalence of burnout was significantly higher for community psychiatric nurses (prevalence 59.2%) than for PHNs engaged in other public health services in this nationwide survey.
- Excessive work demands, particularly for emergency overtime work, and low job control for community psychiatric nurses are work environment factors that appear to contribute to burnout.
- The work characteristics of community psychiatric nurses may be categorized as displaying "high job strain".
- Prevalence of burnout in community psychiatric nurses correlates significantly with frequency of a feeling of "restriction" during work.
- To implement de-institutionalisation that the national government has devised, establishment of a system that can not only accept discharged patients, but also cope with the emergency care needs of discharged patients is indispensable.
- Community psychiatric nurses will play a central role in any such system. Thus, countermeasures to improve the work environment and prevent burnout among nurses should be implemented.

Text

Introduction

The term "burnout" is used to indicate a syndrome characterized by emotional exhaustion, depersonalization and reduced feelings of personal accomplishment[1]. Burnout can be viewed as a response to stressful environmental factors, rather than stressful personal factors[2]. Numerous studies have investigated burnout, revealing that the condition is more likely to develop in human service professions, particularly the medical and educational professions[3,4]. Burnout is considered to result from a long-term accumulation of stressors associated with occupation and working environments[5].

In developed countries like the United Kingdom (UK) and Canada, newly implemented work climates or systems following health reforms and restructuring place considerable stress on district nurses and home care workers[6,7]. For instance, one study reported that many district nurses felt that ongoing changes to the National Health Service represented the largest stressor in the UK[7]. The environments in which medical professionals work are undergoing profound changes, due to increasing demands in medical care, mounting pressure to keep medical costs down, and reforms to medical care systems[8-11]. Changes in medical care systems and working environments can act as stressors on medical professionals, resulting in physical and mental burdens[12,13]. In Japan, the work system for public health nurses (PHNs) in public health centers (PHCs) across the country was fundamentally modified in April 1997, when the Community Health Act came into effect[14-16]. This Act replaced the previous region-specific work system with a job-specific work system. The resulting changes to the work environment of PHNs working in PHCs seem to be contributing to various types of mental stress.

Under the region-specific work system, PHNs were involved with all public health activities in a given region. Under the new job-specific work system, PHNs working in a PHC are involved in one of five major areas of services: (1) health services for adults and the aged; (2) services for mothers and children; (3) services related to infectious diseases; (4) services related to intractable diseases; and (5) mental health services[15]. We focused on PHNs engaged in mental health services (community psychiatric nurses) when conducting this survey. Community psychiatric nurses are said to experience greater physical and mental fatigue due to problems with working conditions (inadequate support systems) and unsatisfactory regional emergency mental health care systems. However, no studies have systematically examined evidence supporting this view. The aim of the present study was therefore to investigate whether prevalence of burnout is higher among community psychiatric nurses working under the recently introduced job-specific work system than among PHNs engaged in other public health services. Factors contributing to burnout were identified, and three major categories related to the work environment (support systems, PHN relationship with physicians, and emergency service systems at PHCs) were examined. In addition, correlations of burnout with emergency patient referral systems and the feelings of PHNs providing mental health services were examined.

Research Methods

In Japan, 448 PHCs are operated by prefectures, which are similar to counties in the UK[16]. Of these, 356 have adopted the job-specific work system, although the number of community psychiatric nurses was unknown at 27 of the 356 PHCs. Community psychiatric nurses working at 329 PHCs were therefore requested to participate in this survey.

A total of 133 PHCs had only one PHN engaged in public mental health services. For these institutions, that PHC selected to participate in the present study. The remaining 196 PHCs had two or more PHNs engaged in public mental health services. Under these circumstances, two PHNs were randomly selected as participants. A total of 525 PHNs primarily engaged in public mental health services were therefore selected, forming the Psychiatric group. The Control group comprised 525 PHNs (one or two nurses selected at random from each of the 327 stations) from the same PHCs and primarily engaged in adult/aged services (n=132), mother/child services (n=132), infectious disease services (n=131) or intractable disease services (n=130). This sample size was sufficient to detect an increased prevalence of burnout in the Psychiatric group of ≥10%, assuming burnout prevalence in the Control group of about 50% as seen in the preliminary survey, with 80% power at the 5% level of significance (two-tailed test). The required sample size was 408 in each group, for a total of 816. On November 5, 2002, a questionnaire was mailed to all 1050 potential subjects. To avoid any potential disadvantage to respondents associated with responses, the questionnaire was anonymous in design and each respondent sealed and mailed the return envelope by themselves. After the initial deadline for responses had passed, all nurses to whom questionnaires had been sent were mailed a request for participation in the survey, to elevate response rate. The questionnaire included a column for obtaining from each respondent informed consent for use of the extracted data in this study.

Instruments for evaluating burnout have been developed by Pines[17], Maslach[18] and Jones[19]. Each of these instruments displays unique characteristics, and selection depends on the specific survey objectives or preferences of the investigator. The Burnout Scale developed by Pines has been translated into Japanese and has been used to study burnout among Japanese nurses and PHNs[23,24]. The present study utilized Pines' Burnout Scale to measure burnout. The scale is a self-diagnosis instrument that includes 21 questions evaluating three factors of burnout: a) physical exhaustion; b) emotional exhaustion; and c) mental exhaustion. Of the 21 items, 17 are negative and 4 are positive[17]. Responses to all items utilize a 7-point scale. Composite burnout score represents the mean response for all items, with scores for positive items reversed. This scale was previously validated based on a sample of more than 5000 individuals, comprising Americans, Canadians, Japanese, Australians, and Israelis. Construct validity was established using discriminant validity methods, which utilize correlational-type analysis of the target test, with several other relevant measures. The Burnout Scale has also shown high test-retest reliability and internal consistency[22].

Respondents were classified by burnout score into three groups: Group A (score ≤2.9; mentally stable, healthy, no burnout); Group B (3≤score≤3.9; positive signs, risk of burnout); and Group C (score ≥4; burnout present, action required)[17,20]. Groups B and C were considered to represent a state of "burn-out" for the purposes of this study. A separate questionnaire was also prepared to investigate factors providing support for PHNs working in PHCs and the adequacy of emergency mental health service systems. This questionnaire included items pertaining to individual characteristics (age of nurses, population of region covered by each PHC, length of nursing career, etc.) and the work environment (actual data on work, work systems, support systems, etc.). Prior to the main survey, a preliminary survey of 104 PHNs at 52 PHCs was conducted. Results of the preliminary survey were utilized to improve the validity and reliability of this separate questionnaire.

Relative risk (RR) of burnout for the Psychiatric group compared to the Control group was presented with 95% confidence interval (CI). Gross differences in burnout prevalence between Psychiatric and Control groups were compared using the Mantel-Haenszel method to adjust for possible confounding effects. Stratified comparisons were performed to adjust for characteristics that differed significantly ($p \leq 0.10$) between Psychiatric and Control groups. Adjusted RRs, associated 95% CIs and p-values were calculated using the Mantel-Haenszel test. The Mantel extension test for trends was used to evaluate correlations between burnout and working conditions (Table3). In order to evaluate the relationship between burnout and risk factors, the significance of monotonic trends was assessed by treating the categorical answers as continuous variables in multiple logistic regression models that included age and number of years in current service (Table4). These analyses were performed for both groups. Values of $p \leq 0.05$ were considered statistically significant. All statistical analyses were based on two-tailed probabilities. SPSS for Windows software (version 10.0.5J, SPSS Japan, Tokyo, Japan) was used for statistical analyses.

Results

Of the 1050 questionnaires sent out, 858 were returned. Responses were received from 423 community psychiatric nurses and 435 nurses engaged in other services (adult/aged services, n=112; mother/child services, n=102; infectious disease services, n=109; intractable disease services, n=112). Overall response rate was 81.7%. Of the 858 responses, 625 were collected by the original deadline (primary responses), and 233 were collected after the reminder letter was sent (secondary responses). No significant differences were observed between primary and secondary responses in terms of response tendencies for any questions in the questionnaire. Some respondents answered that they were involved in two or more of the five service categories mentioned above, rather than specializing in one particular service category. These respondents were excluded from analysis. As a result, 785 respondents were included in the final analysis, including 396 community psychiatric nurses and 389 PHNs not engaged in mental health services. The estimate of internal consistency (Cronbach's α) for the Burnout Scale was 0.94 in the 785 respondents.

Table 1 compares characteristics between Psychiatric and Control groups. Psychiatric and Control groups displayed significant differences in number of years in current service (p=0.009).

Table 2 shows overall prevalence of burnout for the two groups. Relative risk of burnout was significantly increased for the Psychiatric group compared with the Control group. Two factors that differed significantly ($p \leq 0.10$) between Psychiatric and Control groups, age-strata and number of years in current service, were examined to adjust for possible confounding effects. Relative risks for overall, age-strata, and number of years in current service were significantly increased.

Table 1. Characteristics of PHNs

Characteristics	Service area		p [*]
	Psychiatric health care, n=396	Others, n=389	
Age			
-30	35 (9)	49 (13)	
31-35	68 (17)	69 (18)	
36-40	66 (17)	81 (21)	
41-45	106 (27)	80 (21)	
46-50	57 (14)	53 (14)	
51+	64 (16)	57 (15)	0.064
Population covered by health centre (x1000)			
<100	124 (32)	126 (33)	
100-150	90 (23)	89 (23)	
150-200	53 (14)	56 (15)	
200-250	38 (10)	31 (8)	
250-300	29 (7)	26 (7)	
>300	58 (15)	56 (15)	0.968
Time taken to workshop (min)	40 [20, 60]	45 [20, 60]	0.339
Career as PHN (y)	19 [12, 24]	17 [11, 23]	0.125
Number of years in current service			
<1	144 (36)	181 (47)	
1	57 (14)	45 (12)	
2+	195 (49)	163 (42)	0.009

[*] Wilcoxon rank-sum test   No. (%), or median [25th, 75th percentile]

Table 2. Prevalence of burnout according to service area, age and number of years in current service, and relative risks (RRs) of burnout for psychiatric group compared with control group

	Service area				Comparision between psychiatric health care and others		
	Psychiatric health care, n=387		Others, n=377				
	Burnout, %	(95% CI)	Burnout, %	(95% CI)	RR	(95% CI)	p
All	59.2	(54.3-64.1)	51.5	(46.4-56.5)	1.15 [a]	(1.01-1.31) [a]	0.032 [b]
Age(y)							
-30	58.8		61.2				
31-35	65.7		50.7				
36-40	64.1		51.9				
41-45	53.3		41.0				
46-50	57.9		54.0				
51+	58.3		55.8		1.17 [c]	(1.03-1.33) [c]	0.022 [d]
Years in current service							
<1	62.3		50.3				
1	64.8		46.5				
2+	55.4		54.1		1.15 [c]	(1.01-1.31) [c]	0.037 [d]

[a] Crude relative risk and 95% confidence interval
[b] Chi-square test
[c] Adjusted relative risks and 95% confidence intervals using the Mantel-Haenszel method
[d] Mantel-Haenszel test

Table 3 shows the association between prevalence of burnout in each group and answers to questions on PHN relationships with physicians, support systems, and emergency service systems at PHCs. Affirmative responses to "Is success or failure of service largely determined by the physician?" were significantly associated with prevalence of burnout in the Psychiatric group (p=0.008), but not in the Control group (p=0.868). For the question, "How often are emergency overtime services needed per year?", increased annual frequency of emergency overtime services correlated with prevalence of burnout in the Psychiatric group (p=0.014), but not in the Control group (p=0.426).

Table 3. Prevalence of burnout among PHNs, stratified by service area and working conditions

Working conditions	Service area					
	Psychiatric health care, n=387			Others, n=377		
	Total	Burnout (%)	p*	Total	Burnout (%)	p*
Support status						
PHNs in service						
3+	171	57.9		61	52.5	
2	134	57.5		115	48.7	
1	69	63.8	0.531	172	54.7	0.619
Staff members other than PHNs						
2+	107	50.5		75	48.0	
0/1	176	61.9	0.064	136	53.7	0.473
Help by PHNs in other service areas						
Sufficient	85	41.2		99	41.4	
Moderate	221	63.3		199	50.3	
Seldom	62	67.7		67	65.7	
Not at all	15	60.0	0.004	12	75.0	0.001
Emergency services after usual business hours						
Night/holiday duty rotation system						
Present	262	56.9		178	49.4	
Planned/Unknown	19	52.6		70	52.9	
Absent	92	67.4	0.099	76	55.3	0.384
Frequency of emergency overtime work						
None	39	41.0		215	48.4	
Less than 5 times/year	167	58.1		107	56.1	
More than 6 times/year	172	64.0	0.014	49	51.0	0.426
Service schedule disturbed by emergency services						
Never	10	40.0		100	44.0	
Rarely	54	48.1		144	50.7	
Sometimes	180	56.1		83	55.4	
Often	141	68.8	0.002	38	68.4	0.011
Relations to physicians						
Physician needed						
Never	46	47.8		284	51.8	
Rarely	86	58.1		50	52.0	
Sometimes	109	66.1		16	56.3	
Often	135	60.7	0.169	5	60.0	0.730
Physician difficult to secure when needed**						
Never	18	38.9		17	35.3	
Rarely	58	62.1		26	61.5	
Sometimes	108	58.3		20	60.0	
Often	146	67.1	0.051	7	42.9	0.450
Success/failure is dependent on physician						
Never	17	35.3		72	55.6	
Rarely	79	57.0		66	47.0	
Sometimes	214	57.5		151	49.0	
Always	72	72.2	0.008	48	60.4	0.868

* Wilcoxon rank-sum test (for trends)   ** Asked only to those affirming need for physician (i.e. excluding the 46 responding "never" to Physician needed)

Table 4. Percentages of PHNs assigned to Group B (signs of burnout) or C (burnout present) in relation to feeling state

Feeling state	In charge of					
	Psychiatric health care			Others		
	Total	%	P for trend*	Total	%	P for trend*
Total	387	59.2	-	377	51.5	-
Feeling tension during overtime work‡						
Never	17	23.5		42	47.6	
Rarely	64	56.3		51	49.0	
Sometimes	144	63.2		59	59.3	
Always	122	68.0	0.002	29	72.4	0.029
Feeling restrained during overtime work‡						
Never	14	14.3		39	46.2	
Rarely	62	54.8		56	57.1	
Sometimes	147	63.9		56	57.1	
Always	122	68.9	< 0.001	28	64.3	0.169
Feeling work is burdensome						
No	6	16.7		10	10.0	
Little	63	30.2		150	32.7	
Some	206	57.3		155	60.6	
Much	101	82.2	< 0.001	45	80.0	< 0.001

* Adjusted for age and number of years in current service using logistic regression.
‡ Asked only to those with overtime emergency service requirements (i.e., those in psychiatric health care, excluding the 39 participants responding "never" for overtime emergency service requirements).

Table 4 shows the relationship of burnout prevalence in each PHN group to several feeling states. This analysis reveals that prevalence of burnout in psychiatric PHNs correlates significantly with frequency of a feeling of "restriction" during work.

Comments

The key finding of this study was that prevalence of burnout is significantly higher for community psychiatric nurses than for PHNs engaged in other public health services. Prevalence of burnout reached 59.2% for community psychiatric nurses. This is higher than the prevalence reported in a previous survey of physicians engaged in emergency pediatric care (50%), using the same Pines' Burnout Scale[23]. Past studies of burnout among medical professionals have focused on hospital-based staff, and have revealed unresolved problems pertaining to hospital staff[24-26]. The present study, however, reveals that more than half of PHNs engaged in community health services at PHCs display some level of burnout, irrespective of the type of public health services provided. This study also shows that the situation is more serious for community psychiatric nurses, who represented the primary focus of this study. We believe the results of this study display external validity, since the study was carefully and adequately designed, and involved PHNs across the country. Furthermore, no previous study of PHNs has been conducted on such a large scale.

The distribution of burnout among community psychiatric nurses displayed two slow peaks: one for the thirties age group; the other for the fifties age group. Differences in burnout prevalence between Psychiatric and Control groups were particularly noticeable for nurses in their thirties. Community psychiatric nurses in this age bracket have often been pursuing a nursing career for at least a decade, and are in the prime of their life as community psychiatric nurses, possessing large amounts of knowledge and experience. For this reason, high expectations and heavy work demands may be heaped on these nurses by both superiors and subordinates. Levels of expectation and work demands may prove excessive, causing extreme mental and physical exhaustion and contributing to burnout. The apex of the second burnout peak was for nurses in their fifties, and may well reflect the influences of reduced physiological functioning and the increasing development of illness that occurs in the fifties.

With regard to nurse relationships with physicians, the most striking difference observed between the Psychiatric and Control groups was the correlation between prevalence of burnout and percentage of responses indicating that success or failure of services is perceived as largely dependent on the physicians involved. In the Psychiatric group, prevalence of burnout rose significantly with increasing perception of dependence on physicians. No such correlation was noted in the Control group. Of the nurses who stated that the success or failure of service was "always" dependent on the physicians involved, 72.2% experienced burnout. This percentage was higher than that for any other question, meaning that burnout in community psychiatric nurses is closely related to whether the physician needed for a given community psychiatric service satisfies the requests or expectations of nurses. Furthermore, in the Psychiatric group, increased frequency of services requiring emergency overtime work elevated the prevalence of burnout. No such correlation was observed in the Control group. The implication here is that mental health services differ from other public health services in terms of the nature of cases requiring emergency overtime work, and that mental health services more frequently involve difficult cases that are more likely to cause burnout in PHNs.

The prevalence of burnout recorded by this study may slightly overestimate the real situation, since cases with relatively mild symptoms were also included as cases of burnout according to our criteria. That is, Group B (positive signs and risk of burnout) and Group C (burnout present and action required) were both deemed representative of burnout. Although the prevalence of burnout needs to be evaluated more carefully, the present study undoubtedly indicates that the prevalence of burnout is higher among PHNs involved in mental health care than among PHNs in charge of other services. Furthermore, considering a British report that one in every two community psychiatric nurses was seriously emotionally drained by their work[27], the prevalence of burnout revealed in the present study may not be excessively high. It is plausible to imagine from these studies that as work environments for PHNs in developed countries have undergone rapid changes in recent years, more than a few PHNs have been burdened by great physical and mental stress, possibly causing varying degrees of burnout.

The present study focused only on the work environment, whereas burnout can be caused by factors related to both the workplace and personal and social factors. The significant factors identified in the present study cannot completely explain the level of burnout observed in all cases. Relationships between burnout among community psychiatric nurses and personal or social factors must also be examined. Further investigation of the issues surrounding work environment and job stress will add to our understanding of burnout, work environment and potential preventive measures among community psychiatric nurses. Theories on job stress, particularly the demand-control model described by Karasek, have contributed to the study of job stress by supplying theoretical frameworks with which to explain associations between psychosocial characteristics of the work environment and health outcomes[28,29]. The demand-control model suggests that a high demand-low control combination at work can contribute to mental and physical pathology[30,31]. In our study, the work environment factor "increased frequency of emergency overtime work" would presumably represent high job demands, and the factors "Difficulty securing a physician" and "Success/failure is determined by physician" may both represent low job control. The work characteristics of community psychiatric nurses may thus be categorized as displaying "high job strain", and some studies have reported that "high job strain" is associated with mental illness[32]. In future, associations between work environment, stress levels, and mental illness among community psychiatric nurses should be analyzed utilizing approaches including not only burnout theories, but also job stress theories, such as the demand-control model.

The basic difference between the burden of providing psychiatric health services and the burden of providing other health services is said to be the "the existence of overtime for psychiatric health services" [33]. Under the current system, psychiatric PHNs are placed in the situation where they are not free from work even outside their duty hours, which leads to them becoming psychologically exhausted. We tried to clarify a clear difference between psychiatric PHNs and non- psychiatric PHNs in terms of the three major presumable psychological states that lead to psychological exhaustion, namely, feeling tension, feeling restrained, and feeling burdened. When analyzed in relation to several states of feeling of

PHNs, prevalence of burnout among psychiatric PHNs was found to increase significantly as frequency of experiencing a feeling of restriction during work increased. The number of mentally ill patients for whom examination by qualified psychiatrist is requested or who are reported to the PHC pursuant to the provisions of the relevant law has been increasing recently[34]. However, emergency psychiatric service systems able to satisfy urgent needs at night or on holidays are often absent or inadequate[35], and psychiatric PHNs tend to experience difficulty in dealing with urgent cases. Under such circumstances, psychiatric PHNs are understandably anxious about receiving calls for urgent arrangements, and are not free from this anxiety even after normal working hours (e.g., weeknights and off-duty holidays). As a result, psychiatric PHNs have a sensation of continued restriction in their job. Working environments in which individuals must work for prolonged periods or cannot see an end to their work can serve as malignant stressors that have been considered a factor responsible for burnout[36]. Psychiatric PHNs who often experience these sensations of restriction are likely to develop burnout.

Based on the present results, one way to prevent burnout among psychiatric PHNs would appear to involve the establishment of well-functioning emergency mental health service systems that can cope with demands at night and on holidays. The Japanese government started a program to improve emergency mental health service systems in each prefecture recently, and this program has gradually been implemented[37]. Some prefectures, however, still lack systems that are capable of coping with demands on holidays or at night, and other prefectures have systems that do not work efficiently[38]. PHNs are sometimes unable to contact psychiatrists when needed, or have difficulty in finding a hospital able to accept the patient. Establishing well-functioning emergency mental health service systems should therefore be a priority in all prefectures. Examples of potential improvements include organizing independently operated emergency mental health service systems and providing adequate education to psychiatrists so that they can recognize the need for emergency mental health services.

The present study displays several limitations. First, the reliability and validity of the Japanese version of Pines' Burnout Scale, employed in the present study, have yet to be strictly verified. However, a previous study using this version of Pines' Burnout Scale did demonstrate the internal validity of the scale[23]. In the present study, Cronbach's α coefficient was 0.94, indicating a high level of internal consistency for the scale. Secondly, we performed 9 tests for each group in Table 3. To adjust for multiple testing we calculated adjusted p-values of those tests that had displayed significance before adjusting using the Holm method[39]. In analyses of the Psychiatric group, the resulting p-values were 0.032, 0.084, 0.018 and 0.056 for the working conditions "Help by PHNs in other service areas", "Frequency of emergency overtime work", "Service schedule disturbed by emergency services", and "Success/failure is dependent on the physician", respectively. The possibility cannot be excluded that multiple testing might have contributed to spurious significant results for "Frequency of emergency overtime work" and "Success/failure is dependent on the physician".

Conclusion

In conclusion, our study shows that prevalence of burnout is significantly higher for community psychiatric nurses than for PHNs engaged in other services. Excessive work demands, particularly for emergency overtime work, and low job control for community psychiatric nurses appear to represent work environment factors contributing to burnout. Countermeasures to improve the work environment and thus prevent burnout among nurses need to be implemented.

References

[1]   van Dierendonck, D; Schaufeli, WB; Sixma, HJ. Burnout among general practitioners: a perspective from equity theory. *J Soc Clin Psychol.*, 1994, 13, 86-100.

[2]   Maslach, C; Schaufeli, WB; Leiter, MP. Job burnout. *Annu Rev Psychol.*, 2001, 52, 397-422.

[3]   Gundersen, L. Physician burnout. *Ann Intern Med.*, 2001, 135(2), 145-148.

[4]   Cherniss, C. Beyond Burnout: Helping Teachers, Nurses, Therapists, and Lawyers Recover from Stress and Disillusionment. New York: *Routledge*, 1995.

[5]   Maslach, C; Schaufeli, WB; Leiter, MP. Job burnout. *Annu Rev Psychol.*, 2001, 52, 397-422.

[6]   Denton, M; Zeytinoglu, I; Davies, S; Lian, J. Job stress and Job dissatisfaction of home care workers in the context of health care restructuring. *Int J Health Serv.*, 2002, 32, 327-57.

[7]   Evans, L. An exploration of district nurses' perception of occupational stress. *British Journal of Nursing*, 2002, 11, 576-85.

[8]   Matsuda, S. The health and social system for the aged in Japan. *Aging Clin Exp Res.*, 2002, Aug, 14(4), 265-70.

[9]   Lai, OK. Long-term care policy reform in Japan. *J Aging Soc Policy*, 2001, 13(2-3), 5-20.

[10]   Watts, J. Japan starts on health-spending slowdown. *Lancet*, 2001, Aug, 25, 358 (9282), 647.

[11]   Ikegami, N; Campbell, JC. Health care reform in Japan: the virtues of muddling through. *Health Aff (Millwood)*, 1999, May-Jun,18(3), 56-75.

[12]   Blair, A; Littlewood, M. Sources of stress. *J Community Nursing*, 1995, 9, 38-40.

[13]   Traynor, M. The views and values of community nurses and their managers: research in progress--one person's pain, another person's vision. *J Adv Nurs.*, 1994, Jul, 20(1), 101-9.

[14]   Health and Welfare Statistics Association. Community health act. *Journal of Health and Welfare Statistics*, 2000, 47(9), 20-1.

[15]   Ohno, A; Yajima, M; Mori, Y; Yoshida, T; Sato, Y. The role of public health nurses at public health centers after community health act implementation. *Kitakanto Med J*, 2000, 50, 127-37.

[16] Health and Welfare Statistics Association. Activity of public health stations. *Journal of Health and Welfare Statistics*, 2002, 49(9), 18-9.

[17] Pines, A; Aronson, E. Burnout. From tedium to personal growth. New York: The Free Press, 1981.

[18] Maslach, C; Jackson, SE. Burnout in health professions: a social psychological analysis. In: GS; Sanders, J; Suls, (Eds). Social Psychology of Health and Illness. Hillsdale, NJ: *Lawrence Erlbaum Associates*, 1982, 227-51.

[19] Jones, WJ. The staff burnout scale for health professionals (SBS-HP). Park Ridge, IL: London Hourse, 1980

[20] Inaoka, F; Matsuno, K; Miyasato, K. A study of burnout in nurses and its etiology. Nursing, 1984, 36, 81-103.

[21] Matsuno, K. Study of "burn out syndrome" among public health nurses and its causative factors. *Japan Journal of Public Health*, 1983, 30, 503-510.

[22] Pines, AM. The burnout measure. Paper presented at the National Conference on burnout in the human service. *Philadelphia*. November, 1981.

[23] Fields, AI; Cuerdon, TT; Brasseux, CO; et al. Physician burnout in pediatric critical care medicine. *Crit Care Med*, 1995, Aug, 23(8), 1425-9.

[24] Shanafelt, TD; Bradley, KA; Wipf, JE; Back, AL. Burnout and self-reported patient care in an internal medicine residency program. *Ann Intern Med*, 2002, Mar, 5, 136(5), 358-67.

[25] Whippen, DA; Canellos, GP. Burnout syndrome in the practice of oncology: results of a random survey of 1,000 oncologists. *J Clin Oncol*, 1991, Oct, 9(10), 1916-20.

[26] Aiken, LH; Clarke, SP; Sloane, DM. International Hospital Outcomes Research Consortium. Hospital staffing, organization, and quality of care: cross-national findings. *Int J Qual Health Care*, 2002, Feb, 14(1), 5-13.

[27] Fagin, L; Brown, D; Bartlett, H; Leary, J; Carson, J. The Claybury community psychiatric nurse stress study: is it more stressful to work in hospital or the community? *J Adv Nurs.*, 1995, 22, 347-58.

[28] Karasek, RA. Job demands, job decision latitude and mental strain: implications for job redesign. *Adm Sci Q*, 1979, 24, 285-307.

[29] Karasek, RA; Theorell, T. Healthy Work: Stress, Productivity and the Reconstruction of working life. New York, NY: Basic Books, 1990.

[30] Karasek, RA; Theorell, T; Schwartz, JE; Schnall, PL; Pieper, CF; Michela, JL. Job characteristics in relation to the prevalence of myocardial infraction in the US health examination survey (HES) and the health and nutrition examination survey (HANES). *Am J Public Health*, 1988, 78, 910-8.

[31] Karasek, RA; Baker, D; Marxer, F; Ahlbom, A; Theorell, T. Job decision latitude, job demands, and cardiovascular disease: a prospective study of Swedish men. *Am J Public Health*, 1981, 71, 694-705.

[32] Mausner-Dorsch, H; Eaton, WW. Psychosocial work environment and depression: epidemiologic assessment of the demand-control model. *Am J Public Health*, 2000, 90, 1765-70.

[33] Takezawa, K. Distress among public health nurses in charge of emergency mental health care. *Kokoro to Syakai*, 1991, 65, 47-51. (Article in Japanese).

[34] Health and Welfare Statistics Association. Mental health service. *J Health and Welfare Statistics*, 2002, 49(9), 115-117.

[35] Health and Welfare Statistics Association. Psychiatric patient care. *J Health and Welfare Statistics*, 1997, 44(9), 138-140.

[36] Maslach, C. Burned Out. *Human Behavior*, 1976, 5, 16-22.

[37] Health and Welfare Statistics Association. Emergency mental health service. *J Health and Welfare Statistics*, 1995, 42(9), 136.

[38] Toda, Y. Survey III on patient referral and administrative tasks pertaining to Article 34 of the amended Mental Health and Welfare Act: Proceedings of the Conference on Community Health Promotion Studies 2002. Tokyo: *Japan Public Health Association*, 2002, 57-58, (Article in Japanese).

[39] Holm S. A. simple sequentially rejective multiple test procedure. *Scand J Statistics*, 1979, 6, 65-70.

Index

B

E

F

I

J

K

Kant, 210, 236
kappa, 274, 281
Keynes, 57, 190
kidney failure, 158
King, 96, 111, 121, 227, 239

L

labeling, 158
labor, 260, 267
lack of control, 232
lack of personal accomplishment, 198, 272
language, 20, 36, 124, 178, 179, 180, 188, 233, 261
later life, 218, 225
laughter, 12
law, 64, 104, 133, 232, 294
law enforcement, 104
laws, 18
lawsuits, 239
lawyers, 131
leadership, viii, 155, 160, 161, 162, 166, 169, 240
learned helplessness, 219
learners, 244, 245, 247, 248, 249, 250, 251, 252, 253, 254
learning, viii, x, 1, 20, 32, 33, 35, 40, 41, 43, 51, 56, 58, 84, 85, 88, 110, 166, 176, 179, 186, 243, 244, 245, 246, 247, 248, 249, 250, 251, 252, 253, 254, 255
learning activity, 249
learning environment, 245
learning outcomes, 244, 245, 246, 252
learning skills, 88
legal systems, 124
leisure, xi, 272, 273
leisure time, xi, 272, 273
licenses, 105
life cycle, 218
life expectancy, 216, 272
life experiences, 3, 38, 84, 90, 132
life satisfaction, 265, 266, 268
life span, 101, 219, 222
life stressors, 83, 97
life style, 196
lifespan, ix, 115, 213, 216, 218, 224, 225
lifestyle, 39, 97, 128, 132, 163, 216, 228, 282
lifestyle changes, 39
life-threatening, 172, 217

lifetime, 48, 96, 120
likelihood, 87, 88, 96, 100, 128, 132, 157, 160, 162, 163, 164, 216
limitation, 84, 184, 207, 238
limitations, 6, 28, 32, 84, 167, 196, 208, 235, 236, 237, 253, 294
linear, 4, 7, 18, 133, 150
linear regression, 133
links, 27, 68, 164, 215, 230, 248, 273
listening, 12, 23, 24, 43, 53, 99, 182
living conditions, ix, 101, 213
loans, 8, 105
location, 3, 4, 11, 16, 49, 105
locus, 163
logistics, 253
London, 57, 58, 59, 60, 96, 111, 115, 121, 149, 150, 151, 152, 154, 188, 189, 190, 191, 211, 225, 227, 269, 282, 296
loneliness, 97, 189
long work, 157
longitudinal studies, viii, 155, 167
longitudinal study, 116, 170
loss of control, 241
losses, 127, 165
Louisiana, 213
love, 36, 247, 262
low risk, 127
low-income, 218, 227
lying, 97

M

M.I.N.I, 197, 211
machinery, 95
Mackintosh, 282
magnet, 161
magnetic, iv
maintenance, 9, 30, 52, 104
maladaptive, 10, 50, 98, 102, 231, 242, 273, 279
males, 89, 107, 244
malignant, 294
malingering, 121
malpractice, 232, 240
management, vii, viii, 2, 8, 66, 83, 91, 110, 123, 124, 125, 126, 130, 132, 138, 146, 148, 149, 150, 153, 154, 166, 170, 194, 196, 212, 253, 262, 263
manic, 36
manipulation, 18
manners, 129
manpower, vii, 2, 23

N

O

P

Q

R

S

T

U

V

W

Y